WORD BOOKS FROM SAUNDERS

Sloane: THE MEDICAL WORD BOOK, 2nd Edition

Sloane: MEDICAL ABBREVIATIONS AND EPONYMS

De Lorenzo: THE PHARMACEUTICAL WORD BOOK

Tessier: THE SURGICAL WORD BOOK

Sloane: A WORD BOOK IN PATHOLOGY AND
LABORATORY MEDICINE

THE SURGICAL WORD BOOK

CLAUDIA J. TESSIER, R.R.A., C.M.T.
Assistant Professor
Department of Medical Record Administration
College of Associated Health Professions
University of Illinois at the Medical Center, Chicago

W. B. Saunders Company

Philadelphia/London/Toronto/Mexico City/Rio de Janeiro/Sydney/Tokyo

W. B. SAUNDERS COMPANY
Harcourt Brace Jovanovich, Inc.

The Curtis Center
Independence Square West
Philadelphia, PA 19106

Library of Congress Cataloging in Publication Data

Tessier, Claudia J.
  The surgical word book.

  1. Surgery—Dictionaries.   2. Surgical instruments and apparatus—Dictionaries.
I. Title.   [DNLM: 1. Surgery—Nomenclature. WO 15 T339s]
RD 17.T47   617'.003'21   81-40486
ISBN 0-7216-8805-5   AACR2

The Surgical Word Book   ISBN 0-7216-8805-5

Last digit is the print number: 12

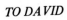

PREFACE

Throughout my career, first as a medical secretary, then as a medical transcriptionist, and finally as a medical records administrator and educator, I have relished working with medical terminology. Its formation and usage fascinate me, and I enjoy the challenge of confronting a new term and seeking its confirmation through medical references and other health professionals.

It was during my tenure as a medical transcriptionist for a national transcription service that I first became aware of the need for a simple-to-use, comprehensive, and inexpensive surgical terminology reference text. I had available at that time the standard array of terminology references (as well as some not so standard), and as new terms were encountered I would work my way through the references in hopes of finding confirmation of the term's spelling and/or usage. Most of these texts included surgical terms only to a limited extent. The few available surgical terminology books were either bulky (not from extent of entries but from extraneous material), and/or expensive (I wanted my own reference copy, not one to pass around from desk to desk), and/or of poor format (listings by surgical specialty or type of operation did me little good, since surgeons used the terms across specialties). All such texts were poorly cross-indexed; I could not retrieve information simply, directly, and quickly.

So I decided to write a surgical terminology reference text without these shortcomings, and *The Surgical Word Book* is the result. It is compact, with no extraneous text or information. Yet it is comprehensive (over 35,000 entries). It is priced so that individuals can afford their own copies if they so desire, and institutions can afford multiple copies.

Most important of all, its general alphabetized format and cross-indexing by category make it easy to use. Eponymic names are emphasized, since these are generally difficult to find in other references.

Although the idea for this text grew out of my experience as a medical transcriptionist, it is not only the transcriptionist and the supervisor who will find this book useful. It is also appropriate for use by other health care professionals and employees, including nurses, operating room personnel and ward clerks; medical record administrators, technicians, and employees; purchasing, supply, and billing personnel; and health insurance personnel. Certainly, educators and students in the allied health professions will also find it useful.

Recognizing that surgical terminology is dynamic, not static, it will be necessary in the years to come to revise and update this text. Your suggestions for its improvement and expansion will be welcomed.

Claudia Tessier

ACKNOWLEDGMENTS

I am grateful to all those who have given me the opportunity to learn — teachers, colleagues, and students — so that I may now share what I have learned; to the staff of W. B. Saunders for their assistance in the preparation of this text; and most especially to my husband, family, and friends for their encouragement and support throughout its development.

ACKNOWLEDGMENTS

HOW TO USE THIS TEXT

The Surgical Word Book requires no table of contents or index. Its format is based on that of a standard dictionary, with all entries in alphabetical order for easy retrieval. To further assist its users, it is extensively cross indexed, thereby serving as its own index.

Over 275 categories are listed both as primary entries and as cross-indexed sub-entries by category. Most of these categories are types of surgical instruments (abraders, clamps, forceps, etc.), but also included are such categories as anesthetics, positions, and sutures. Eponymic names are particularly evident in this cross-indexing. For example, the entry "Allis forceps" is found in alphabetical order under A:

Allis dissector
Allis forceps
Allis hemostat

It is likewise found under the categorical entry "forceps":

forceps
alligator
Allis
anastomosis

The cross-indexing feature of this text is of particular use in checking for alternative spellings or uses. Again taking "Allis forceps" as an example, if one thought the spelling to be "Alice," a quick check through the forceps category entries for the letter A would yield "Allis" as the correct spelling. Alternatively, if "Allis forceps" simply was not listed, a check of the general alphabetical listings would turn up "Allis clamp," "Allis dissector," etc. Such findings would support the use of the name Allis with forceps as well. It is important to remember that neither your initial spelling nor the surgeon's usage should restrict you from checking alternatives.

In this cross-indexing of entries by category, the category name is not repeated in each sub-entry. Thus:

forceps
alligator
Allis
anastomosis

NOT:

forceps
alligator forceps
Allis forceps
anastomosis forceps

When the category name starts the sub-entry phrase, it is noted in abbreviated form (forceps = f.; muscle = m., etc.). Thus,

forceps
DeLee
f. extraction
Glassman

The possessive form is generally not used in the text, since its use varies from dictating surgeon to dictating surgeon, from transcriptionist to transcriptionist, from institution to institution. Certainly, it can be added by those who wish to do so. In some instances, the possessive form is included for clarity's sake; e.g. New's instruments, to avoid confusion of the eponymic "New" with the adjective "new." When the possessive form is included, it has no influence on the alphabetizing of the entries.

Parenthetical entries are likewise ignored in alphabetizing:

EMG (electromyogram)
EMG electrode

Abbreviations are listed alphabetically, with their meanings in parentheses. Many of these are also cross-referenced:

electromyogram (EMG)

AND

EMG (electromyogram)

Hyphenated *word parts* (prefixes, suffixes, roots) are alphabetized as if the word parts were joined:

multiholed tube

multi-lead electrode

multilocular

On the other hand, hyphenated *whole words* (including eponymic names) are alphabetized as if the two words were separated by a space instead of a hyphen:

Nelson rib stripper

Nelson-Roberts stripper

Nelson scissors

Plurals formed by standard English language rules are not included. Plurals formed by Latin, Greek, etc. rules are noted in parentheses; many are cross-indexed:

falx (pl. falces)

AND

falces (sing. falx)

Numerals are alphabetized as if they were spelled out:

fountain syringe

4-A Magovern prosthesis

fourchette

Anatomical terms for veins, muscles, nerves, etc. are entered both in Latin form and in English form. Since many surgeons mix the Latin and English words within a phrase, this is reflected in the cross-indexing of the Latin entries. Thus, the categorical entry appears:

musculus

m. pubovaginalis

Whereas the general alphabetical entry appears:

pubovaginalis muscle

NOT

pubovaginalis musculus

a

A-a gradient
A&P colporrhaphy (anterior and
    posterior repair)
A-S-E bandage (axilla, shoulder
    and elbow)
Aaron sign
ab-externo incision
Abadie clamp
Abbe condenser
Abbe-Estlander operation
Abbe intestinal anastomosis
Abbe neurectomy
Abbe operation for esophageal
    stricture
Abbe ring
Abbe stage I cheiloplasty
Abbe stage II cheiloplasty
Abbott elevator
Abbott gouge
Abbott-Lucas approach
Abbott-Miller tube
Abbott operation
Abbott-Rawson tube
Abbott scoop
Abbott table
Abbott tube
ABD dressing
ABD pads
abdomen
abdominal
abdominal aneurysm
abdominal aorta

abdominal aortogram
abdominal aortography
abdominal ballottement
abdominal bandage
abdominal contents
abdominal hernia
abdominal hysterectomy
abdominal incision
abdominal needle
abdominal nephrectomy
abdominal paracentesis
abdominal-perineal resection
abdominal retractor
abdominal scissors
abdominal scoop
abdominal-vascular retractor
abdominal version
abdominal wall
abdominocentesis
abdominohysterectomy
abdominoparacentesis
abdominopelvic amputation
abdominoperineal
abdominoperineal resection
abdominoplasty
abdominoscopy
abdominothoracic incision
abdominouterotomy
abducens nerve (cranial nerve VI)
abducent nerve
abduction
abduction splint

abductor digiti minimi manus
    muscle
abductor digiti minimi pedis
    muscle
abductor hallucis muscle
abductor muscle
abductor pollicis brevis muscle
abductor pollicis longus muscle
Abell uterine suspension
Abelson adenotome
Abelson cannula
Aberhart disposable urinal
Abernethy operation
aberrant
aberrant artery
aberrant thyroid
aberrant vessel
ablation
abortion
above-elbow amputation
above-knee amputation
abrader
       cartilage
       corneal
       Dingman
       Howard
       Lieberman
       Montague
Abraham cannula
Abraham elevator
Abraham enterotome
Abraham knife
Abrams biopsy punch
Abrams needle
Abrams punch
Abramson tube
abrasion
abruptio placenta

abscess
abscission needle
absorbable
absorbable gauze
absorbable surgical sutures
absorbable sutures
absorbent
absorbent gauze
absorption anesthesia
Aburel operation
abutment
accessorius nerve
accessory
accessory duct
accessory ligament
accessory nerve (cranial nerve XI)
accessory spleen
accessory structures
accessory thyroid glands
accompanying artery of sciatic
    nerve
accompanying vein of hypoglossal
    nerve
accordion drain
accordion graft
accumulation
Ace adherent bandage
Ace bandage
acetabula (*sing.* acetabulum)
acetabular component
acetabular cup
acetabular cup positioner
acetabular cup template
acetabular guide
acetabular knife
acetabular reamer
acetabular seating holes
acetabulectomy

acetabuloplasty
acetabulum (*pl.* acetabula)
acetylcholine
achalasia
Achilles reflex
Achilles tendon
achillorrhaphy
achillotenotomy
achillotomy
achlorhydria
acidosis
acini (*sing.* acinus)
acinous gland
acinus (*pl.* acini)
ACMI antroscope
ACMI bronchoscope
ACMI catheter
ACMI cystoscope
ACMI forceps
ACMI gastroscope
ACMI hysteroscope
ACMI laparoscope
ACMI nasopharyngoscope
ACMI proctoscope
ACMI proctosigmoidoscope
ACMI telescope
ACMI-Valentine tube
ACMI valve
ACMI urethroscope
Acmistat catheter
acorn-shaped eye implant
acorn-tipped bougie
acorn-tipped catheter
acoustic nerve
acoustic neurotomy
acquired hernia
acral anesthesia
Acrax prosthesis

Acrel ganglion
acromial process
acromioclavicular articulation
acromioclavicular ligament
acromiocoracoid ligament
acromion
acromion process
acromionectomy
acromioplasty
acromiothoracic artery
acrylic ball eye implant
acrylic bone cement
acrylic conformer
acrylic eye implant
acrylic implant
acrylic splint
ACTH (adrenocorticotropic
    hormone)
actinomycosis
actinotherapy
actual cautery
acuminatum (*pl.* acuminata)
acupuncture
acupuncture anesthesia
acute
acute angle
Acutrol sutures
Adair-Allis forceps
Adair forceps
Adair procedure
Adair tenaculum
Adams aspirator
Adams ectropion operation
Adams hip operation
Adams operation
Adams position
Adams retractor
Adams saw

adapted instruments
adapter
    Air-Lon
    T-adapter
    universal T-adapter
Adaptic dressing
Adaptic gauze
Adaptic gauze dressing
Adaptic gauze pack
Adaptic gauze packing
Adaptic needle holder
Adasoy procedure
adduction
adductor brevis muscle
adductor canal
adductor hallucis muscle
adductor longus muscle
adductor magnus muscle
adductor muscle
adductor pollicis muscle
Adelmann finger disarticulation
Adelmann operation
adenectomy
adenitis
adenocarcinoma
adenofibroma
adenoid curet
adenoid forceps
adenoid punch
adenoidectomy
adenoids
adenoma (*pl.* adenomas,
    adenomata)
adenomammectomy
adenomata (*sing.* adenoma)
adenomatosis
adenomatous
adenomatous goiter

adenomatous polyp
adenomyosis
adenopathy
adenotome
    Abelson
    Box
    Box-DeJager
    Breitman
    Cullom-Mueller
    direct-vision
    guillotine
    Kelly
    Laforce
    Laforce-Grieshaber
    Laforce-Stevenson
    Mueller-Laforce
    Myles
    Shambaugh
adenotomy
adenotonsillectomy
adequate
adherent bandage
adhesiolysis
adhesion
adhesiotomy
adhesive
adhesive absorbent dressing
adhesive aluminum splint
adhesive bandage
adhesive bands
adhesive cement
adhesive dressing
adhesive needle holder
adhesive plastic drape
adhesive silicone implant
adhesive tape
adhesive tape strips
adipectomy

adipocele
adipose
adipose ligament
adipose renal capsule
adipose tissue
adiposis
adjacent
adjustable cross splint
adjustable cup reamer
adjustable nail
adjustable splint
adjustment
adjustment of cardiac pacemaker
Adler forceps
Adler punch
adnexa
adnexal structures
adnexopexy
adolescent cataract
adrenal
adrenal glands
adrenal veins
adrenalectomize
adrenalectomy
adrenalorrhaphy
adrenalotomy
adrenocorticotropic hormone
  (ACTH)
Adson-Beckman retractor
Adson brain suction tip
Adson-Brown forceps
Adson bur
Adson cannula
Adson chisel
Adson clip
Adson conductor
Adson drill
Adson elevator

Adson forceps
Adson headrest
Adson hemostat
Adson hook
Adson knife
Adson-Murphy needle
Adson needle
Adson needle holder
Adson periosteal elevator
Adson retractor
Adson rongeur
Adson saw guide
Adson scissors
Adson sign
Adson speculum
Adson suction tube
Adson tube
adult laryngoscope
advancement
advancement forceps
advancement of muscle
advancement of ocular muscle
advancement of round ligament
advancement of tendon
adventitia
adventitious
adynamic ileus
AE amputation (above-elbow)
Aebli scissors
aerate
aeration
aerogram
aerography
Aeroplast dressing
afferent
afterloading screw
afterloading tandem
agenesis

agenetic fracture
agglutination
Agnew keratome
Agnew knife
Agnew needle
Agnew operation
Agnew splint
Agnew-Verhoeff incision
agraffe
agraffe clamp
Agrikola retractor
Ahlquist-Durham clip
Ainsworth punch
air bubble
air cannula
air cells
air cystogram
air cystography
air dermatome
air drill
air injection cannula
Air-Lon adapter
Air-Lon plug
Air-Lon tube
air myelography
air-puff tonometer
air pyelogram
air syringe
air tube
airfoam splint
airplane splint
airtight
airway
    disposable
    Guedel
AK amputation (above-knee)
Akerlund deformity
Akin bunionectomy

akinesia
akinesis
akinetic
Akiyama prosthesis
AL tandem (afterloading)
ala (*pl.* alae)
Alanson amputation
alar
alar incision
alar osteotome
alar retractor
Albarran gland
Albee bone graft
Albee-Delbet operation
Albee hip operation
Albee osteotome
Albee saw
Albee spinal fusion
Albee table
Albert-Andrews laryngoscope
Albert bronchoscope
Albert operation
Albert position
Albert sutures
albuginea
Alcock canal
Alcock catheter
Alcock hemostatic bag
Alcock-Hendrickson lithotrite
Alcock lithotrite
Alcock obturator
Alcock plug
Alcock syringe
Alcock-Timberlake obturator
alcohol
Alcon cautery
Alcon cryophake
Alcon sutures

Alden retractor
Aldrich operation
Aldridge-Studdefort urethral
     suspension
Alexander-Adams uterine
     suspension
Alexander chisel
Alexander-Farabeuf elevator
Alexander-Farabeuf periosteo-
     tome
Alexander gouge
Alexander incision
Alexander needle
Alexander operation
Alexander osteotome
Alexander periosteotome
Alexander prostatectomy
Alexander punch
Alexander raspatory
Alfred M. Large clamp
alignment
alimentary
alimentary canal
alimentary tract
alimentation
alkaline battery cautery
Allarton operation
Allen applicator
Allen-Barkan knife
Allen-Brown shunt
Allen clamp
Allen eye implant
Allen forceps
Allen pliers
Allen retractor
Allen screw
Allen trocar
Allen wrench

alligator forceps
alligator grasping forceps
alligator scissors
Allingham colotomy
Allingham excision of rectum
Allingham operation
Allingham speculum
Allingham ulcer
Allis-Adair forceps
Allis clamp
Allis-Coakley forceps
Allis dissector
Allis-Duval forceps
Allis forceps
Allis hemostat
Allis-Ochsner forceps
Allis periosteal elevator
Allison clamp
Allison herniorrhaphy
Allison retractor
Allison sutures
allograft
allotransplantation
alloy
Allport-Babcock retractor
Allport-Babcock searcher
Allport bur
Allport hook
Allport operation
Allport retractor
Allport searcher
Alm retractor
Almoor operation
Alouette amputation
alpha-chymotrypsin cannula
alpha-chymotrypsin solution
alphaprodine
Alsus-Knapp operation

Altemeier operation
alternating
alternating sutures
Alumafoam splint
aluminum bridge splint
aluminum cortex retractor
aluminum eye shield
aluminum finger cot splint
aluminum mallet
aluminum splint
Alvarez prosthesis
Alvarez-Rodriguez catheter
alveolar
alveolar artery
alveolar duct
alveolar nerve
alveolar process
alveolares superiores anteriores
    arteries
alveolares superiores nerves
alveolaris inferior artery
alveolaris inferior nerve
alveolaris superior posterior artery
alveolectomy
alveoli (*sing.* alveolus)
alveolodental membrane
alveoloplasty
alveolotomy
alveolus (*pl.* alveoli)
alveoplasty
Alvis curet
Alvis operation
Alyea clamp
amalgam
amalgam carrier
ambient oxygen
amblyopia
Ambu bag

amebic
amebic abscess
amenable
amenorrhea
Americaine
American Optical Company
    instruments
American umbilical scissors
Ames shunt
amethocaine
Amico drill
Amico extractor
Ammon blepharoplasty
Ammon canthoplasty
Ammon dacryocystotomy
Ammon operation
amniocentesis
amniogram
amniography
amnion
amnioscopy
amniotic
amniotic hernia
amniotic sac
amniotic trocar
amniotome
amniotomy
amobarbital
Amoils cryoextractor
Amoils cryoprobe
Amoils retractor
amphidiarthrodial joint
Amplatz catheter
ampulla
ampulla of Vater
ampullaris anterior nerve
ampullaris lateralis nerve
ampullaris posterior nerve

ampullary nerve
amputating knife
amputating saw
amputation
amputation by transfixion
amputation in contiguity
amputation knife
amputation of breast
amputation of cervix
amputation of clitoris
amputation of ear
amputation of penis
amputation rake
amputation retractor
amputation saw
amputation stump
Amsler grid
Amsler needle
Amsler sclera marker
Amtech-Killeen pacemaker
Amussat operation
Amussat probe
amygdaloid fossa
amygdaloidectomy
amygdalotomy
Amytal
Anagnostakis operation
anal
anal canal
anal fissure
anal retractor
anal speculum
anal verge
analgesia
Anametric prosthesis
anasarca
anasarca trocar
anastomosis

anastomosis apparatus
anastomosis arteriovenosa
anastomosis clamp
anastomosis forceps
anastomosis of epididymis to vas
anastomosis of nerves
anastomosis of vas deferens
anastomotic
anastomotic vein
anastomotica inferior vein
anastomotica superior vein
anatomical closure
anatomical position
anatomically
Ancap silk suture
anchor band
anchor plate
anchor splint
anchorage
anchorage procedure
anchoring sutures
anconeus muscle
Anderson-Adson retractor
Anderson curet
Anderson operation
Anderson splint
Anderson suction tube
Andrews applicator
Andrews chisel
Andrews forceps
Andrews gouge
Andrews-Hartmann forceps
Andrews-Hartmann rongeur
Andrews operation
Andrews-Pynchon tube
Andrews retractor
Andrews tongue depressor
Anectine

Anel lacrimal dilation
Anel lacrimal probe
Anel lacrimal syringe
anemia
Anestacon
anesthesia
    absorption
    acral
    acupuncture
    angiospastic
    assisted respiration
    Atkinson lid block
    axillary
    axillary block
    balanced
    basal
    Bier
    Bier block
    Bier local
    bilateral mandibular block
    block
    block technique
    brachial
    brachial plexus block
    caudal
    caudal block
    cerebral
    cervical
    chemical
    circle absorption
    circular block
    closed
    colonic
    combined sacral and caudal
      block
    compression
    conduction
    continuous caudal

anesthesia *(continued)*
    continuous epidural
    continuous peridural
    continuous spinal
    controlled respiration
    Corning
    dental
    differential spinal
    digital block
    electric
    electricity-induced
    electroanesthesia
    endobronchial
    endotracheal
    endotracheal general
    endotracheal insufflation
    epidural
    extradural
    field block
    fractional
    fractional epidural
    fractional spinal
    frost
    general
    general endotracheal
    general inhalation
    general insufflation
    Gwathmey oil-ether
    high-pressure
    hyperbaric
    hyperbaric spinal
    hypobaric
    hypobaric spinal
    hypotensive
    hypothermic
    infiltration
    infraorbital block
    inhalation

anesthesia *(continued)*
    insufflation
    intercostal
    intramedullary
    intranasal
    intraoral
    intraosseous
    intrapulpal
    intraspinal
    intratracheal
    intravenous
    intravenous regional
    intubation
    isobaric
    isobaric spinal
    Kulenkampff
    lingual block
    local
    low spinal
    lumbar epidural
    mandibular block
    Meltzer
    midfemoral block
    mixed
    naso-endotracheal
    nasotracheal intubation
    nerve block
    nerve blocking
    no-absorption
    nonbreathing
    O'Brien block
    open
    open drop
    open endotracheal inhalation
    open inhalation
    orbicularis block
    paracervical block
    paraneural

anesthesia *(continued)*
    parasacral
    paravertebral
    partial
    partial rebreathing
    peridural
    perineural
    periodontal
    permeation
    pharyngeal insufflation
    plexus
    presacral
    pressure
    pudendal
    pudendal block
    pupillary block
    rebreathing
    rectal
    refrigeration
    regional
    regional block
    respiration assisted
    respiration unassisted
    retrobulbar
    retrobulbar block
    sacral
    sacral block
    saddle-block
    saddle-block spinal
    semi-closed
    semi-closed endobronchial
    semi-closed endotracheal
    semi-open
    semi-open endotracheal
        inhalation
    single injection
    spinal
    spinal subarachnoid block

anesthesia *(continued)*
    splanchnic
    splanchnic block
    stellate block
    subarachnoid
    surface
    surgical
    sympathetic block
    therapeutic
    to-and-fro
    topical
    total
    total spinal
    transsacral
    transsacral block
    transtracheal
    twilight
    twilight sleep
    unassisted respiration
    Van Lint and Atkinson block
    Van Lint block
    vein
anesthesiologist
anesthesiology
anesthetic
anesthetic agents
    alcohol
    alphaprodine
    Americaine
    amethocaine
    amobarbital
    Amytal
    Anectine
    Anestacon
    anticholinesterase
    Avertin
    benoxinate hydrochloride
    benzocaine

anesthetic agents *(continued)*
    benzoquinonium chloride
    Blockain
    Brevital
    Brevital sodium
    bupivacaine hydrochloride
    butacaine
    butethamine hydrochloride
    Butyn
    Carbocaine hydrochloride
    carbon dioxide
    Cetacaine
    chloramine
    chloroform
    chloroprocaine hydro-
        chloride
    cinchocaine
    Citanest
    cocaine
    cocaine hydrochloride
    curare
    Cyclaine
    cyclomethycaine sulfate
    cyclopentane
    cyclopropane
    decamethonium bromide
    decamethonium iodide
    Demerol
    dibucaine hydrochloride
    diethyl oxide
    Dilaudid
    divinyl ether
    Duranest
    Dyclone
    dyclonine hydrochloride
    edrophonium chloride
    ether
    ether in oil

anesthetic agents *(continued)*
- ethocaine
- Ethrane
- ethyl chloride
- ethyl ether
- ethyl oxide
- ethyl vinyl ether
- ethylene
- etidocaine hydrochloride
- Evipal
- Fluoromar
- Fluothane
- Forane
- gallamine
- halothane
- helium
- hexobarbital
- hexylcaine hydrochloride
- Holocaine
- Innovar
- Ketaject
- Ketalar
- ketamine hydrochloride
- lidocaine hydrochloride
- lignocaine
- Lorfan
- Marcaine hydrochloride
- meperidine
- mepivacaine hydrochloride
- methohexital sodium
- methoxyflurane
- Metycaine hydrochloride
- morphine
- nadbath
- Nalline
- narcotic agents
- narcotic antagonists
- Nembutal

anesthetic agents *(continued)*
- Nesacaine
- Nesacaine-CE
- Nisentil
- nitrous oxide
- Novocain
- Nupercaine hydrochloride
- Ophthaine
- Oxaine
- oxethazaine
- Penthrane
- pentobarbital
- Pentothal
- Percaine
- piperocaine hydrochloride
- Pontocaine
- pramoxine hydrochloride
- prilocaine hydrochloride
- procaine hydrochloride
- Proctodon
- proparacaine hydrochloride
- propoxycaine hydrochloride
- secobarbital
- Seconal
- sodium pentothal
- succinyl choline
- Surfacaine
- Tensilon
- tetracaine hydrochloride
- thialbarbitone
- thiamylal sodium
- thiopental sodium
- topical cocaine
- trichloroethylene
- Trilene
- Trimar
- Tronothane hydrochloride
- Vinamar

anesthetic agents *(continued)*
    Vinethene
    vinyl ether
    vinyl ethyl ether
    Xylocaine
    Xylocaine jelly
    Xylocaine with epinephrine
anesthetist
anesthetize
anesthetizing agents (see *anesthetic agents*)
aneuroplasty
aneurysm
aneurysm clamp
aneurysm clip
aneurysm forceps
aneurysm needle
aneurysmal
aneurysmectomy
aneurysmoplasty
aneurysmorrhaphy
aneurysmotomy
Angelchik anti-reflux prosthesis
Angell curet
Angelucci operation
Anger camera
angiectomy
angiitis
Angio-Conray
angiocardiogram
angiocardiography
angiocatheter
angiogram
angiographic catheter
angiography
angiography needle
angiolith
angioma (*pl.* angiomas, angiomata)

angiopancreatitis
angioplasty
angiorrhaphy
angiosclerotic
angioscope
angioscopy
angiospasm
angiospastic
angiotomy
angiotribe
angiotribe forceps
angiotripsy
angiitis
angle band
angle drain
angle knife
Angle splint
angle suture
angled clamp
angled curet
angled director
angled probe
angled scissors
angled stone forceps
angled suction tube
angular artery
angular forceps
angular incision
angular knife
angular needle
angular needle holder
angular oval punch
angular rongeur
angular saw
angular scissors
angular tip electrode
angular vein
angularis artery

angularis vein
angulated blade electrode
angulated forceps
angulated needle holder
angulation
anisometropia
ankle bone
ankle joint
ankle mortise
ankyloproctia
ankylosis
Ann Arbor clamp
Ann Arbor retractor
Annandale operation
annular
annular ligament
annuli (*sing.* annulus)
annuloplasty
annulorrhaphy
annulus (*pl.* annuli)
anococcygeal nerves
anococcygei nerves
anoperineal
anoplasty
anorectal dressing
anorectocolonic
anorectum
anorexia
anoscope
    a. speculum
    a. with obturator
    Bacon
    Bodenheimer
    Boehm
    Brinkerhoff
    Buie-Hirschman
    Fansler
    Goldbacher

anoscope *(continued)*
    Hirschman a. with obturator
    Ives
    Muer
    Otis
    Pratt
    Pruitt
    rotating
    Sims
    Welch Allyn
anoscopy
anosigmoidoscopic
anosigmoidoscopy
anospinal
Anson-McVay herniorrhaphy
Anson-McVay operation
antalgic gait
antebrachial vein
antecolic
antecolic gastrojejunostomy
antecolic jejunostomy
antecubital
antecubital fossa
anteflexion
antegonial angle
antegonial notch
antegrade flow
antepartum
anterior and posterior colpor-
    rhaphy (A&P repair)
anterior and posterior repair of
    cystocele and rectocele
anterior cervical lip
anterior chamber
anterior chamber cannula
anterior chamber irrigator
anterior colporrhaphy
anterior commissure

anterior commissure laryngoscope
anterior commissurotomy
anterior forceps
anterior fusion operation
anterior gastrectomy
anterior gastrojejunostomy
anterior iridodialysis
anterior jejunostomy
anterior ligament
anterior pillar
anterior pillar incision
anterior rectus sheath
anterior resection clamp
anterior resection of sigmoid and
    rectum
anterior retractor
anterior segment forceps
anterior splint
anterolateral approach
anteromedial
anteversion
Anthony compressor
Anthony-Fisher balloon
Anthony retractor
Anthony suction tube
Anthony tube
antibiotics
anticholinesterase
anticoagulants
anticus
anti-embolism stockings
antiglaucoma peripheral
    iridectomy
anti-incontinence penile prosthesis
antimesenteric
antimesenteric border
antiperistalsis
antiperistaltic

antiperistaltic anastomosis
antiperistaltic jejunostomy
antiseptic dressing
antitragus muscle
Antole-Condale elevator
antra (*sing.* antrum)
antral
antral balloon
antrectomy
antroscope
antroscopy
antrostomy
antrostomy punch
antrotomy
antrum (*pl.* antra)
antrum balloon
antrum bur
antrum cannula
antrum chisel
antrum curet
antrum gouge
antrum irrigator
antrum needle
antrum of Willis
antrum perforator
antrum punch
antrum pyloricum
antrum rasp
antrum retractor
antrum rongeur
antrum trephine
antrum trocar
antrum wash tube
antrum window operation
anuli (*sing.* anulus)
anuloplasty
anulus (*pl.* anuli)
anuria

anus
any-angle splint
aorta
aorta abdominalis
aorta ascendens
aorta clamp
aorta descendens
aorta forceps
aorta retractor
aorta thoracica
aortic anastomosis
aortic aneurysm
aortic aneurysm clamp
aortic aneurysm forceps
aortic aneurysm graft
aortic arch
aortic arch arteriogram
aortic arch arteriography
aortic cannula
aortic catheter
aortic curet
aortic dilator
aortic insufficiency
aortic occluder
aortic occlusion clamp
aortic occlusion forceps
aortic scissors
aortic valve
aortic valve brush
aortic valve prosthesis
aortic valve retractor
aortic valve rongeur
aortic valvotomy
aortic valvulotomy
aortic vent needle
aorticocoronary bypass
aorticopulmonary shunt
aorticopulmonary window operation

aorticorenal
aortocoronary
aortocoronary bypass
aortogram
aortogram needle
aortographic catheter
aortographic suction tip
aortography
aortography needle
aortoiliac
aortoiliac bypass
aortoiliac endarterectomy
aortoplasty
aortopulmonary
aortopulmonary fenestration
aortorrhaphy
aortotomy
aortotomy incision
ape-hand deformity
apepsia
aperiosteal supracondylar
    tendoplastic amputation
apertognathia
aperture
apex (*pl.* apices)
apex cardiogram
apex cardiography
Apgar score
aphagia
aphakia
aphasia
aphonic bruits
apical
apices (*sing.* apex)
apicectomy
apicoectomy
apicolysis

apicolysis retractor
apicostomy
aplasia
aplastic
Apley grind test
Apley maneuver
Apley sign
apocrine gland
aponeurectomy
aponeurorrhaphy
aponeurosis (*pl.* aponeuroses)
aponeurotic falx
aponeurotic fascia
aponeurotomy
apophyseal fracture
apparatus
    anastomosis
    aspiration
    Barany
    Belzer
    cryosurgery
    Dietrich
    Doppler
    extension
    Fell-O'Dwyer
    ICLH (Imperial College, London Hospital)
    Jaquet
    Killian
    Kirschner
    Lewy suspension
    Light-Veley
    Lynch suspension
    Malgaigne
    McAtee
    pneumothorax
    Potain
    Roger Anderson

apparatus *(continued)*
    Sayre
    suction
    suspension
    Tallerman
    Taylor
    Tobold
    traction
    vacuum aspiration
    Volutrol
    Waldenberg
    Wangensteen
appendalgia
appendectomy
appendectomy retractor
appendectomy spoon
appendical
appendiceal
appendiceal abscess
appendicealgia
appendicectasis
appendicectomy
appendices (*sing.* appendix)
appendicism
appendicitis by contiguity
appendicitis granulosa
appendicitis larvata
appendicitis obliterans
appendiclausis
appendicocecostomy
appendicocele
appendicoenterostomy
appendicolithiasis
appendicolysis
appendicopathia
appendicopathy
appendicosis
appendicostomy

appendicotomy
appendicular
appendicular artery
appendicular vein
appendicularis artery
appendicularis vein
appendiculoradiogram
appendiculoradiography
appendix (*pl.* appendices or
   appendixes)
appendix cerebri
appendix inverter
appendix tapes
appendix vermiformis
appendolithiasis
appendoroentgenogram
appendoroentgenography
appendotome
appendotome knife
applanation tonometer
applanation tonometry
appliance
application
application of cast
application of obstetric forceps
application of splint
application of therapeutic agent
application of traction device
applicator
     Allen
     Andrews
     a. forceps
     aural
     Brown
     Buck
     Chaoul
     corneal
     cotton

applicator *(continued)*
     cotton-tipped
     Dean
     Ernst
     Fletcher loading
     Gifford
     Holinger
     Jackson
     Kyle
     laryngeal
     Lathbury
     Lejeune
     metal
     nasopharyngeal
     Plummer-Vinson radium
     Pynchon
     radioactive
     radioisotope
     radium
     Ralks
     Roberts
     Sawtell
     sonic
     Uebe
Appolito operation
Appolito sutures
apposition
apposition sutures
approximate
approximated
approximation
approximation forceps
approximation sutures
approximator (see *sternal approxi-
    mator*)
aqueduct
aqueduct of Sylvius
aqueductus vestibuli vein

aqueous
aqueous humor
aqueous Zephiran
arachnoid
arachnoid membrane
Arbuckle probe
arch
arch angiogram
arch angiography
arch aortogram
arch aortography
arch arteriogram
arch arteriography
arch bar
arch of aorta
arch wire
Archer forceps
Arco lithium pacemaker
arcuata pedis artery
arcuatae renis arteries
arcuatae renis veins
arcuate arteries of kidney
arcuate artery of foot
arcuate incision
arcuate ligaments
arcuate veins of kidney
arcus aortae
ARD bandage
areola (*pl.* areolae)
areolar
areolar glands
areolar incision
areolitis
argon laser
argon laser photocoagulator
Argyle catheter
Argyle chest tube
Argyle-Salem sump tube

Argyle tube
Argyll Robertson pupil
Argyll Robertson strap operation
    for ectropion of eyelid
Argyll Robertson sutures
Aries-Pitanguy breast reduction
    technique
Aristocort
Arlt-Jaesche operation
Arlt loupe
Arlt operation
Arlt scoop
Arlt sutures
arm extension position
arm rests
arm splint
Armour knife
Armour tube
Armsby operation
Army bone gouge
Army-Navy retractor
Army osteotome
Army retractor
Arnott dilator
Aron Alpha adhesive
arrector muscles of hair
arrectores pilorum muscles
arrhythmia
Arruga expressor
Arruga eye implant
Arruga forceps
Arruga-Gill forceps
Arruga lens expressor
Arruga operation
Arruga retractor
Arruga saw
Arruga speculum
Arruga trephine

Arslan operation
arteria (*pl.* arteriae)*
    aa. alveolares superiores
      anteriores
    a. alveolaris inferior
    a. alveolaris superior
      posterior
    a. angularis
    a. appendicularis
    a. arcuata pedis
    aa. arcuatae renis
    a. arcus aortae
    aa. arteriolae rectae renis
    a. auricularis posterior
    a. auricularis profunda
    a. axillaris
    a. basilaris
    a. brachialis
    a. brachialis superficialis
    a. buccalis
    a. bulbi penis
    a. bulbi vestibuli vaginae
    a. canalis pterygoidei
    a. carotis communis
    a. carotis interna
    a. centralis retinae
    a. cerebelli inferior anterior
    a. cerebelli inferior posterior
    a. cerebelli superior
    a. cerebri anterior
    a. cerebri media
    a. cerebri posterior
    a. cervicalis ascendens
    a. cervicalis profunda
    a. choroidea anterior

*a. = arteria [L.].
 aa. = arteriae [L., pl.].

arteria (*pl.* arteriae)* *(continued)*
    aa. ciliares anteriores
    aa. ciliares posteriores breves
    aa. ciliares posteriores longae
    a. circumflexa femoris
      lateralis
    a. circumflexa femoris
      medialis
    a. circumflexa humeri
      anterior
    a. circumflexa humeri
      posterior
    a. circumflexa ilium pro-
      funda
    a. circumflexa ilium super-
      ficialis
    a. circumflexa scapulae
    a. colica dextra
    a. colica media
    a. colica sinistra
    a. collateralis media
    a. collateralis radialis
    a. collateralis ulnaris inferior
    a. collateralis ulnaris superior
    a. comitans nervi ischiadici
    a. communicans anterior
      cerebri
    a. communicans posterior
      cerebri
    aa. conjunctivales anteriores
    aa. conjunctivales posteri-
      ores
    a. coronaria dextra
    a. coronaria sinistra
    a. cortis externa
    a. cremasterica
    a. cystica
    a. deferentialis

arteria (*pl.* arteriae)* *(continued)*
    aa. digitales dorsales manus
    aa. digitales dorsales pedis
    aa. digitales palmares
      communes
    aa. digitales palmares
      propriae
    aa. digitales plantares
      communes
    aa. digitales plantares
      propriae
    a. dorsalis clitoridis
    a. dorsalis nasi
    a. dorsalis pedis
    a. dorsalis penis
    a. ductus deferentis
    a. epigastrica inferior
    a. epigastrica superficialis
    a. epigastrica superior
    aa. episclerales
    a. ethmoidalis anterior
    a. ethmoidalis posterior
    a. facialis
    a. femoralis
    a. gastrica dextra
    a. gastrica sinistra
    aa. gastricae breves
    a. gastroduodenalis
    a. gastroepiploica dextra
    a. gastroepiploica sinistra
    a. genus descendens
    a. genus inferior lateralis
    a. genus inferior medialis
    a. genus media
    a. genus superior lateralis

ᵏa. = arteria [L.].
 aa. = arteriae [L., pl.].

arteria (*pl.* arteriae)* *(continued)*
    a. genus superior medialis
    a. glutea inferior
    a. glutea superior
    aa. helicinae penis
    a. hepatica communis
    a. hepatica propria
    a. hyaloidea
    aa. ilei
    a. ileocolica
    a. iliaca communis
    a. iliaca externa
    a. iliaca interna
    a. iliolumbalis
    a. infraorbitalis
    aa. intercostales posteriores
    a. intercostalis suprema
    aa. interlobares renis
    aa. interlobulares hepatis
    aa. interlobulares renis
    a. interossea anterior
    a. interossea communis
    a. interossea posterior
    a. interossea recurrens
    aa. jejunales
    a. labialis inferior
    a. labialis superior
    a. labyrinthi
    a. lacrimalis
    a. laryngea inferior
    a. laryngea superior
    a. lienalis
    a. ligamenti teretis uteri
    a. lingualis
    aa. lumbales
    a. lumbalis ima
    a. malleolaris anterior
      lateralis

arteria (*pl.* arteriae)* *(continued)*
   a. malleolaris anterior
     medialis
   a. masseterica
   a. maxillaris
   a. mediana
   a. meningea anterior
   a. meningea media
   a. meningea posterior
   a. mentalis
   a. mesenterica inferior
   a. mesenterica superior
   aa. metacarpeae dorsales
   aa. metacarpeae palmares
   aa. metatarseae dorsales
   aa. metatarseae plantares
   a. musculophrenica
   aa. nasales posteriores
     laterales et septi
   aa. nutriciae humeri
   a. obturatoris
   a. obturatoris accessoria
   a. occipitalis
   a. ophthalmica
   a. ovarica
   a. palatina ascendens
   a. palatina descendens
   a. palatina major
   aa. palatinae minores
   aa. palpebrales laterales
   aa. palpebrales mediales
   aa. pancreaticoduodenales
     inferiores
   aa. perforantes
   a. pericardiacophrenica

arteria (*pl.* arteriae)* *(continued)*
   a. perinealis
   a. peronea
   a. pharyngea ascendens
   aa. phrenicae inferiores
   aa. phrenicae superiores
   a. plantaris lateralis
   a. plantaris medialis
   a. poplitea
   a. princeps pollicis
   a. profunda brachii
   a. profunda clitoridis
   a. profunda femoris
   a. profunda linguae
   a. profunda penis
   a. pudenda interna
   aa. pudendae externae
   a. pulmonalis dextra
   a. pulmonalis sinistra
   a. radialis
   a. radialis indicis
   a. rectalis inferior
   a. rectalis media
   a. rectalis superior
   a. recurrens radialis
   a. recurrens tibialis anterior
   a. recurrens tibialis posterior
   a. recurrens ulnaris
   a. renalis
   aa. renis
   aa. sacrales laterales
   a. sacralis mediana
   aa. sigmoideae
   a. sphenopalatina
   a. spinalis anterior
   a. spinalis posterior
   a. stylomastoidea
   a. subclavia

*a. = arteria [L.].
 aa. = arteriae [L., pl.].

arteria (*pl.* arteriae)* *(continued)*
- a. subcostalis
- a. sublingualis
- a. submentalis
- a. subscapularis
- a. supraorbitalis
- aa. suprarenales superiores
- a. suprarenalis inferior
- a. suprarenalis media
- a. suprascapularis
- a. supratrochlearis
- aa. surales
- a. tarsea lateralis
- aa. tarseae mediales
- aa. temporales profundae
- a. temporalis media
- a. temporalis superficialis
- a. testicularis
- a. thoracica interna
- a. thoracica lateralis
- a. thoracica suprema
- a. thoracoacromialis
- a. thoracodorsalis
- a. thyroidea ima
- a. thyroidea inferior
- a. thyroidea superior
- a. tibialis anterior
- a. tibialis posterior
- a. transversa colli
- a. transversa facieci
- a. tympanica anterior
- a. tympanica inferior
- a. tympanica posterior
- a. tympanica superior
- a. ulnaris

arteria (*pl.* arteriae)* *(continued)*
- a. umbilicalis
- a. urethralis
- a. uterina
- a. vaginalis
- a. vertebralis
- aa. vesicales superiores
- a. vesicalis inferior
- a. zygomaticoorbitalis

arterial anastomosis
arterial cannula
arterial catheter
arterial cutdown
arterial graft
arterial needle
arterial prosthesis
arterial puncture
arterial scissors
arterial silk sutures
arterial transfusion of blood
arteriectomy
arteriogram
arteriogram needle
arteriography
arteriolae rectae renis arteries
arteriole
arterioplasty
arteriorrhaphy
arteriosclerosis
arteriosclerotic
arteriotomy
arteriotomy incision
arteriotomy scissors
arteriovenostomy
arteriovenous anastomosis
arteriovenous aneurysm
arteriovenous fistula

*a. = arteria [L.].
aa. = arteriae [L., pl.].

arteriovenous malformation
  (AVM)
arteriovenous shunt
artery(ies)*
    accompanying a. of sciatic
      nerve
    acromiothoracic
    alveolar
    angular
    appendicular
    arcuate a. of foot
    arcuate a's of kidney
    a. clamp
    a. forceps
    a. needle
    a. of bulb of penis
    a. of bulb of urethra
    a. of bulb of vestibule of
      vagina
    a. of ductus deferens
    a. of labyrinth
    a. of pterygoid canal
    a. of round ligament of
      uterus
    a. scissors
    auditory
    auricular
    axillary
    basilar
    brachial
    brachiocephalic
    buccal
    carotid
    caudal
    celiac

artery(ies)* *(continued)*
    central a. of retina
    cerebellar
    cerebral
    cervical
    choroid
    ciliary
    circumflex a. of scapula
    circumflex femoral
    circumflex humeral
    circumflex iliac
    coccygeal
    colic
    collateral
    common carotid
    communicating
    conjunctival
    coronary
    cremasteric
    cystic
    deep a. of clitoris
    deep a. of penis
    deep brachial
    deep femoral
    deep lingual
    deferential
    dental
    diaphragmatic
    digital
    dorsal a. of clitoris
    dorsal a. of foot
    dorsal a. of nose
    dorsal a. of penis
    dorsalis pedis
    duodenal
    epigastric
    episcleral

*a. = artery.
 a's = arteries.

artery(ies)* *(continued)*

ethmoidal
external carotid
facial
fallopian
femoral
fibular
frontal
funicular
gastric
gastroduodenal
gastroepiploic
genicular
gluteal
helicine a's of penis
hemorrhoidal
hepatic
hyaloid
hypogastric
ileal
ileocolic
iliac
iliolumbar
infraorbital
innominate
intercostal
interlobar a's of kidney
interlobular a's of kidney
interlobular a's of liver
internal carotid
interosseous
intestinal
jejunal
labial
lacrimal

artery(ies)* *(continued)*

laryngeal
left coronary
lingual
lumbar
malleolar
mammary
mandibular
masseteric
maxillary
median
meningeal
mental
mesenteric
metacarpal
metatarsal
musculophrenic
nasal
nutrient a's of humerus
obturator
occipital
ophthalmic
ovarian
palatine
palpebral
pancreaticoduodenal
perforating
pericardiacophrenic
perineal
peroneal
pharyngeal
phrenic
plantar
popliteal
principal a. of thumb
pudendal
pulmonary
radial

*a. = artery.
 a's = arteries.

artery(ies)* *(continued)*
    radial a. of index finger
    radiate a's of kidney
    ranine
    rectal
    recurrent
    renal
    sacral
    scapular
    sciatic
    sigmoid
    spermatic
    sphenopalatine
    spinal
    splenic
    stylomastoid
    subclavian
    subcostal
    sublingual
    submental
    subscapular
    supraorbital
    suprarenal
    suprascapular
    supratrochlear
    sural
    sylvian
    tarsal
    temporal
    testicular
    thoracic
    thoracoacromial
    thoracodorsal
    thyroid
    tibial

*a. = artery.
 a's = arteries.

artery(ies)* *(continued)*
    transverse a. of face
    transverse a. of neck
    transverse a. of scapula
    tympanic
    ulnar
    umbilical
    urethral
    uterine
    vaginal
    vertebral
    vesical
    zygomaticoorbital
arthrectomy
arthritis
arthrocentesis
arthrodesis
arthrodesis screw
arthroendoscopy
arthrogram
arthrography
arthrolysis
arthroplasty
arthroplasty gouge
arthroscopy
arthrostomy
arthrotomy
articular capsule
articular fracture
articular muscle
articular osteotome
articular surface
articularis cubiti muscle
articularis genus muscle
articulation (see also *joint*)
    acromioclavicular
    a. osteotome
    atlantoaxial

articulation *(continued)*
    brachiocarpal
    brachioulnar
    calcaneocuboid
    capitular
    carpal
    carpometacarpal
    chondrosternal
    condylar
    costosternal
    costotransverse
    costovertebral
    humeroradial
    humeroulnar
    incudomalleolar
    incudostapedial
    intercarpal
    interchondral
    intercostal
    intermetacarpal
    intermetatarsal
    interphalangeal
    intertarsal
    mandibular
    maxillary
    mediocarpal
    metacarpocarpal
    metacarpophalangeal
    metatarsophalangeal
    occipitoatlantal
    phalangeal
    radiocarpal
    radioulnar
    sacrococcygeal
    sacroiliac
    scapuloclavicular
    sternoclavicular
    sternocostal

articulation *(continued)*
    subtalar
    talocalcaneonavicular
    talonavicular
    tarsometatarsal
    temporomandibular
    temporomaxillary
    tibiofibular
artifact
artificial insemination
artificial joint implant
artificial pacemaker
artificial respiration
artificial rupture of membranes
Artmann chisel
aryepiglottic
aryepiglottic muscle
aryepiglotticus muscle
arytenoid
arytenoid abduction
arytenoid muscle
arytenoid process
arytenoidectomy
arytenoideus obliquus muscle
arytenoideus transversus muscle
arytenoidopexy
arytenoids
Asai operation
ascending aorta
ascending colon
ascending pyelogram
ascending pyelography
ascending urogram
ascending urography
Asch forceps
Asch operation
Asch splint
Asch straightener

ascites
asepsis
aseptic
Asepto syringe
Ashby forceps
Ashford mamilliplasty
Ashhurst splint
askew
aspermia
aspirate
aspirating dissector
aspirating needle
aspirating tip
aspirating trocar
aspirating tube
aspiration
aspiration apparatus
aspiration biopsy
aspiration cannula
aspiration curettage
aspiration of bronchus
aspiration of lung
aspiration of sinuses
aspiration of vitreous
aspirator
    Adams
    a. cannula
    blue-tip
    bronchoscopic
    Broyles
    Carabelli
    Carmody
    cataract
    clamp-on
    Clerf
    Cook County Hospital
    Dieulafoy
    electric

aspirator *(continued)*
    Fritz
    gallbladder
    Gottschalk
    Lukens
    middle ear
    Potain
    red-tip
    soft cataract
    Stedman
    suction pump
    Taylor
    Thorek
    universal
    Vabra
    vacuum
    yellow-tip
ASR blade
ASR scalpel
assimilation
assisted respiration
astragalectomy
astragalus
astrocytoma
asymmetrical
asymmetry
asymptomatic
asynchronous pacemaker
ataractic
ataraxia
ataxia
atelectasis
atheromatosis
atheromatosis cutis
atheromatous
atheromatous plaque
atherosclerosis
athyreosis

Atkins-Cannard tube
Atkins knife
Atkins-Tucker laryngoscope
Atkinson lid block
atlantoaxial articulation
atlas
Atlee clamp
Atlee dilator
atonia
atonic
atonicity
atony
atraumatic
atraumatic clamp
atraumatic forceps
atraumatic needle
atraumatic suture needle
atraumatic sutures
atraumatic tissue forceps
atresia
atretic
atria (*sing.* atrium)
atrial
atrial electrode
atrial fibrillation
atrial flutter
atrial retractor
atriocommissuropexy
atrioplasty
atrioseptal defect
atrioseptopexy
atrioseptoplasty
atrioseptostomy
atriotomy
atrioventricular block
atrioventricular canal
atrioventricular node
atrioventriculostomy

atrium (*pl.* atria)
Atroloc sutures
atrophic
atrophic fracture
atrophy
atropine
attenuation
attic adhesion
attic cannula
attic dissector
attic ear punch
atticoantral
atticoantrostomy
atticoantrotomy
atticotomy
atticus punch
atypical
audiography
audiometer
audiometry
auditory artery
auditory nerve
auditory veins
Aufranc awl
Aufranc dissector
Aufranc gouge
Aufranc groin apron
Aufranc hip prosthesis
Aufranc hook
Aufranc periosteal elevator
Aufranc reamer
Aufranc retractor
Aufranc-Turner hip prosthesis
Aufrecht sign
Aufricht elevator
Aufricht-Lipsett rasp
Aufricht rasp
Aufricht retractor

Aufricht speculum
augmentation
augmentation mammaplasty
Augustine nail
Ault clamp
aural applicator
aural forceps
aural microscope
aural speculum
Aureomycin
Aureomycin gauze
auricle
auricle clamp
auricular appendage catheter
auricular artery
auricular artery clamp
auricular ligation
auricular muscle
auricular nerve
auricular veins
auriculares anteriores nerves
auriculares anteriores veins
auricularis anterior muscle
auricularis magnus nerve
auricularis posterior artery
auricularis posterior muscle
auricularis posterior nerve
auricularis posterior vein
auricularis profunda artery
auricularis superior muscle
auriculectomy
auriculomastoid line
auriculotemporalis nerve
auriscope
auscultation
Austin clip
Austin knife
Austin Moore arthroplasty

Austin Moore extractor
Austin Moore hip prosthesis
Austin Moore impactor
Austin Moore pin
Austin Moore rasp
Austin Moore reamer
Austin retractor
autoclave
autoclip
autogenous graft
autograft
autologous
automatic corneal trephine
automatic cranial drill
automatic rotating tourniquet
automatic screwdriver
automatic skin retractor
automatic tourniquet
autopsy
autosuture instrument
autotransfusion
Auvard cranioclast
Auvard-Remine speculum
Auvard speculum
Auvray incision
AV (arteriovenous, atrioventric-
    ular)
AV (arteriovenous) aneurysm
AV (arteriovenous) fistula
avascular
avascular space
avascularization
Aveline Gutierrez parotidectomy
Avertin
Avila approach
AVM (arteriovenous malforma-
    tion)
avulsion
avulsion fracture

avulsion of nerve
awl
    Aufranc
    bone
    curved
    DePuy
    Rochester
    trochanteric
    Wangensteen
    Wilson
    Zuelzer
Axenfeld sutures
axial cataract
axilla (*pl.* axillae)
axillaris artery
axillaris nerve
axillaris vein
axillary
axillary adenopathy
axillary anesthesia

axillary artery
axillary artery catheterization
axillary block anesthesia
axillary glands
axillary nerve
axillary node
axillary vein
axis
axis traction
axis-traction forceps
Ayer forceps
Ayers T-piece
Ayerst knife
Ayre brush
Ayre knife
Ayre-Scott knife
Ayre tube
azygogram
azygography
azygos vein

b

B-seam ultrasound machine
Babcock clamp
Babcock forceps
Babcock inguinal herniorrhaphy
Babcock needle
Babcock operation
Babcock raspatory
Babcock retractor
Babcock suture wire
Babcock trocar
Babcock vein stripper
baby retractor
bacitracin
back-and-forth sutures
back-bleeding
back brace
back manipulation
backache
backcut incision
Backhaus clamp
Backhaus dilator
Backhaus forceps
backward cutting scissors
Bacon anoscope
Bacon forceps
Bacon raspatory
Bacon retractor
Bacon rib shears
Bacon rongeur
Badal operation
Badgley nail
Badgley operation

Badgley plate
Badgley retractor
Baffes operation
baffle
bag catheter
Bahnson clamp
Bahnson retractor
Bailey bur
Bailey cannula
Bailey catheter
Bailey clamp
Bailey conductor
Bailey contractor
Bailey-Cowley clamp
Bailey dilator
Bailey forceps
Bailey-Gibbon rib contractor
Bailey Gigli-saw guide
Bailey-Glover-O'Neil commis-
    surotomy
Bailey-Glover-O'Neil knife
Bailey-Glover-O'Neil valvulotome
Bailey leukotome
Bailey-Morse clamp
Bailey-Morse knife
Bailey pliers
Bailey rib contractor
Bailey rongeur
Bailey-Williamson forceps
Bailliart ophthalmodynamometer
Bailliart tonometer
Bainbridge clamp

Bainbridge forceps
Baird forceps
Bakamjian pedicle flap
bakelite mallet
bakelite resectoscope sheath
Baker cyst
Baker forceps
Baker tube
Bakes dilator
Bakes probe
balanced anesthesia
balanced suspension
balanitis
balanoplasty
Baldwin operation
Baldy operation
Baldy-Webster uterine suspension
Balfour blade
Balfour gastrectomy
Balfour gastroenterostomy
Balfour retractor
Balkan fracture frame
Balkan splint
ball-and-socket joint
ball electrode
ball-end hook
Ball operation
ball reamer
ball tip electrode
ball-tipped scissors
ball-type prosthesis
ball-type valve
ball valve
ball valve prosthesis
Ballantine clamp
Ballantine-Drew coagulator
Ballen-Alexander retractor
Ballenger bur

Ballenger chisel
Ballenger curet
Ballenger electrode
Ballenger elevator
Ballenger forceps
Ballenger-Forster forceps
Ballenger gouge
Ballenger-Hajek chisel
Ballenger-Hajek elevator
Ballenger knife
Ballenger-Lillie bur
Ballenger periosteotome
Ballenger raspatory
Ballenger-Sluder tonsillectome
Ballenger urethroscope
Ballentine forceps
Ballentine-Peterson forceps
ballistocardiography
balloon
    Anthony-Fisher
    antral
    antrum
    b. catheter
    b. septostomy
    Brighton
    epistaxis
    Fox
    postnasal
    Rushkin
    Sengstaken
    Shea-Anthony
    sinus
ballooning
ballotable
ballottement
ballpoint scissors
Bamby clamp
Bancroft-Plenk gastrectomy

band
    anchor
    angle
    belly
    clamp
    Magill
    Matas
    matrix
    metal
    orthodontic
    Parham
    Parham-Martin
    tooth
    vessel
Band-Aid dressing
bandage (see also *dressing*)
    A-S-E (axilla, shoulder and
      elbow)
    abdominal
    Ace
    Ace adherent
    adherent
    adhesive
    ARD
    b. scissors
    barrel
    Barton
    Baynton
    Bennell
    binocle
    binocular
    Borsch
    Buller
    Capeline
    circular
    compression
    cotton elastic
    cotton-wool

bandage *(continued)*
    cravat
    crepe
    crucial
    Curad plastic
    demigauntlet
    Desault
    elastic
    elastic adhesive
    Elasticon
    Elastoplast
    Esmarch
    figure-of-eight
    fixation
    four-tailed
    Fricke
    Galen
    Garretson
    gauntlet
    gauze
    Genga
    Gibney
    Gibson
    Hamilton
    hammock
    Heliodorus
    Hippocrates
    Hueter
    immobilizing
    immovable
    Kerlix
    Kiwisch
    Kling
    Larrey
    Maissonneuve
    many-tailed
    Marlex
    Martin

bandage *(continued)*
    monocular
    oblique
    perineal
    plaster
    pressure
    Priessnitz
    protective
    reverse
    reversed
    Ribble
    Richet
    roller
    Sayre
    scarf
    Scultetus
    Seutin
    spica
    spiral
    spiral reverse
    spray
    starch
    stockinette
    Surgiflex
    suspensory
    T-bandage
    Theden
    thermophore
    triangular
    Tuffnell
    Velpeau
    Webril
    wet
    Y-bandage
banding
Bane forceps
Bane hook
Bane rongeur

banjo splint
Bankart operation for shoulder
    dislocation
Bankart retractor
Banner snare
Bantam coagulator
bar
    acrylic
    arch
    clasp
    connector
    dental arch
    Erich arch
    intramedullary
    Jelanko
    Kazanjian T-bar
    Kennedy
    labial
    lingual
    Livingston
    major connector
    minor connector
    occlusal rest
    palatal
    strut
Bar incision
Barany apparatus
Barbara pelvimeter
barbed broach
barbiturate antagonists
barbiturates
Bard catheter
Bard cystoscope tip
Bard dilator
Bard electrode
Bard-Parker blade
Bard-Parker dermatome
Bard-Parker forceps

Bard-Parker knife
Bard-Parker knife handle
Bard-Parker scissors
Bard-Parker sterilizer
Bard resectoscope
Bard tip
Bardam catheter
Bardelli operation
Bardenheuer incision
Bardex catheter
Bardex Foley catheter
Bardex hemostatic bag
Bardic cannula
Bardic catheter
Bardic curet
Bardic tube
barium
barium enema
barium swallow
Barkan forceps
Barkan goniotomy
Barkan goniotomy lens
Barkan knife
Barker needle
Barker operation
Barker Vacu-tome dermatome
Barker Vacu-tome knife
Barlow forceps
Barlow syndrome
Barnes compressor
Barnes dilator
Barnes-Dormia stone basket
Barnes-Simpson forceps
Barnes speculum
Barnes trocar
Barnhill curet
Baron elevator
Baron knife

Baron retractor
Baron suction tube
Barr bolt
Barr hook
Barr nail
Barr operation
Barr probe
Barr retractor
Barr speculum
Barraquer brush
Barraquer-Colibri eye speculum
Barraquer-DeWecker scissors
Barraquer erysiphake
Barraquer forceps
Barraquer knife
Barraquer needle holder
Barraquer operation
Barraquer scissors
Barraquer silk sutures
Barraquer speculum
Barraquer trephine
Barraquer-Zeiss microscope
Barraya forceps
barrel bandage
barrel dressing
barrel-type chest
Barrett-Adson retractor
Barrett-Allen forceps
Barrett forceps
Barrett inverter
Barrett knife
Barrett-Murphy forceps
Barrett needle
Barrett tenaculum
Barrio operation
Barsky cleft lip repair
Barsky elevator
Barsky operation

Barsky pharyngoplasty
Barth hernia
Bartholin's glands
Bartlett stripper
Barton bandage
Barton-Cone tongs
Barton dressing
Barton forceps
Barton fracture
Barton operation for ankylosis
Barton tongs
Barton traction handle
Baruch scissors
Barwell operation
basal
basal anesthesia
basal cell carcinoma
basal ganglia
basal ganglia guide
basal hypnotic agents
basal iridectomy
basal skull fracture
basal vein
basalis vein
base
baseball finger splint
baseball sutures
Basedow paralysis
basement membrane
basilar
basilar artery
basilar membrane
basilar process
basilaris artery
Basile screw
basilic vein
basilica vein
basiotribe

basiotripsy
basivertebral veins
basivertebrales veins
basket (see also *stone basket*)
basket forceps
Basset operation
Bassini herniorrhaphy
Basterra operation
basting stitch
basting stitch anastomosis
Bastow raspatory
Batch-Spittler-McFadden amputation
Bateman operation
Bateman prosthesis
Bates operation for urethral stricture
bath
Battle incision
Battle-Jalaguier-Kammerer incision
Battle operation
Baudelocque operation for extrauterine pregnancy
Bauer forceps
Bauer-Trusler-Tondra cleft lip repair
Baum operation
Baumrucker resectoscope
Bausch & Lomb instruments
Bavarian splint
Baylor splint
Baynton bandage
Baynton operation
bayonet forceps
bayonet incision
bayonet osteotome
bayonet rongeur

bayonet saw
bayonet separator
BE amputation (below-elbow)
Beall mitral valve prosthesis
beam splitter
bean forceps
Beard-Cutler operation
Beard cystotome
Beard knife
Beard speculum
Beardsley clamp
Beardsley dilator
Beardsley forceps
Beardsley trocar
Beardsley tube
Beatson ovariotomy
Beaulieu camera
Beaupre forceps
Beaver blade
Beaver curet
Beaver-DeBakey blade
Beaver dissector
Beaver electrode
Beaver keratome
Beaver knife
Beaver retractor
Beaver saw
Bechtel prosthesis
Bechtel screw
Beck cardiopericardiopexy
Beck clamp
Beck forceps
Beck gastrostomy
Beck-Jianu gastrostomy
Beck knife
Beck loop
Beck-Mueller tonsillectome
Beck I operation

Beck II operation
Beck rasp
Beck raspatory
Beck-Satinsky clamp
Beck-Schenck tonsillectome
Beck scoop
Becker operation
Becker retractor
Becker scissors
Becker screwdriver
Becker trephine
Beckman-Adson retractor
Beckman-Colver speculum
Beckman-Eaton retractor
Beckman retractor
Beckman speculum
Beckman-Weitlaner retractor
Béclard amputation
Béclard hernia
Béclard sutures
bed
        Gatch
        Hough
bedside suction tube
bedsore
Beebe forceps
Beer cataract flap operation
Beer forceps
Beer knife
Belfield vasotomy
Bell erysiphake
Bell operation
Bell sutures
Bellocq cannula
Bellocq sound
Bellocq tube
Bellows cryoextractor
bellows suction

Bellucci scissors
belly band
Belmas operation
below-elbow amputation (BE)
below-knee amputation (BK)
Belsey esophagoplasty
Belsey herniorrhaphy
Belsey perfusor
belt
      Posey
      safety
Belzer apparatus
Benaron forceps
bending fracture
Benedict gastroscope
Beneventi retractor
Bengolea forceps
benign prostatic hypertrophy
Bénique sound
Bennell bandage
Bennett elevator
Bennett forceps
Bennett fracture
Bennett operation
Bennett respirator
Bennett retractor
Bennett spud
benoxinate hydrochloride
Benson separator
bent blade plate
bent fracture
bent hook
Bent shoulder excision
Bentley filter
benzocaine
benzoquinonium chloride
Berbecker pliers
Berbecker wire cutter

Berbridge scissors
Berens clamp
Berens compressor
Berens dilator
Berens eye implant
Berens forceps
Berens hook
Berens implant
Berens keratome
Berens knife
Berens lens expressor
Berens lid everter
Berens loupe
Berens operation
Berens punch
Berens retractor
Berens-Rosa eye implant
Berens scissors
Berens scoop
Berens spatula
Berens speculum
Bergenhem implantation of ureter
      into rectum
Berger interscapular amputation
Bergmann hydrocele repair
Bergmann incision
Bergmann-Israel incision
Berke clamp
Berke forceps
Berke-Motais ptosis correction
Berke ptosis correction
Berlind-Auvard speculum
Berman clamp
Berman magnet
Berman metal locator
Berman-Moorhead metal locator
Bermenam-Werner probe
Berna retractor

Bernard operation
Bernay retractor
Bernberg bow intrauterine device
  (IUD)
Berndt hip ruler
Berne forceps
Berne rasp
Bernstein gastroscope
Bernstein test
berry aneurysm
Berry clamp
Berry forceps
Berry raspatory
Bertrandi sutures
Berwick's dye
Best clamp
Best forceps
Best operation
Best telescope
beta-lactose pack
beta ray microscope
Betadine
betatron irradiation
Bethune clamp
Bethune-Coryllos rib shears
Bethune elevator
Bethune hook
Bethune periosteal elevator
Bethune retractor
Bethune rib shears
Bethune shears
Bethune tourniquet
Bevan forceps
Bevan incision
Bevan operation
Bevan-Rochet operation
bevel
beveled, bevelled

Beyea operation
Beyer forceps
Beyer needle
Beyer punch
Beyer rongeur
bezoar
bias-cut stockinette
bias stockinette
biaxial joint
Bicek retractor
biceps brachii muscle
biceps femoris muscle
biceps muscle
bicipital
bicornuate uterus
bicoudate catheter
bicoudé catheter
bicuspid valve
bicuspidate
bicuspidization
bident retractor
Bielschowsky operation
Bier amputation
Bier anesthesia
Bier block
Bier local anesthesia
Biesenberger reduction mammaplasty
bifid retractor
bifrontal
bifrontal craniotomy
bifurcated seamless prosthesis
bifurcation graft
bifurcation osteotomy
bifurcation prosthesis
Bigelow clamp
Bigelow litholapaxy
Bigelow lithotrite

bilateral mandibular block anesthesia
bilateral procedure
bile
bile canaliculi
bile duct
Bilhaut-Celoquet wedge resection
biliary catheter
biliary duct
biliary dyskinesia
biliary retractor
biliary tract
Bililite
Bill traction handle
Billeau curet
Billroth I anastomosis
Billroth II anastomosis
Billroth forceps
Billroth I gastrectomy
Billroth II gastrectomy
Billroth I gastroenterostomy
Billroth II gastroenterostomy
Billroth operation
Billroth tongue excision
Billroth tube
bilobate
bilobed
bilocular joint
bimanual examination
bimanual version
binangle
binangled chisel
Binkhorst eye implant
Binnie operation
binocle bandage
binocular bandage
binocular dressing
binocular loupe

binocular microscope
binocular ophthalmoscope
biohazard operating technique
biopsy
biopsy by curettage
biopsy curet
biopsy forceps
biopsy loop electrode
biopsy needle
biopsy punch
biopsy punch forceps
biopsy specimen forceps
biopsy telescope
biopsy tongs
biotome
Biotronik pacemaker
biparietal
biparietal craniotomy
biparietal diameter
bipartite
bipolar catheter
bipolar catheter electrode
bipolar cautery
bipolar coagulation forceps
bipolar coagulator
bipolar electrode
bipolar forceps
bipolar Medtronic pacemaker
bipolar needle
bipolar pacemaker
bipolar version
Bircher operation
Bird respirator
Birkett forceps
Birkett hernia
Birtcher cautery
Birtcher coagulator
Birtcher electrode

Birtcher hyfrecator
birth canal
birthmark
Bischoff operation
bisect
bisection
Bishop-Black tendon tucker
Bishop chisel
Bishop-Coop enterostomy
Bishop-DeWitt tendon tucker
Bishop gouge
Bishop-Harmon cannula
Bishop-Harmon forceps
Bishop-Harmon irrigator
Bishop-Harmon tip
Bishop perforator
Bishop-Peter tendon tucker
Bishop saw
Bishop tendon tucker
Bissell operation
bistoury
bistoury blade
bistoury knife
bite biopsy
bite block
bitemporal
bitemporal craniotomy
biting forceps
biting punch
bivalve retractor
bivalve speculum
bivalve tube
bivalved elliptical incision
bivalved speculum
Bizzarri-Guiffrida knife
Bizzarri-Guiffrida laryngoscope
Björk drill
Björk-Shiley mitral valve prosthesis

Björk-Shiley valve
BK amputation (below-knee)
black braided sutures
Black clamp
Black retractor
black silk sutures
black twisted sutures
Black-Wylie dilator
blackout
bladder
bladder blade
bladder calculus (calculi)
bladder catheter
bladder dilator
bladder evacuator
bladder flap
bladder forceps
bladder neck
bladder neck contracture
bladder neck spreader
bladder pacemaker
bladder retractor
bladder specimen forceps
bladder suspension
bladder syringe
bladder trocar
bladder tube
blade
    ASR
    Balfour
    Bard-Parker
    Beaver
    Beaver-DeBakey
    bistoury
    bladder
    b. electrode
    b. holder
    b. plate

blade *(continued)*
    center
    cervical
    cervical biopsy
    circular
    Cloward
    Cooley-Pontius
    Crile
    DeBakey
    Dixon
    double-angle
    Epstein
    Gill
    Guedel
    hemilaminectomy
    Hopp
    Horgan
    Lundsgaard
    MacIntosh
    McPherson-Wheeler
    scalpel
    Swiss
    Taylor
    tubular
bladebreaker knife
Blair-Brown knife
Blair-Brown needle
Blair-Brown operation
Blair-Brown retractor
Blair-Byars operation
Blair chisel
Blair elevator
Blair hook
Blair knife
Blair operation
Blair retractor
Blair saw guide
Blake curet

Blake forceps
Blake rake
Blakemore-Sengstaken tube
Blakemore tube
Blakesley forceps
Blakesley retractor
Blakesley tongue depressor
Blakesley trephine
Blalock anastomosis
Blalock clamp
Blalock forceps
Blalock-Hanlon operation
Blalock-Niedner clamp
Blalock procedure
Blalock-Taussig anastomosis
Blalock-Taussig operation
Blanchard clamp
Blanchard cryptotome
Blanchard forceps
blanching
Blandy urethroplasty
blanket sutures
Blasius lid operation
Blaskovics operation
Blaskovics ptosis correction
Blasucci catheter
Blasucci tip
Blatt operation
bleeder
bleeding points
blepharectomy
blepharochalasis
blepharoplasty
blepharoptosis
blepharorrhaphy
blepharostat
blepharotomy
blister

block anesthesia
block dissection
block technique
Blockain
Blocker operation
blood clots
blood-flow probe
blood supply
blood transfusion
Bloodgood inguinal herniorrhaphy
Bloodgood operation
bloodless
bloodless amputation
bloodless circumcision clamp
Bloodwell forceps
bloody stool
Blot perforator
blotchy
Blount bone spreader
Blount operation
Blount osteotome
Blount osteotomy
Blount plate
Blount retractor
Blount staple
blow-out fracture
blow-up gloves
blue cotton sutures
blue dome cyst
blue nevus
blue-tip aspirator
blue twisted cotton sutures
Blumer's shelf
Blundell-Jones operation
blunt dissection
blunt dissection and snare technique
blunt dissector

blunt hook
blunt needle
blunt periosteal elevator
blunt probe
blunt rake retractor
blunt retractor
blunt scissors
blurred vision
Boari button
Boari operation
Boariplasty
boat nail
Bobb operation
bobbins
Bobroff operation
Bochdalek foramen
Bodenheimer anoscope
Bodenheimer speculum
bodkin
body cavity
Boehm anoscope
Boehm proctoscope
Boehm sigmoidoscope
Boettcher forceps
Boettcher hemostat
Boettcher hook
Boettcher scissors
Boettcher trocar
boggy uterus
Bogue operation
Böhler-Braun splint
Böhler clamp
Böhler fracture frame
Böhler pin
Böhler splint
Böhler tongs
Bohlman pin
Bohm operation

Boies elevator
Boies forceps
Boiler trephine
Bolex camera
bolster
bolster operation
bolster sutures
bolt
    Barr
    cannulated
    DePuy
    Fenton
    Hubbard
    Nylok
    Webb
    Wilson
    Zimmer
bolus
bolus dressing
Bonaccolto forceps
Bonaccolto scleral ring
Bond forceps
Bond splint
bone(s)
    acetabulum
    acromion
    ankle
    astragalus
    atlas
    axis
    b. awl
    b. biopsy needle
    bone-biting forceps
    b. block
    bone-breaking forceps
    b. bur
    b. clamp
    b. chisel

bone(s) *(continued)*
    b. curet
    b. cutter
    bone-cutting forceps
    bone-cutting rongeur
    b. drill
    b. elevator
    b. extractor
    b. file
    b. forceps
    b. gouge
    b. graft
    bone-grasping forceps
    b. guttering
    bone-holding clamp
    bone-holding forceps
    b. hook
    b. implant
    b. mallet
    bone-nibbling rongeur
    b. osteotome
    b. plate
    b. punch
    b. rasp
    b. reamer
    b. rongeur
    b. saw
    b. screw
    b. screwdriver
    b. septum forceps
    b. skid
    bone-splitting forceps
    b. spreader
    b. tamp
    b. trephine
    b. tube
    b. wax (see separate listing)
breast

bone(s) *(continued)*
- calcaneus
- capitate
- carpal
- cervical vertebrae
- clavicle
- coccygeal vertebrae
- coccyx
- collar
- concha
- condyle
- cribriform process
- cuboid
- cuneiform
- dorsal vertebrae
- epistropheus
- ethmoid
- fabella
- femur
- fibula
- foot
- frontal
- gladiolus
- greater multangular
- hamate
- heel
- hip
- humerus
- hyoid
- ilium
- incus
- innominate
- ischium
- knee
- lacrimal
- lateral condyle
- lateral meniscus
- lesser multangular

bone(s) *(continued)*
- lumbar vertebrae
- lunate
- malar
- malleus
- mandible
- manubrium
- mastoid
- maxilla
- medial condyle
- medial meniscus
- meniscus
- metacarpal
- metatarsal
- multangular
- nasal
- navicular
- occipital
- orbital
- palatine
- parietal
- patella
- pelvic
- petrous
- phalanx *(pl.* phalanges)
- pisiform
- pubic
- radius
- ramus
- ribs
- sacral vertebrae
- sacrum
- scaphoid
- scapula
- semilunar
- sesamoid
- shin
- shoulder blade

bone(s) *(continued)*
    sphenoid
    squamous
    stapes
    sternum
    subperiosteal
    talus
    tarsal
    temporal
    thigh
    thoracic vertebrae
    tibia
    toe
    trapezium
    trapezoid
    triangular
    triquetral
    turbinate
    tympanic
    ulna
    unciform
    uncinate
    vertebra *(pl.* vertebrae)
    vomer
    wrist
    xiphoid
    zygomatic
bone wax
    b. w. sutures
    casting
    Horsley
    Mosetig-Moorhof
Bonina-Jacobson tube
Bonn forceps
Bonnano tube
Bonner position
Bonnet enucleation of eyeball

Bonney clamp
Bonney forceps
Bonney hysterectomy
Bonney needle
Bonney-type sutures
Bonta knife
bony ridge
Bonzel iridodialysis
boomerang needle holder
boot brace
borborygmus
Boros esophagoscope
Borsch bandage
Borthen operation
Bose hook
Bose tracheotomy
Bosher knife
Bossalino operation
bosselated
Bossi dilator
Boston Lying-In cervical forceps
Bosworth drill
Bosworth operation
Bosworth retractor
Bosworth screw
Bosworth-Shawler incision
Bosworth snare
Bosworth speculum
Bosworth tongue depressor
Bottini operation
bottle hernia operation
bottle repair
bottle operation
Botvin forceps
Boucheron speculum
Bouchut tube

bougie

    acorn-tipped

    b. à boule

    Buerger

    bulbous

    caustic

    Chevalier Jackson

    common duct

    conic

    Cooper

    cylindrical

    dilatable

    dilating

    Dourmashkin

    ear

    elastic

    elbowed

    esophageal

    eustachian

    exploratory

    filiform

    Fort

    French

    Friedman-Otis

    fusiform

    Gabriel Tucker

    Gruber

    Guyon

    Holinger

    Holinger-Hurst

    Hurst

    infant

    Jackson

    LeFort

    Maloney

    medicated

    mercury-filled esophageal

    olive-tip

bougie *(continued)*

    olive-tipped

    Otis

    Phillips

    Plummer

    rectal

    retrograde

    rosary

    Ruschelit

    soluble

    spiral-tip

    tapered

    tracheal

    Trousseau

    tunneled

    Tucker

    Urbantschitsch

    ureteral

    urethral

    urethral whip

    Wales

    wax

    wax-tipped

    whalebone filiform

    whip

    whistle

    woven

bougienage

Bouilly operation

Bourns respirator

boutonniere deformity

Bovie

    B. cautery

    B. coagulation tip

    B. coagulator

    B. current

    B. electrode

    B. electrosurgical unit

Bovie *(continued)*
  B. knife
  B. needle
  B. unit
  clinic
  coagulating current
  liquid conductor
bovied
bovine graft
bow intrauterine device (IUD)
bowel
bowel obstruction
bowel pattern
bowel retractor
bowel sounds
Bowen chisel
Bowen gouge
Bowen-Grover meniscotome
Bowen osteotome
Bowen periosteal elevator
Bowlby splint
bowling-pin incision
Bowman's capsule
Bowman dilator
Bowman's glands
Bowman's membrane
Bowman needle
Bowman operation
Bowman probe
Bowman scissors
Bowman slitting of canaliculus
Box adenotome
Box-DeJager adenotome
box-joint forceps
boxer fracture
Boyce position
Boyd amputation
Boyd incision

Boyd operation
Boyd scissors
Boyden's sphincter
Boyes clamp
Boyes-Goodfellow hook
Boyes-Goodfellow hook retractor
Boyle Davis mouth gag
Boynton needle holder
Boys-Allis forceps
Bozeman catheter
Bozeman clamp
Bozeman forceps
Bozeman-Frisch catheter
Bozeman operation
Bozeman position
Bozeman speculum
Bozeman sutures
Bozeman-Wertheim needle holder
BPD (biparietal diameter)
BPH (benign prostatic hyper-
    trophy)
Braasch catheter
Braasch cystoscope
Braasch forceps
Braastad retractor
brace
    back
    boot
    cervical
    cervical collar
    chairback
    collar
    Cook walking
    drop foot
    Forrester
    four-point cervical
    four-poster cervical
    Hudson

brace *(continued)*
  hyperextension
  ischial weightbearing
  Jewett
  King
  Knight
  Kuhlman
  long leg
  Lyman-Smith
  Milwaukee
  Murphy
  non-weightbearing
  Oppenheim
  Schanz
  scoliosis
  short leg
  snap-lock
  SOMI
  stirrup
  Taylor
  Teufel
  Thomas
  toedrop
  walking
  Warm Springs
  weightbearing
  Wilke
  Williams
brachial anesthesia
brachial artery
brachial muscle
brachial plexus block
brachial plexus nerve
brachial veins
brachiales veins
brachialis artery
brachialis muscle
brachialis superficialis artery

brachiocarpal articulation
brachiocephalic artery
brachiocephalic trunk
brachiocephalic veins
brachiocephalicae (dextra et
    sinistra) veins
brachioradial ligament
brachioradial muscle
brachioradialis muscle
brachioulnar articulation
Bracken forceps
bracketed splint
Brackett operation
Brackett probe
Brackin incision
Braden reservoir
Bradford forceps
Bradford fracture frame
Bradford-Young Y-V plasty
Bradshaw-O'Neill clamp
bradyarrhythmia
bradycardia
bradykinesia
braided nylon sutures
braided silk sutures
braided sutures
braided wire sutures
Brailey operation
Brailey stretching of supra-
    trochlear nerve
brain biopsy needle
brain cannula
brain clip
brain-exploring cannula
brain-exploring trocar
brain forceps
brain hook
brain knife

brain retractor
brain scan
brain scissors
brain spatula
brain speculum
brain spoon
brain stem
brain suction tip
brain suction tube
brain tumor forceps
branch
branchial
branchial cyst
Brand tendon passer
Brand tendon stripper
Brandt technique
Bransford-Lewis dilator
Brant splint
Brantley-Turner retractor
brassiere-type dressing
Brauer cardiolysis
Brauer operation
Braun anastomosis
Braun and Jaboulay gastrectomy
Braun and Jaboulay gastro-
    enterostomy
Braun cranioclast
Braun forceps
Braun frame
Braun hook
Braun-Jardine-DeLee hook
Braun ligature carrier
Braun operation
Braun scissors
Braun tenaculum
Braun-Wangensteen operation
Braunwald-Cutter prosthesis
Brawley rasp

Brawley retractor
brawny edema
Braxton-Hicks contraction
Braxton-Hicks version
breast biopsy
breast bone
breast plate
breast prosthesis
breast tenaculum
Breck pin
breech delivery
breech extraction
Breisky-Navratil speculum
Breisky pelvimeter
Breitman adenotome
Brenner forceps
Brenner inguinal herniorrhaphy
Brenner operation
Brent eyebrow reconstruction
Brescio-Cimino arteriovenous
    fistula
Brett operation
Brevital sodium
Brewer operation
Brewer speculum
Brewster retractor
Bricker ileal conduit
Bricker ileoureterostomy
Bricker ureteroileostomy
Brickner position
bridge
bridge clamp
bridge forceps
bridge telescope
bridging
bridle sutures
Briggs operation
Briggs transilluminator

Brigham forceps
Brighton balloon
Brinkerhoff anoscope
Brinkerhoff speculum
brisement forcé
brisk
Bristow periosteal elevator
Bristow procedure
Brittain arthrodesis
Brittain chisel
brittle
broach
    barbed
    femoral
    femoral prosthesis
    Harris
    root canal
    smooth
broaching
broad-blade forceps
broad ligament
broad ligament of uterus
Brock clamp
Brock dilator
Brock incision
Brock knife
Brock probe
Brock punch
Brock valvotomy
Brock valvulotome
Brockenbrough needle
Brockman operation
Brodie probe
Brodney cannula
Brodney clamp
Brodney hemostatic bag
Bromptom Hospital retractor
bronchi (*sing.* bronchus)

bronchial biopsy forceps
bronchial catheter
bronchial dilator
bronchial glands
bronchial tree
bronchial veins
bronchial washings
bronchiales veins
bronchiectasis
bronchiole
bronchocele sound
bronchocutaneous fistula
bronchodilation
bronchodilator
bronchoesophageal muscle
bronchoesophageus muscle
bronchogenic
bronchogram
bronchography
bronchoplasty
bronchopleural fistula
bronchopneumonia
bronchorrhaphy
bronchoscope
    ACMI
    Albert
    Broyles
    Bruening
    Chevalier Jackson
    coagulation
    costophrenic
    Davis
    double channel irrigating
    Emerson
    Foregger
    Haslinger
    Holinger
    Holinger-Jackson

bronchoscope *(continued)*
    hook-on
    irrigating
    Jackson
    Jesberg
    Kernan-Jackson
    Killian
    Michelson
    Moersch
    Negus
    Overholt Jackson
    pediatric
    Pilling
    respiration
    Riecker
    Safar
    slotted
    standard
    staple
    Storz
    telescope
    Tucker
    ventilation
    Waterman
    Yankauer
bronchoscopic aspirator
bronchoscopic brush
bronchoscopic forceps
bronchoscopic magnet
bronchoscopic probe
bronchoscopy
bronchospasm
bronchospirometric catheter
bronchospirometry
bronchostomy
bronchotomy
bronchus *(pl.* bronchi)
bronchus clamp

bronchus forceps
Bronson magnet
Bronson-Turz retractor
bronze wire sutures
Brooks punch
Brooks scissors
Brophy bistoury
Brophy cleft palate operation
Brophy-Deschamps needle
Brophy elevator
Brophy forceps
Brophy knife
Brophy mouth gag
Brophy needle
Brophy operation
Brophy periosteal elevator
Brophy periosteotome
Brophy plate
Brophy scissors
Brophy tenaculum
Broviac catheter
Brown-Adson forceps
Brown applicator
Brown-Blair dermatome
Brown-Blair operation
Brown-Buerger cystoscope
Brown-Buerger forceps
Brown chisel
Brown clamp
Brown dermatome
Brown-Dohlman eye implant
Brown electrodermatome
Brown elevator
Brown forceps
Brown hook
Brown knife
Brown needle
Brown operation

Brown periosteotome
Brown-Pusey trephine
Brown rasp
Brown retractor
Brown saw
Brown scissors
Brown-Sequard lesion
Brown snare
Brown splint
Brown tonsillectome
Browne hypospadias repair
Browne-McHardy dilator
Browne stone basket
Browne urethral reconstruction
Broyles aspirator
Broyles bronchoscope
Broyles dilator
Broyles esophagoscope
Broyles forceps
Broyles laryngoscope
Broyles nasopharyngoscope
Broyles telescope
Broyles tube
Bruch's membrane
Bruening bronchoscope
Bruening cannula
Bruening chisel
Bruening-Citelli rongeur
Bruening electroscope
Bruening esophagoscope
Bruening forceps
Bruening otoscope
Bruening punch
Bruening snare
Bruening speculum
bruit
bruit de clapotement
Brun curet

Bruner vaginal speculum
brunescent cataract
Brunetti chisel
Brunner chisel
Brunner forceps
Brunner glands
Brunner goiter dissector
Brunner incision
Brunner raspatory
Brunner retractor
Brunner rib shears
Bruns chisel
Brunschwig forceps
Brunschwig pancreato-
    duodenectomy
Brunschwig retractor
Brunschwig total pelvic exentera-
    tion
Brunton otoscope
Bruser incision
brush
        aortic valve
        Ayre
        Barraquer
        bronchoscopic
        b. biopsy
        denture
        Edwards-Carpentier aortic
            valve
        Glassman
        Haidinger
        Kurten wire
        polishing
        stomach
        wire
brushings
Bryant lumbar colotomy
Bryant traction

buccal artery
buccal glands
buccal mucosa
buccal nerve
buccalis artery
buccalis nerve
buccinator muscle
Bucholz prosthesis
Buck applicator
Buck curet
Buck hook
Buck knife
Buck operation
Buck osteotome
Buck probe
Buck splint
Buck traction
Buck tractor
bucket-handle fracture
bucket-handle tear
buckling
buckling operation
Buckstein insufflator
Bucy-Frazier cannula
Bucy-Frazier suction tube
Bucy knife
Bucy retractor
Bud bur
Budinger operation
Buerger bougie
Buerger disease
Buerger-McCarthy forceps
Buerger-McCarthy scissors
Buerger snare
Bugbee electrode
Buie cannula
Buie clamp
Buie electrode

Buie forceps
Buie hemorrhoidectomy
Buie-Hirschman anoscope
Buie-Hirschman clamp
Buie-Hirschman speculum
Buie irrigator
Buie operation
Buie position
Buie probe
Buie scissors
Buie sigmoidoscope
Buie-Smith retractor
Buie-Smith speculum
Buie suction tube
Buie tube
build-up eye implant
bulb catheter
bulb retractor
bulb ureteral catheter
bulbi penis artery
bulbi penis vein
bulbi vestibuli vaginae
    artery
bulbi vestibuli vein
bulbocavernosus muscle
bulbocavernous glands
bulbocavernous muscle
bulbomembranous
bulbospongiosus muscle
bulbourethral glands
bulbous bougie
bulge
bulky compressive dressing
bulky dressing
bulky pressure dressing
bulla (pl. bullae)
bulldog clamp
bulldog forceps

bulldog scissors
Buller bandage
bullet forceps
bullet probe
bullet tenaculum
bullous
Bumm curet
Bumper fracture
Bumpus forceps
Bumpus resectoscope
bunching sutures
bundle branch block
Bunge amputation
Bunge meatotome
Bunge spoon
Bunim forceps
bunion
bunion dissector
bunion operation
bunionectomy
Bunnell drill
Bunnell needle
Bunnell operation
Bunnell probe
Bunnell pull-out wire
Bunnell splint
Bunnell sutures
Bunnell tendon passer
Bunnell tendon repair
Bunnell tendon stripper
Bunts catheter
bupivacaine hydrochloride
bur
    Adson
    Allport
    antrum
    Bailey
    Ballenger

bur *(continued)*
    Ballenger-Lillie
    bone
    bud
    b. drill
    b. hole
    bur-hole incision
    Burwell
    Caparosa
    carbide
    cataract
    Cavanaugh
    choanal
    cone
    conical
    corneal
    cranial
    cross-cut
    curetting
    Cushing
    cutting
    Davidson
    dental
    D'Errico
    diamond
    Doyen
    electric
    electrically driven
    enlarging
    eustachian
    fenestration
    Ferris Smith-Halle
    fissure
    Frey-Freer
    Halle
    House
    Hudson
    inverted cone

bur *(continued)*
    Jordan
    Jordan-Day
    Kopetzky
    Lempert
    Marin
    mastoid
    McKenzie
    Mueller
    neurosurgical
    perforating
    round
    Sachs
    Shea
    sinus
    skull
    slotting
    Somerset
    sphenoid
    Wachsberger
    Wilkerson
    Wullstein
    Yazujian
Burch caliper
Burch evisceration
Burch forceps
Burch-Greenwood tendon tucker
Burch pick
Burckhardt operation
Burdick cautery
Burdick electrosurgical unit
Burdizzo vasectomy
Burford-Finochietto retractor
Burford-Finochietto rib spreader
Burford-Finochietto spreader
Burford retractor
Burford rib spreader
Burford spreader

Burger technique for scapulo-
    thoracic disarticulation
Burgess operation
buried sutures
Burnham forceps
Burnham scissors
Burns chisel
Burns telescope
Burow blepharoplasty
Burow operation
bursa *(pl.* bursae)
bursectomy
bursocentesis
bursotomy
bursting fracture
Burwell bur
burying of fimbriae in uterine wall
Busch scissors
butacaine
Butcher saw
butethamine hydrochloride
Butterfield cystoscope
butterfly clip
butterfly dressing
butterfly fracture
buttock
button
    Boari
    b. cautery
    button-end knife
    b. knife
    b. sutures
    Chlumsky
    collar
    Jaboulay
    Kazanjian
    Kistner
    Lardennois

button *(continued)*
  Moore
  Murphy
  peritoneal
  polyethylene collar
  Reuter
  Todd
  tracheostomy
  Villard
buttonhole
buttonhole fracture
buttonhole incision
buttonhook
buttonhook retractor
buttress
Butyn
Buxton clamp
Buzzi operation
Byford retractor
bypass
bypass graft
bypass prosthesis
bypass tube
bypass vein graft

C

C-clamp
C-P suction (Chaffin-Pratt)
CAB (coronary artery bypass)
CABG (coronary artery bypass
    graft)
cable wire sutures
Cabot splint
CAD prosthesis (computerized
    assisted design)
cadaver
café-au-lait
Cairns forceps
Cairns retractor
Cairns rongeur
calcaneal tendon
calcaneocuboid articulation
calcaneofibular ligament
calcaneonavicular ligament
calcaneus
calcar
calcareous
calcific
calcification
calcified
calculus (*pl.* calculi)
Caldwell-Luc incision
Caldwell-Luc operation
Caldwell-Luc window operation
Caldwell operation
Caldwell position
Calhoun-Merz needle
Calhoun needle

calibrated guide pin
calibration
Calibri forceps
calicectasis
calicectomy
calices (*sing.* calix)
calipers
    Burch
    Castroviejo
    Cone
    Cottle
    electric
    eye
    Green
    ice-tong
    Jameson
    Ladd
    skinfold
    Thorpe
    tonsil
    Townley
calix (*pl.* calices)
Callahan flange
Callahan forceps
Callahan operation
Callander amputation
Callender clip
Callisen operation
callus
caloric testing
Calot node
Calot operation

Calot triangle
Caltagirone chisel
Caltagirone knife
calvarial hook
calvarium clamp
Calve cannula
camera
    Anger
    Beaulieu
    Bolex
    cine-camera
    Nikon
    Polaroid
Cameron electrosurgical unit
Cameron fracture appliance
Cameron gastroscope
Cameron-Haight elevator
Cameron-Haight periosteal
    elevator
Cameron-Lorenz cautery
Cameron-Miller cautery
Cameron periosteal elevator
Campbell catheter
Campbell elevator
Campbell forceps
Campbell-Goldthwait patella
    dislocation operation
Campbell gouge
Campbell needle
Campbell operation
Campbell osteotome
Campbell periosteal elevator
Campbell retractor
Campbell rongeur
Campbell sound
Campbell splint
Campbell trocar
Camper's fascia

canal
    adductor
    Alcock's
    alimentary
    anal
    atrioventricular
    birth
    c. knife
    c. of Corti
    c. of Nuck
    carotid
    cervical
    condylar
    femoral
    Guyon's
    haversian
    Hunter's
    hypoglossal
    infraorbital
    inguinal
    medullary
    optic
    pulp
    root
    sacral
    Schlemm's
    semicircular
    spinal
    vertebral
    Volkmann's
canalicular scissors
canaliculi (*sing.* canaliculus)
canaliculi vein
canaliculodacryocystostomy
canaliculoplasty
canaliculorhinostomy
canaliculus (*pl.* canaliculi)
canaliculus knife

canaliculus punch
canaliculus vein
canalis pterygoidei artery
canalis pterygoidei nerve
canalis pterygoidei vein
canalization
canaloplasty
cancellous bone
cancellous bone graft
cancer cell collector
Cane forceps
Canfield knife
canine muscle
canine teeth
canine-to-canine lingual splint
Cannon endarterectomy loop
Cannon-Rochester elevator
Cannon stripper
cannula
    Abelson
    Abraham
    Adson
    air
    air injection
    alpha-chymotrypsin
    anterior chamber
    antrum
    aortic
    arterial
    aspiration
    aspirator
    attic
    Bailey
    Bardic
    Bellocq
    biopsy
    Bishop-Harmon
    brain

cannula *(continued)*
    brain-exploring
    Brodney
    Bruening
    Bucy-Frazier
    Buie
    Calve
    c. scissors
    c. tip
    Carabelli
    Casselberry
    Castroviejo
    caval
    cerebral
    chemopallidectomy
    Chilcott
    Clagett
    clysis
    Coakley
    Cohen-Eder
    Colt
    Cone
    Cone-Bucy
    Cooper
    coronary perfusion
    cricothyrotomy
    curved
    cyclodialysis
    Day
    DeWecker
    Dorsey
    double lumen
    Dow Corning
    drainage
    Duke
    Dupuis
    Elsberg
    esophagoscopic

cannula *(continued)*
    exploring
    eye and ear
    fallopian
    femoral artery
    Fisher
    Frazier
    frontal sinus
    gallbladder
    Gass
    Goldstein
    Goodfellow
    Hahn
    Hasson-Eder
    Haverfield
    Haynes
    Hepacon
    Hoen
    Holinger
    hollow
    Holman-Mathieu
    Hudgins
    Huse
    Ingals
    injection
    intrauterine
    irrigating
    Jarcho
    Kahn
    Kanavel
    Killian
    Killian-Eichen
    Kos
    Krause
    Kreutzmann
    lacrimal
    laparoscopic
    laryngeal

cannula *(continued)*
    Lillie
    Lindeman
    Lukens
    Luongo
    Mayo
    mediastinal
    metal
    mirror
    Moncreiff
    monitoring
    Morris
    Myles
    Neal
    New York Eye and Ear
    Paterson
    Patton
    Pereyra
    perfusion
    Pierce
    plastic
    polyethylene
    Pritchard
    Pynchon
    Randolph
    rectal injection
    return flow
    Rigg
    Robb
    Rockey
    Rolf
    Roper
    Rubin
    "S"
    Sachs
    Sarns
    Scott
    Seletz

cannula *(continued)*
    Sewall
    Silastic
    silicone
    sinus
    Skillern
    SMI
    Soresi
    Southey
    Spencer
    sphenoid
    Strauss
    suprapubic
    syringe
    Teflon
    Tenner
    tracheal
    tracheostomy
    Trendelenburg
    urethrographic
    uterine
    vabra
    vacuum intrauterine
    Van Alyea
    venoclysis
    ventricular
    Verres
    Von Eichen
    washout
    Wells
cannulate
cannulated bolt
cannulated drill
cannulated forceps
cannulated nail
cannulated reamer
cannulation
cannulation of venae cavae

cannulization
canthectomy
canthi *(sing.* canthus)
cantholysis
canthoplasty
canthorrhaphy
canthotomy
canthus *(pl.* canthi)
cantilevered
Cantor tube
cap splint
Caparosa bur
Caparosa wire crimper
Cape Town prosthesis
Capeline bandage
capillary
capillary fracture
capillary microscope
capital
capitate bone
capitonnage sutures
capitular articulation
capitulum
capsular adhesions
capsular ligament
capsule
    adipose renal
    articular
    Bowman's
    c. forceps
    c. fragment forceps
    c. grasping forceps
    c. knife
    c. of lens
    c. retractor
    c. scissors
    external
    fibrous renal

capsule *(continued)*
    Glisson's
    glomerular
    internal
    joint
    malpighian
    renal
    Tenon's
capsulectomy
capsulolenticular
capsuloplasty
capsulorrhaphy
capsulotome
capsulotomy
capsulotomy scissors
caput medusae
caput succedaneum
Carabelli aspirator
Carabelli cannula
Carabelli collector
Carabelli lumen finder
Carabelli tube
carbide bur
Carbocaine hydrochloride
carbolize
carbon dioxide
carbon dioxide cautery
carbuncle
carcinoid
carcinoma *(pl.* carcinomas *or*
    carcinomata)
carcinoma in situ
Carden amputation
cardia
cardia of stomach
cardiac arrest
Cardiac Care Unit (CCU)
cardiac catheter

cardiac catheterization
cardiac dilator
cardiac glands
cardiac massage
cardiac monitor
cardiac nerve
cardiac pacemaker
cardiac resuscitation
cardiac revascularization
cardiac scissors
cardiac tamponade
cardiac valve dilator
cardiac veins
cardiaci thoracici nerves
cardiacus cervicalis inferior nerve
cardiacus cervicalis medius nerve
cardiacus cervicalis superior nerve
cardiectomy
Cardillo retractor
cardinal ligament
cardiocentesis
cardioesophageal
cardiogram
cardiography
cardiolysis
cardiomegaly
cardiomyopexy
cardiomyotomy
cardio-omentopexy
cardiopericardiopexy
cardioplasty
cardioplegia
cardiopneumonopexy
cardiopulmonary arrest
cardiopulmonary bypass
cardiorrhaphy
cardioschisis
cardioscope

cardiospasm
cardiospasm dilator
cardiosplenopexy
cardiotomy
cardiovalvulotome
cardiovalvulotomy
cardiovascular
cardiovascular forceps
cardiovascular tourniquet
cardioversion
Cargile membrane
Cargile sutures
carina
Carlens catheter
Carlens curet
Carlens forceps
Carlens mediastinoscope
Carlens tube
Carmack curet
Carmalt clamp
Carmalt forceps
Carmalt hemostat
Carmalt tube
Carman tube
Carmel clamp
Carmody aspirator
Carmody-Brophy forceps
Carmody drill
Carmody forceps
Carmody pump
carotici externi nerves
caroticotympanic nerve
caroticotympanici nerve
caroticus internus nerve
carotid angiogram
carotid angiography
carotid arteriogram
carotid arteriography

carotid artery
carotid artery clamp
carotid canal
carotid endarterectomy
carotid nerve
carotid pulse tracing
carotid sheath
carotid triangle
carotid vein
carotis communis artery
carotis interna artery
carpal articulations
carpal bones
carpal prosthesis
carpal tunnel release
carpectomy
Carpenter dissector
Carpenter knife
Carpentier anuloplasty
Carpentier-Edwards aortic valve
        replacement
Carpentier-Edwards valve
Carpentier valve
carpometacarpal articulations
carpometacarpal ligament
Carpue rhinoplasty
Carr tourniquet
Carrel clamp
Carrel sutures
Carrel tube
Carrell operation
Carrell patch
carrier
        amalgam
        Braun ligature
        cotton
        Deschamps
        Fitzwater ligature

carrier *(continued)*
    foil
    Kilner suture
    Lahey
    Lahey ligature
    ligature
    Madden ligature
    Mayo
    sponge
    Wangensteen
Carrion penile prosthesis
Carroll-Legg osteotome
Carroll-Legg periosteal elevator
Carroll osteotome
Carroll periosteal elevator
Carroll-Smith-Petersen osteotome
Carson catheter
Carter clamp
Carter curet
Carter elevator
Carter knife
Carter operation
Carter retractor
Carter speculum
Carter sphere introducer
Carter splenectomy
Carter splint
cartilage abrader
cartilage clamp
cartilage forceps
cartilage graft
cartilage guide
cartilage implant
cartilage knife
cartilage punch
cartilage scissors
cartilage stripper
cartilaginous

cartilaginous arthroplasty
cartilaginous joint
Cartwright heart prosthesis
Cartwright valve prosthesis
Cartwright vascular prosthesis
caruncle
caruncle forceps
Casanellas operation
caseous
Cassel operation
Casselberry cannula
Casselberry position
Cassidy-Brophy forceps
cast cutter
Castallo retractor
Castallo speculum
Castellani paint
Castelli-Paparella collar-button
    tube
Castelli-Paparella myringotomy
    tube
Castelli tube
casting bone wax
castration
Castroviejo-Arruga forceps
Castroviejo caliper
Castroviejo cannula
Castroviejo clamp
Castroviejo dermatome
Castroviejo dilator
Castroviejo forceps
Castroviejo-Kalt needle holder
Castroviejo-Kalt traction handle
Castroviejo keratome
Castroviejo knife
Castroviejo needle holder
Castroviejo operation
Castroviejo punch

Castroviejo retractor
Castroviejo scissors
Castroviejo snare
Castroviejo spatula
Castroviejo speculum
Castroviejo trephine
CAT scan (computerized axial tomography)
catamenia
cataract aspirator
cataract bur
cataract extraction
cataract extractor
cataract flap operation
cataract knife
cataract lamp
cataract lens
cataract needle
cataract operation
cataract probe
cataract scissors
cataract spoon
cataract suction unit
catarrh
catarrhal
catgut ligatures
catgut plain ties
catgut sutures
Cathelin segregator
catheter
    ACMI
    Acmistat
    acorn-tip
    acorn-tipped
    Alcock
    Alvarez-Rodriguez
    Amplatz
    angiocatheter

catheter *(continued)*
    angiographic
    aortic
    aortographic
    Argyle
    arterial
    auricular appendage
    bag
    Bailey
    balloon
    Bard
    Bardam
    Bardex
    Bardex Foley
    Bardic
    bicoudate
    bicoudé
    biliary
    bipolar
    bladder
    Blasucci
    Bozeman
    Bozeman-Fritsch
    Braasch
    bronchial
    bronchospirometric
    Broviac
    bulb
    bulb ureteral
    Bunts
    Campbell
    cardiac
    Carlens
    Carson
    c. à demeure
    c. coudé
    c. en chemise
    c. needle

catheter *(continued)*

- c. plug
- c. tip
- c. trocar
- caval
- cecostomy
- central venous
- cerebral
- Chaffin
- cholangiography
- conical
- conical tip
- Constantine
- coudé
- coudé tip
- Councill
- Cournand
- Coxeter
- Cummings
- Cummings-Pezzer
- curved
- cut-down
- Davol
- DeLee
- de Pezzer
- Deseret
- Desilet
- Devonshire
- disposable
- Dormia stone-basket
- double-current
- double-lumen
- drainage
- Drew-Smythe
- Easy
- Edwards
- elbowed
- embolectomy

catheter *(continued)*

- esophagoscopic
- eustachian
- fallopian
- faucial
- faucial eustachian
- female
- fenestrated
- filiform
- filiform-tipped
- flexible
- flexible metal
- floating
- flow-directed
- Fogarty
- Foley
- Foley-Alcock
- four-wing Malecot retention
- French
- French Foley
- French Robinson
- Friend
- Fritsch
- Furniss
- Garceau
- gastroenterostomy
- Gilbert
- Gouley
- Goutz
- Hagner
- Hakion
- Hanafee
- Hartmann
- Hatch
- hemostatic
- Hepacon
- Higgins
- Hryntschak

catheter *(continued)*

- indwelling
- infant
- infant female
- infant male
- intercostal
- intracardiac
- intrauterine
- intravenous
- irrigating
- Itard
- IV (intravenous)
- Jaeger-Whiteley
- Javid
- Jelco
- Jelm
- Kimball
- Lane
- Lapides
- latex
- LeFort
- Lehman
- Lloyd
- lobster-tail
- Longdwel
- Malecot
- Maloney
- mastoid
- McCaskey
- McIver
- Mercier
- metal
- Metras
- Morris
- mushroom
- nasotracheal
- Neal
- Nelaton

catheter *(continued)*

- nephrostomy
- NIH
- Odman-Ledin
- olive-tip
- Owens
- pacemaker
- pacing
- Paparella
- Pezzer
- Pharmaseal
- Phillips
- pigtail
- Pilcher
- plastic
- polyethylene
- polystan
- prostatic
- pulmonary artery
- railway
- rectal
- red Robinson
- red rubber
- retention
- return flow hemostatic
- Robinson
- Rodriguez-Alvarez
- Ross
- round tip
- rubber
- Rusch
- Rusch-Foley
- Ruschelit
- Salmon
- Schrotter
- Seletz
- self-retaining
- Silastic

catheter *(continued)*
    Skene
    soft
    solid-tip
    Sones
    spiral-tip
    Squire
    Stitt
    stone-basket
    straight
    styletted
    suction
    Suggs
    suprapubic
    Swan-Ganz
    Tauber
    Teflon
    Tenckhoff
    Texas
    Thompson
    three-way
    Tiemann
    Tiemann-coudé
    Tomac
    tracheal
    transseptal
    transthoracic
    transvenous pacemaker
    Trattner
    triple lumen
    Tuohy
    two-way
    umbilical
    umbilical artery
    umbilical vein
    ureteral
    ureterographic
    urethral

catheter *(continued)*
    urinary
    urologic
    vabra
    Vacurette
    Venocath
    venous
    vertebrated
    Virden
    Walther
    Weber
    whalebone filiform
    whistle-tip
    Winer
    winged
    Wishard
    Wolf
    Woodruff
    woven-silk
    Wurd
    Yankauer
    Zavod
catheterization
catheterization of bladder
catheterization of duct
catheterization of eustachian tube
catheterization of heart
catheterize
cathode
catling amputation knife
Cattell operation
Cattell T-tube
cauda equina
caudad
caudal
caudal anesthesia
caudal artery
caudal block

caudal ligament
caudal needle
caudate process
Caulk punch
Causse-Shea prosthesis
caustic bougie
cauterization
cauterization of cervix
cauterization of nose
cauterize
cautery
    actual
    Alcon
    alkaline battery
    bipolar
    Birtcher
    Bovie
    Burdick
    button
    Cameron-Lorenz
    Cameron-Miller
    carbon dioxide
    c. clamp
    c. hook
    c. knife
    c. of retinal detachment
    chemical
    chemocautery
    coagulation
    cold
    Corrigan
    cryocautery
    Downes
    electric
    electrocautery
    fine
    galvanic
    gas

cautery *(continued)*
    Geiger-Downes
    hand
    heat
    Hildreth
    linear
    Magielski
    micropoint
    Mira
    monopolar
    Mueller
    National
    Op-Temp
    ophthalmic
    Paquelin
    Parker-Heath
    penlight
    Percy
    potential
    Prince
    retinal puncture
    Rommel
    Rommel-Hildreth
    Scheie
    silver nitrate
    solar
    Souttar
    spot
    steam
    straight
    sun
    Todd
    valvanocautery
    virtual
    von Graefe
    Wadsworth-Todd
    Wappler
    wet-field

cautery *(continued)*
   wound
   Ziegler
caval cannula
caval catheter
caval snare
caval tourniquet
Cavanaugh bur
Cave gouge
Cave incision
Cave knife
Cave operation
Cave retractor
Cave-Rowe operation
Cave spatula
cavernosae penis veins
cavernoscopy
cavernosi clitoridis nerves
cavernosi penis nerves
cavernostomy
cavernotomy
cavernous
cavernous nerves of clitoris
cavernous nerves of penis
cavernous urethra
cavernous veins of penis
Cavin osteotome
Cavin shunt
Cavitron dissector
Cavitron-Kelman phacoemulsification
Cavitron-Kelman surgical unit
cavity
cavogram
cavography
Caylor scissors
CCT (computerized cranial
   tomography)

CCU (coronary care unit; cardiac
   care unit)
cecal
cecal appendix
cecal hernia
cecectomy
Cecil operation
Cecil urethral stricture operation
cecocele
cecocolic
cecocolon
cecocoloplicopexy
cecocolostomy
cecofixation
cecoileostomy
cecopexy
cecoplication
cecoptosis
cecorectal
cecorrhaphy
cecosigmoidostomy
cecostomy
cecostomy catheter
cecostomy retractor
cecostomy trocar
cecotomy
cecum
Celestin prosthesis
Celestin tube
celiac
celiac artery
celiac axis
celiac glands
celiac trunk
celiectomy
celiocentesis
celioenterotomy
celiogastrotomy

celiohysterectomy
celioparacentesis
celiopyosis
celiorrhaphy
celioscopy
celiotomy
celiotomy incision
cellophane dressing
cellulitis
cellulocutaneous
cellulocutaneous flap
celluloid implant
celluloid sutures
celsian amputation
celsian lithotomy
celsian operation
Celsus lithotomy
Celsus operation
cement
cement restrictor
cementoma
cementum fracture
center blade
centering collar
centering drill
centering ring
centesis
centimeter (cm)
central amputation
central artery of retina
central iridectomy
central tendon of diaphragm
central tendon of perineum
central terminal electrode
central vein of retina
central vein of suprarenal gland
central veins of liver
central venous catheter

central venous pressure (CVP)
central vision
centrales hepatis veins
centralis glandulae suprarenalis
    vein
centralis retinae artery
centralis retinae vein
centrifuge microscope
cephalad
cephalic
cephalic triangle
cephalic vein
cephalic version
cephalica accessoria vein
cephalica vein
cephalogram
cephalography
cephalometry
cephalopelvic disproportion
cephalotomy
ceratocricoid muscle
ceratocricoideus muscle
cerclage
cerebellar artery
cerebellar veins
cerebelli inferior anterior artery
cerebelli inferior posterior artery
cerebelli inferiores veins
cerebelli superior artery
cerebelli superiores veins
cerebellum
cerebellum retractor
cerebral anesthesia
cerebral angiogram
cerebral angiography
cerebral angiography needle
cerebral arteriogram
cerebral arteriography

cerebral artery
cerebral cannula
cerebral catheter
cerebral epidural space
cerebral fossa
cerebral nerves
cerebral palsy
cerebral retractor
cerebri anterior artery
cerebri anterior vein
cerebri inferiores veins
cerebri internae veins
cerebri magna vein
cerebri media artery
cerebri media profunda vein
cerebri media superficialis vein
cerebri posterior artery
cerebri superiores veins
cerebrospinal fluid
cerebrum
cerulean cataract
ceruminous glands
cervical adenopathy
cervical amputation
cervical anesthesia
cervical artery
cervical biopsy
cervical biopsy blade
cervical biopsy curet
cervical blade
cervical brace
cervical canal
cervical cerclage
cervical cesarean section
cervical chain
cervical collar brace
cervical cordotomy
cervical cordotomy knife

cervical curet
cervical dilator
cervical drill
cervical fascia
cervical foraminal punch
cervical forceps
cervical glands
cervical incision
cervical knife
cervical laminectomy punch
cervical needle
cervical node
cervical os
cervical plexus nerve block
cervical punch
cervical punch forceps
cervical radium insertion
cervical retractor
cervical tenaculum
cervical traction
cervical traction forceps
cervical vein
cervical vertebrae
cervicales nerves
cervicalis ascendens artery
cervicalis profunda artery
cervicalis profunda vein
cervicectomy
cervicitis
cervicoplasty
cervitome
cervix
cervix-holding forceps
cesarean forceps
cesarean hysterectomy
cesarean section
Cetacaine
Chaffin catheter

Chaffin-Pratt suction tube
Chaffin-Pratt suction unit
Chaffin-Pratt tube
Chaffin suction tube
Chaffin sump tube
Chaffin tube
chain saw
chain sutures
chairback brace
chalazion
chalazion clamp
chalazion curet
chalazion excision
chalazion forceps
chalazion knife
chalazion punch
chalazion retractor
chalazion trephine
Chamberlain incision
Chamberlain mediastinotomy
Chamberlen forceps
Chambers pessary
chamfer reamer
chancroid
Chandelier sign
Chandler elevator
Chandler forceps
Chandler hip fusion
Chandler mallet
Chandler retractor
Chandler splint
Chaoul tube
Chaput operation
Chardack-Greatbatch pacemaker
Chardack pacemaker
Charles needle
Charles operation
Charlton needle

Charlton trocar
Charnley arthrodesis
Charnley arthroplasty
Charnley clamp
Charnley compressor
Charnley cup
Charnley drill
Charnley forceps
Charnley-Mueller arthroplasty
Charnley-Mueller prosthesis
Charnley-Mueller rasp
Charnley prosthesis
Charnley reamer
Charnley retractor
Charriere saw
Chatfield-Girdlestone splint
Chauffeur fracture
Chaussier tube
Chayes handpiece
Cheatle forceps
Cheatle-Henry incision
Cheatle-Henry operation
check ligaments
checkup
cheek retractor
cheesy cataract
Cheever tonsillectomy
cheilectomy
cheiloplasty
cheilorrhaphy
cheilostomatoplasty
cheilotomy
Chelsea-Eaton speculum
chemical anesthesia
chemical burn
chemical cautery
chemical hysterectomy
chemical pallidectomy

chemocauterization
chemocautery
chemodectomy
chemolysis
chemoneurolysis
chemonucleolysis
chemopallidectomy
chemopallidectomy scissors
chemopeel
chemosurgery
chemothalamectomy
chemotherapy
Cherney incision
Chernez incision
Cheron forceps
Cherry-Adson forceps
Cherry-Austin drill
Cherry drill
Cherry extractor
Cherry-Kerrison forceps
Cherry osteotome
Cherry probe
Cherry retractor
Cherry scissors
cherry sponge
Cherry tongs
chessboard graft
chest position
chest tube
Chevalier Jackson bougie
Chevalier Jackson bronchoscope
Chevalier Jackson esophagoscope
Chevalier Jackson forceps
Chevalier Jackson gastroscope
Chevalier Jackson laryngoscope
Chevalier Jackson operation
Chevalier Jackson scissors
Chevalier Jackson speculum

Chevalier Jackson tube
Cheyne dissector
Cheyne operation
Cheyne periosteal elevator
Chiazzi operation
chicken-bill rongeur
chicken-bill rongeur forceps
Chiene incision
Chiene operation
Chilcott cannula
Child forceps
Child pancreatectomy
Child-Phillips forceps
Child-Phillips needle
child's rib spreader
Children's Hospital clip
Children's Hospital forceps
Children's Hospital screwdriver
Children's Hospital spatula
chin muscle
chin strap
Chinese twisted silk sutures
chip syringe
chisel
    Adson
    Alexander
    Andrews
    antrum
    Artmann
    Ballenger
    Ballenger-Hajek
    binangled
    Bishop
    Blair
    bone
    Bowen
    Brittain
    Brown

chisel *(continued)*
- Bruening
- Brunetti
- Brunner
- Bruns
- Burns
- Caltagirone
- c. elevator
- c. fracture
- Cinelli
- Cinelli-McIndoe
- Clawicz
- Cloward
- Compere
- Converse
- corneal
- costotome
- Cottle
- Councilman
- Crane
- crurotomy
- Derlacki
- Derlacki-Shambaugh
- D'Errico
- disarticulation
- dissecting
- Eicher
- ethmoidal
- Faulkner
- Faulkner-Browne
- Fomon
- footplate
- Freer
- frontal sinus
- Gardner
- gooseneck
- guarded
- Hajek

chisel *(continued)*
- Halle
- Heerman
- Henderson
- Hibbs
- hollow
- House
- Joseph
- Katsch
- Keyes
- Kezerian
- Killian
- Killian-Reinhard
- Kreischer
- Lambotte
- laminectomy
- Lebsche
- Lexer
- MacAusland
- Magielski
- mastoid
- Metzenbaum
- Meyerding
- Moore
- Murphy
- nasal
- Rish
- Roberts
- Schuknecht
- septum
- Sewall
- Shambaugh-Derlacki
- Sheehan
- sinus
- Smith-Petersen
- spinal fusion
- splitting
- stapes

chisel *(continued)*
    sternum
    Stille
    tri-fin
    trocar
    Troutman
    twin-pattern
    Virchow
    West
    White
    Wilmer
    Worth
chloramine
chloroform
chloromycetin
chloroprocaine hydrochloride
Chlumsky button
choana (*pl.* choanae)
choanal bur
cholangiectasis
cholangiocholangiostomy
cholangiocholecystocholedochectomy
cholangioenterostomy
cholangiogastrostomy
cholangiogram
cholangiography
cholangiography catheter
cholangiojejunostomy
cholangiopancreatogram
cholangiopancreatography
cholangiostomy
cholangiotomy
cholangitis
cholecyst
cholecystectomy
cholecystelectrocoagulectomy
cholecystendysis

cholecystenteric
cholecystenteroanastomosis
cholecystenterorrhaphy
cholecystenterostomy
cholecystgastrostomy
cholecystic
cholecystitis
cholecystnephrostomy
cholecystocecostomy
cholecystocholangiogram
cholecystocholangiography
cholecystocolostomy
cholecystocolotomy
cholecystoduodenostomy
cholecystoenterostomy
cholecystogastric
cholecystogastrostomy
cholecystogram
cholecystography
cholecystoileostomy
cholecystojejunostomy
cholecystokinetic
cholecystolithiasis
cholecystolithotripsy
cholecystopancreatostomy
cholecystopexy
cholecystoptosis
cholecystopyelostomy
cholecystorrhaphy
cholecystostomy
cholecystotomy
choledochal
choledochal sphincterotomy
choledochectomy
choledochitis
choledochocholedochorrhaphy
choledochocholedochostomy
choledochoduodenostomy

choledochoenterostomy
choledochogastrostomy
choledochogram
choledochography
choledochohepatostomy
choledochoileostomy
choledochojejunostomy
choledocholith
choledocholithiasis
choledocholithotomy
choledocholithotripsy
choledochopancreatostomy
choledochoplasty
choledochorrhaphy
choledochoscopy
choledochosphincterotomy
choledochostomy
choledochotomy
choledochus
Cholegrafin
cholelithiasis
cholelithotomy
cholelithotrity
cholesteatoma
chondrectomy
chondritis
chondroglossus muscle
chondroplasty
chondrosternal articulation
chondrosternoplasty
chondrotomy
chop amputation
Chopart amputation
Chopart cheiloplasty
Chopart's joint
chordae tendinae
chordectomy
chordotomy

chorion
chorionic
choroid artery
choroid plexus
choroid vein
choroidal cataract
choroidea anterior artery
choroidea vein
choroidectomy
Choyce eye implant
Choyce Mark VIII eye implant
chromic catgut sutures
chromic gut sutures
chromic sutures
chronic
chuck drill
chuck handle
chuck key
Chun-gun transillumination
Church scissors
Chvostek sign
chyle
chylectasis
chylous
cicatrectomy
cicatrices (*sing.* cicatrix)
cicatricial
cicatricial entropion
cicatricotomy
cicatrix (*pl.* cicatrices)
cicatrization
Cicherelli forceps
Cicherelli rongeur
cigarette drain
cilia
cilia base
cilia forceps
Cilco extractor

ciliares anteriores arteries
ciliares breves nerves
ciliares longi nerves
ciliares posteriores breves arteries
ciliares posteriores longae arteries
ciliares veins
ciliaris muscle
ciliarotomy
ciliary arteries
ciliary glands
ciliary ligament
ciliary muscle
ciliary nerves
ciliary processes
ciliary veins
ciliectomy
circumflexa ilium superficialis
    artery
Cimino arteriovenous fistula
cinchocaine
cineangiocardiogram
cineangiocardiography
cineangiogram
cineangiography
cine-camera
Cinelli chisel
Cinelli-McIndoe chisel
cinematic amputation
cineplastic amputation
cineplasty
cineradiogram
cineradiography
cingulectomy
cingulumotomy
circle absorption anesthesia
CircOlectric bed
circular amputation

circular bandage
circular blade
circular block anesthesia
circular guillotine incision
circular incision
circular punch
circular saw
circular sutures
circular twin saw
circulation
circulatory
circulatory embarrassment
circumanal glands
circumareolar incision
circumcision
circumcision clamp
circumcision scissors
circumcision shield
circumcision sutures
circumcisional incision
circumcorneal incision
circumferential
circumferential incision
circumferentiating skin incision
circumflex artery of scapula
circumflex femoral artery
circumflex femoral veins
circumflex humeral artery
circumflex iliac artery
circumflex iliac vein
circumflex vessel
circumflexa femoris lateralis
    artery
circumflexa femoris medialis
    artery
circumflexa humeri anterior
    artery

circumflexa humeri posterior
  artery
circumflexa ilium profunda artery
circumflexa ilium profunda vein
circumflexa ilium superficialis
  artery
circumflexa ilium superficialis
  vein
circumflexa scapulae artery
circumflexae femoris laterales
  veins
circumflexae femoris mediales
  veins
circumlimbar incision
circumoral incision
circumscribed
circumscribing incision
circumvent
cirrhosis
cirrhotic
cirrhotic gastritis
cirsectomy
cirsenchysis
cirsodesis
cirsotome
cirsotome knife
cirsotomy
cistern
cisterna
cisterna chyli
cisterna magna
cisternal puncture
Citanest
Citelli forceps
Citelli-Meltzer punch
Citelli punch
Citelli rongeur
Civiale lithotrity

Clado anastomosis
Clagett cannula
Clagett needle
Clagett operation
Clairborne clamp
clammy
clamp
  Abadie
  agraffe
  Alfred M. Large
  Allen
  Allis
  Allison
  Alyea
  anastomosis
  aneurysm
  angled
  Ann Arbor
  anterior resection
  aorta
  aortic aneurysm
  aortic occlusion
  artery
  Atlee
  atraumatic
  Ault clamp
  auricle
  auricular artery
  Babcock
  Backhaus
  Bahnson
  Bailey
  Bailey-Cowley
  Bailey-Morse
  Bainbridge
  Ballantine
  Bamby
  Beardsley

clamp *(continued)*
- Beck
- Beck-Satinsky
- Berens
- Berke
- Berman
- Berry
- Best
- Bethune
- Bigelow
- Black
- Blalock
- Blalock-Niedner
- Blanchard
- bloodless circumcision
- Böhler
- bone
- bone-holding
- Bonney
- Boyes
- Bozeman
- Bradshaw-O'Neill
- bridge
- Brock
- Brodney
- bronchus
- Brown
- Buie
- Buie-Hirschman
- bulldog
- Buxton
- C-clamp
- calvarium
- Carmalt
- Carmel
- carotid artery
- Carrel
- Carter

clamp *(continued)*
- cartilage
- Castroviejo
- cautery
- chalazion
- Charnley
- circumcision
- Claiborne
- c. and cautery
- c. band
- c. forceps
- c. method vasectomy
- clamp-on aspirator
- clamp-on telescope
- cloth-shod
- coarctation
- Codman
- Collins
- colon
- colostomy
- columella
- Cooley
- Cope
- Cope-DeMartel
- cordotomy
- Cottle
- cotton-roll rubber-dam
- Crafoord Clamp
- Crile
- Crile-Crutchfield
- cross-action
- crossclamp
- Cruickshank
- crushing
- Crutchfield
- Cunningham
- Cushing
- Daems

clamp *(continued)*
- Daniel
- Davidson
- Davis
- Dean-MacDonald
- Deaver
- DeBakey
- DeBakey-Bahnson
- deCourcy
- DeMartel
- DeMartel-Wolfson
- Dennis
- Derra
- Desmarres
- Dieffenbach
- Diethrich
- Dingman
- dissecting
- Dixon-Thomas-Smith
- Dobbie-Trout
- Doctor Collins
- Doctor Long
- Dogliotti-Guglielmini
- Donald
- double towel
- Downing
- Doyen
- duckbill
- ductus
- duodenal
- Earle
- Eastman
- Edebohls
- Edwards
- enterostomy
- entropion
- Erhardt
- Falk

clamp *(continued)*
- Farabeuf-Lambotte
- Fehland
- femoral
- ferrule
- fine-toothed
- Finochietto
- flow-regulator
- Fogarty
- Forrester
- Foss
- fracture
- Frahur
- Frazier-Adson
- Frazier-Sachs
- Freeman
- Friedrich
- Friedrich-Petz
- full-curved
- Furniss
- Furniss-Clute
- Furniss-McClure-Hinton
- Gandy
- Gant
- Garland
- Gaskell
- gastric
- gastroenterostomy
- gastrointestinal
- Gavin-Miller
- Gemini
- GI
- gingival
- Glassman
- Glassman-Allis
- Glover
- goiter
- Goldblatt

clamp *(continued)*
> Gomco
> Goodwin
> grasping
> Gray
> Green
> Gross
> Gussenbauer
> Guyon
> Guyon-Pean
> Halstead
> Harken
> Harrington
> Harrington-Carmalt
> Harrington-Mixter
> Haseltine
> Haverhill
> Hayes
> Heaney
> Heitz-Boyer
> hemoclip
> hemorrhoidal
> hemostatic
> Hendren
> Herbert Adams
> Herff
> Herrick
> Hibbs
> Hirschman
> Hopkins
> Hudson
> Hufnagel
> Hume
> Humphries
> Hunt
> Hurwitz
> Hyams
> hydraclip

clamp *(continued)*
> hysterectomy
> incontinence
> infant vascular
> intestinal
> intestinal occlusion
> intestinal ring
> Jackson
> Jacobs
> Jacobson
> Jahnke-Cook-Seeley
> Jarvis
> Javid
> Jesberg
> Johns Hopkins
> Johnston
> Jones
> Joseph
> Judd
> Judd-Allis
> Juevenelle
> Julian-Fildes
> K-Gar
> Kane
> Kantor
> Kantrowicz
> Kapp
> Kapp-Beck
> Kelly
> Kelsey
> kidney
> kidney pedicle
> Kinsella-Buie
> Kocher
> Kolodny
> Ladd
> Lahey
> Lambert-Lowman

clamp *(continued)*

Lambotte
Lane
laryngectomy
Lees
Lem-Blay
Lewin
lid
Linnartz
Linton
lion-jaw
lip
locking
Lockwood
Lowman
Lulu
lung
lung exclusion
MacDonald
Madden
marginal
Martel
Martin
Mason
Masterson
Mastin
Mayo
Mayo-Guyon
Mayo-Lovelace
McCleery-Miller
McDonald
McGuire
McKenzie
McLean
McNealy-Glassman
McNealy-Glassman-Mixter
McQuigg
meatal

clamp *(continued)*

meatus
metal
Michel
Mikulicz
Miles
Millin
Mixter
Mohr
Moorehead
Moreno
mosquito
Moynihan
Mueller
Muir
muscle
Myles
myocardial
nephrostomy
Nichols
Nicola
Niedner
non-crushing
Nunez
Nussbaum
occluding
occlusion
Ochsner
Ockerblad
O'Connor
O'Neill
os calcis
O'Shaughnessy
osteoplastic flap
padded
parametrium
Parham-Martin
Parker

clamp *(continued)*
- partially occluding
- Partipilo
- patent ductus
- Payr
- Pean
- pedicle
- pelvic
- Pemberton
- penile
- penis
- Pennington
- peritoneal
- Petz
- Phaneuf
- Phillips
- pile
- pin
- pinchcock
- placenta
- Poppen
- Poppen-Blalock
- Poppen-Blalock-Salibi
- Potts
- Potts-Niedner
- Potts-Satinsky
- Potts-Smith
- Poutasse
- Preshaw
- Price-Thomas
- Prince
- Pringle
- Providence
- Providence Hospital
- ptosis
- pulmonary
- pulmonary artery
- pulmonary embolism

clamp *(continued)*
- pulmonary vessel
- pulmonic
- pylorus
- Ralks
- Rankin
- Ranzewski
- Reich-Nechtow
- renal
- renal pedicle
- resection
- reverse-curve
- Reynolds
- Rhinelander
- Richards
- Rienhoff
- right-angle
- ring
- Rochester
- Rochester-Pean
- Rockey
- Roe
- Roeder
- Roosevelt
- rubber-dam
- rubber-shod
- Rubin
- Rubovits
- Rumel
- Rush
- Salibi
- Santulli
- Sarnoff
- Sarot
- Satinsky
- Schmidt
- Schoemaker
- Schutz

clamp *(continued)*

- Scudder
- Sehrt
- Sellor
- Selman
- Selverstone
- Senning
- septum
- serrefine
- Shoemaker
- Shunt
- side-biting
- sigmoid
- Singley
- Smith
- Smithwick
- Somers
- Southwick
- spur-crushing
- Stanton
- stenosis
- Stepita
- Stevenson
- Stille
- Stockman
- stomach
- Stone
- Stone-Holcombe
- straight
- Stratte
- Strauss
- Sumner
- Surgi-Med
- Swan
- swan-neck
- Swiss
- Sztehlo
- tangential

clamp *(continued)*

- Tatum
- tendon
- Thomson
- thoracic
- three-bladed
- tonsil
- tourniquet
- towel
- Trendelenburg-Crafoord
- trochanter-holding
- Trusler
- umbilical
- umbiliclamp
- urethrographic
- vaginal cuff
- Vanderbilt
- vas
- Vasconcelos-Baretto
- vascular
- vena cava
- Verbrugge
- vessel
- vestibular
- voltage
- von Petz
- W. Dean McDonald
- Walther
- Walther-Crenshaw
- Wangensteen
- Warthen
- Watts
- Weaver
- Weck
- wedge resection
- Wells
- Wertheim
- Wertheim-Cullen

clamp *(continued)*
    Wertheim-Reverdin
    Wester
    Whitver
    Willet
    Williams
    Wilman
    Wilson
    wire tightening
    Wolfson
    Yasargil
    Yellen
    Young
    Zachary-Cope-DeMartel
    Ziegler-Furniss
    Zimmer
    Zipser
    Zutt
clamped, cut and ligated
clamped, cut and tied
clamping and tying
Clark dilator
Clark forceps
Clark-Guyton forceps
Clark operation
Clark speculum
Clark vein stripper
Clark-Verhoeff forceps
Clark's level (of malignant
    melanoma)
clasp bar
classic cesearean section
classic incision
classical approach
classical incision
Classon scissors
claudication
clavicle

clavicle splint
clavicotomy
clavicular
clavicular cross splint
clavicular notch
claw foot
claw hand
claw toe
Clawicz chisel
Clayton operation
Clayton osteotome
Clayton shears
Clayton splint
clean and dry incision
clear acrylic template splint
cleavage fracture
cleavage plane
cleft
cleft lip
cleft lip repair
cleft palate
cleft palate elevator
cleft palate forceps
cleft palate knife
cleft palate needle
cleft palate operation
cleft palate prosthesis
cleft palate repair
cleft palate tenaculum
cleidotomy
cleidotripsy
Clerf-Arrowsmith safety pin closer
Clerf aspirating tip
Clerf aspirator
Clerf cancer cell collector
Clerf dilator
Clerf forceps
Clerf laryngoscope

Clerf saw
Clerf tube
Clevis dressing
clinic Bovie
clinoid process
clip
    Adson
    Ahlquist-Durham
    aneurysm
    Austin
    autoclip
    brain
    butterfly
    Callender
    Children's Hospital
    c.-applying forceps
    c. forceps
    c.-removing forceps
    Cushing
    Dandy
    Duane
    Edwards
    Ethicon
    Friedman
    Heifitz
    hemoclip
    hemostasis
    hemostatic
    Hesseltine umbiliclip
    Hoxworth
    hydraclip
    Liga
    Mayfield
    McDermott
    McKenzie
    metal
    Michel
    Olivecrona

clip *(continued)*
    parallel-jaw spring
    Penfield
    Raney
    scalp
    Schutz
    Schwartz
    Scoville-Lewis
    Selman
    Serature
    silver
    skin
    Smith
    Smithwick
    spring
    Sugar
    Sundt
    Surgiclip
    tantalum
    Totco
    towel
    traction
    umbilical
    umbiliclip
    vascular
    vena cava
    von Petz
    Wachtenfeld
    Weck
    wing
    Yasargil
clipping of frenum linguae
clitoridectomy
clitoridotomy
clitorotomy
clivogram
clivography
cloaca *(pl.* cloacae)

Cloquet fascia
Cloquet hernia
closed anesthesia
closed-angle glaucoma
closed drain
closed drainage
closed drainage tube
closed flap amputation
closed fracture
closed reduction
closed reduction and internal
    fixation
closed reduction of dislocation
closed reduction of fracture
closed reduction of fracture-
    dislocation
closed skull fracture
closed suction drainage tube
closed valvotomy
closing forceps
closure (see also *sutures*)
closure of defect
closure of fistula
clot evacuator
clot stripper
cloth-shod clamp
cloverleaf counterbore
cloverleaf excision
cloverleaf nail
cloverleaf pin
cloverleaf pin extractor
Cloward blade
Cloward chisel
Cloward curet
Cloward drill
Cloward guide
Cloward hammer
Cloward-Hoen retractor

Cloward hook
Cloward operation
Cloward osteotome
Cloward periosteal elevator
Cloward punch
Cloward retractor
Cloward rongeur
Cloward vertebral spreader
clubfoot splint
clunial nerves
clunium inferiores nerves
clunium medii nerves
clunium superiores nerves
Clute incision
clysis cannula
cm (centimeter)
CMG (cystometrogram)
coagulate
coagulating current
coagulating current Bovie
coagulating electrode
coagulating forceps
coagulating knife
coagulation
coagulation bronchoscope
coagulation cautery
coagulation electrode
coagulation forceps
coagulator
    Ballantine-Drew
    Bantam
    bipolar
    Birtcher
    Bovie
    c. Bovie
    electricator
    electrocoagulator
    hyfrecator

coagulator *(continued)*
    light
    Magielski electrocoagulator
    Malis
    Poppen
    Ritter
    wet-field
coagulum
coagulum pyelolithotomy
Coakley cannula
Coakley curet
Coakley forceps
Coakley hemostat
Coakley probe
Coakley sinus operation
Coakley speculum
Coakley sutures
Coakley trocar
coapt
coaptation
coaptation plate
coaptation splint
coaptation sutures
coarctation
coarctation clamp
coarctation forceps
coarctotomy
coarse
coat-sleeve amputation
Coats ring
cobalt
cobalt-60 therapy
Coban dressing
Coban wrap
Cobb curet
Cobb elevator
Cobb gouge
Cobb osteotome

Cobb periosteal elevator
Cobbett knife
cobbler's sutures
Cobelli's glands
cobra retractor
cocaine hydrochloride
coccygeal artery
coccygeal glands
coccygeal muscle
coccygeal nerve
coccygeal vertebrae
coccygectomy
coccygeus muscle
coccygeus nerve
coccygodynia
coccygotomy
coccyx
cochlear duct
cochlear implant
cochlear nerve
cock-up hand splint
Cock urethrotomy
cocoon dressing
cod liver oil soaked strips
Codivilla operation
Codman clamp
Codman drill
Codman incision
Codman vein stripper
Cody tack
Coffey incision
Coffey technique I
Coffey technique II
Coffey technique III
Coffey uterine suspension
cogwheel
Cohen-Eder cannula
Cohen-Eder tongs

Cohen elevator
Cohen forceps
Cohen rasp
coil
coil intrauterine device (IUD)
coiled position
coin lesion
cold blade biopsy
cold cautery
cold-cone knife
cold conization
cold conization of cervix
cold-knife conization
cold nodule
cold-punch resectoscope
cold snare
Coldlite-Graves speculum
Coldlite speculum
Cole fracture frame
Cole operation
Cole retractor
Cole vein stripper
colectomy
Colibri forceps
Colibri speculum
colic
colic artery
colic vein
colica dextra artery
colica dextra vein
colica media artery
colica media vein
colica sinistra artery
colica sinistra vein
colicky
colitis
collagen sutures
collagen tape prosthesis

collapse
collar
collar bone
collar brace
collar button
collar-button tube
collar dressing
collar incision
collateral
collateral artery
collateral circulation
collateralis media artery
collateralis radialis artery
collateralis ulnaris inferior artery
collateralis ulnaris superior artery
collecting tube
collector
    cancer cell
    Carabelli
    Clerf cancer cell
    Davidson
    Lukens
Coller forceps
Colles fracture
Colles splint
Collier needle holder
Collin dissector
Collin-Duvall forceps
Collin forceps
Collin osteoclast
Collin pelvimeter
Collin speculum
Collings electrode
Collings knife
Collins clamp
Collins tube
Collis mouth gag
Collis-Nissen operation

Collis technique
Collison drill
Collison screw
Collison screwdriver
collodion dressing
colloid
colloid goiter
colloid milium
collum
collum vesicae felleae
Collyer pelvimeter
coloboma
colocentesis
coloclysis
colocolostomy
colocutaneous
colocystoplasty
colofixation
colohepatopexy
coloileal
coloileotomy
cololysis
colon
colon ascendens
colon clamp
colon descendens
colon resection
colon sigmoideum
colon transversum
colonic anesthesia
colonic insufflator
Colonna arthroplasty
Colonna operation
colonorrhagia
colonorrhea
colonoscope
colonoscope syringe
colonoscopy

colopexostomy
colopexotomy
colopexy
coloplast bag
coloplication
coloproctectomy
coloproctostomy
coloptosis
color contrast microscope
colorectosigmoidostomy
colorectostomy
colorrhaphy
coloscopy
colosigmoidostomy
colostomy
colostomy bag
colostomy clamp
colostomy loops
colostomy pouch
colostomy rod
colostomy tube
colostrum
colotomy
Colp-Hofmeister operation
colpectomy
colpocele
colpoceliocentesis
colpoceliotomy
colpocentesis
colpocleisis
colpocystotomy
colpohysterectomy
colpoperineoplasty
colpoperineorrhaphy
colpopexy
colpoplasty
colpopoiesis
colporectopexy

colporrhaphy
colposcopy
colpostat
colpotomy
Colt cannula
columella
columella clamp
columellar type II tympanoplasty
Colver-Coakley forceps
Colver dissector
Colver forceps
Colver hook
Colver knife
Colver needle
Colver retractor
comatose
combined frontal, ethmoid, and
    sphenoid sinusotomy
combined femoral-inguinal
    herniorrhaphy
combined hemorrhoids
combined internal and external
    version
combined sacral and caudal block
    anesthesia
combined version
comedo (*pl.* comedones)
comedo extractor
comedocarcinoma
comedomastitis
comedones (*sing.* comedo)
comitans nervi hypoglossi vein
comitans nervi ischiadici artery
Commando operation
comminuted fracture
comminution
commissure
commissurorrhaphy

commissurotomy
commissurotomy knife
common bile duct
common carotid artery
common duct
common duct bougie
common duct dilator
common duct probe
common duct scoop
common tendon
communicans anterior cerebri
    artery
communicans posterior cerebri
    artery
communicating artery
comparison microscope
compartmental total knee
    prosthesis
Compere chisel
Compere gouge
Compere operation
Compere osteotome
Compere pin
complete abortion
complete amputation
complete ethmoidectomy
complete excision
complete fracture
complete gastrectomy
complete hysterectomy
complete iridectomy
complete mastectomy
complex simple fracture
complicated fracture
component
component pusher
composite fracture
composite graft

composite joint
composite operation
compound dressing
compound fracture
compound joint
compound microscope
compound nevus
compound skin flap
compound skull fracture
compound sutures
compress
compression anesthesia
compression arthrodesis
compression bandage
compression dressing
compression forceps
compression fracture
compression hook
compression rod
compression screw
compression splint
compressor
    Anthony
    Barnes
    Berens
    Charnley
    Deschamps
    DeVilbiss
    enucleation
    orbital enucleation
    screw
    Sehrt
    shot
    tonsil
computerized axial tomography
    (CAT)
computerized cranial tomography
    (CCT)

concave
concha (*pl.* conchae)
conchectomy
conchotomy
concomitant
concretion
condenser
conduction nerve study
conductor
    Adson
    Bailey
    Davis
    Kanavel
    saw
conduit
conduitogram
conduitography
condylar articulation
condylar canal
condylar fossa
condylar fracture
condyle
condylectomy
condyloid fossa
condyloid process
condyloma (*pl.* condylomata or
    condylomas)
condyloma acuminatum
condylomata (*sing.* condyloma)
condylotomy
cone biopsy
Cone-Bucy cannula
Cone bur
Cone caliper
Cone cannula
Cone curet
cone-down view
Cone forceps

Cone guide
cone knife
Cone needle
Cone punch
Cone retractor
Cone suction tube
Cone wire twister
confirmatory incision
confluent
conformer
    acrylic
    eye implant
    Fox
    plastic
    universal
congenital dislocation
congenital fracture
congenital subluxation
congestion
conglobate gland
conic bougie
conical bur
conical catheter
conical eye implant
conical tip catheter
conical tip electrode
conical trocar
conization electrode
conization instrument
conization knife
conization of cervix
conization technique
conjoined tendon
conjunctiva (*pl.* conjunctivae)
conjunctival arteries
conjunctival flap
conjunctival forceps
conjunctival incision

conjunctival veins
conjunctivales anteriores arteries
conjunctivales posteriores arteries
conjunctivales veins
conjunctivocystorhinostomy
conjunctivodacryocysto-
    rhinostomy
conjunctivodacryocystostomy
conjunctivoplasty
conjunctivorhinostomy
Conn operation
Conn tourniquet
connector bar
Connell incision
Connell operation
Connell sutures
conoid ligament
Conrad-Crosby needle
consecutive amputation
conspicuous
Constantine catheter
constipation
constricted
constriction
constrictor muscle
constrictor pharyngis inferior
    muscle
constrictor pharyngis medius
    muscle
constrictor pharyngis superior
    muscle
construction
contact splint
contiguous
Continent operation
continuous caudal anesthesia
continuous epidural anesthesia
continuous interlocking sutures

continuous over-and-over sutures
continuous peridural anesthesia
continuous running sutures
continuous spinal anesthesia
continuous suction
continuous suction tube
continuous sutures
contour retractor
contractor (see *rib contractor*)
contracture
contraindication
contralateral
contrast medium (*pl.* media)
    Cholegrafin
    Cystokon
    Hypaque
    Pantopaque
    Pilopaque
    Renografin
    Retrografin dye
    technetium pyrophosphate
    Telepaque
contrast medium
contrecoup fracture
controlled drain
controlled respiration
contused
contusion
contusion cataract
conventional reform eye implant
conventional shell-type eye
    implant
convergence
convergent
Converse chisel
Converse curet
Converse hook
Converse knife

Converse-MacKenty elevator
Converse operation
Converse osteotome
Converse rasp
Converse retractor
Converse rongeur
Converse saw
Converse scissors
Converse speculum
conversion
conversion of position
convertible cystoscope
convex
convexity
convolution
convulsion
Conzett goniometer
Cook County aspirator
Cook County suction tube
Cook retractor
Cook speculum
Cook walking brace
Cooley-Bloodwell-Cutter
    prosthesis
Cooley clamp
Cooley-Cutter prosthesis
Cooley dilator
Cooley forceps
Cooley graft
Cooley-Pontius blade
Cooley-Pontius shears
Cooley retractor
Cooley scissors
Cooley suction tube
Coolidge tube
Cooper bougie
Cooper cannula
Cooper elevator

Cooper gouge
Cooper guide
Cooper hernia
Cooper ligament
Cooper needle
Cooper operation
coordinates
Cope clamp
Cope-DeMartel clamp
Cope needle
Copeland retinoscope
copious
Coppridge forceps
cor pulmonale
coracoacromial ligament
coracobrachial muscle
coracobrachialis muscle
coracoclavicular ligament
coracoclavicular screw
coracohumeral ligament
coracoid process
coralliform cataract
Coratomic pacemaker
Corbett forceps
Corbett spud
cord bladder
cordectomy
Cordes forceps
Cordes-New elevator
Cordes-New forceps
Cordes-New punch
Cordes punch
cordiform tendon of diaphragm
cordis anteriores veins
Cordis Atricor pacemaker
Cordis Ectocor pacemaker
Cordis fixed-rate pacemaker
Cordis pacemaker

cordis magna vein
cordis media vein
cordis minimae veins
cordis para vein
Cordis Ventricor pacemaker
Cordonnier ureteroileal loop
cordopexy
cordotomy
cordotomy clamp
cordotomy hook
cordotomy knife
core mold stent
corectomy
corelysis
coreoplasty
coretomy
Corey forceps
Corey tenaculum
corkscrew
cornea knife
cornea scissors
corneal abrader
corneal applicator
corneal bur
corneal chisel
corneal curet
corneal debrider
corneal dissector
corneal eye implant
corneal graft
corneal incision
corneal knife
corneal loupe
corneal microscope
corneal needle
corneal rasp
corneal scissors
corneal section

corneal transplant
corneal transplant forceps
corneal transplant scissors
corneal trephine
corneal tube
corneoconjunctivoplasty
corneoscleral forceps
corneoscleral incision
corneoscleral junction
corneoscleral punch
corneoscleral scissors
corneoscleral sutures
corneoscleral trephination
corneoscleroconjunctival sutures
corner retractor
Cornet forceps
Corning anesthesia
Cornish wool dressing
cornu (*pl.* cornua)
corollary incision
corona (*pl.* coronae)
coronal incision
coronal sulcus
coronal suture
coronaria dextra artery
coronaria sinistra artery
coronary arteriogram
coronary arteriography
coronary artery
coronary artery bypass
coronary artery perfusion
Coronary Care Unit (CCU)
coronary cataract
coronary cusps
coronary perfusion
coronary perfusion cannula
coronary sinus suction tube
coronary tendon

coronary veins
coronoid fossa
coronoid process
corpora (*sing.* corpus)
corporeal cesarean section
corpus (*pl.* corpora)
corpus callosum
corpus luteum
corpus luteum cyst
correction for strabismus
corrective operation
Corrigan cautery
corrugator muscle
corrugator supercilii muscle
cortex (*pl.* cortices)
cortex retractor
Corti rod
cortical cataract
cortical incision
cortical screw
cortical step drill
cortices (*sing.* cortex)
corticosteroids
cortis externa artery
cortisone
Cortisporin
Corwin forceps
Corwin hemostat
Coryllos-Bethune rib shears
Coryllos-Doyen periosteal elevator
Coryllos-Moure rib shears
Coryllos periosteal elevator
Coryllos raspatory
Coryllos retractor
Coryllos-Shoemaker rib shears
Coryllos thoracoscope
cosmetic
costa (*pl.* costae)

costal arch retractor
costal elevator
costal margin
costal periosteal elevator
costal periosteotome
costectomy
costocervical trunk
costochondral joint
costochondrectomy
costoclavicular ligament
costophrenic
costophrenic angle
costophrenic bronchoscope
costoprostatectomy
costosternal articulation
costosternoplasty
costotome
costotome chisel
costotomy
costotransverse articulation
costotransverse ligament
costotransversectomy
costovertebral
costovertebral angle
costovertebral articulation
Cotte neurectomy
Cotting operation
Cottle-Arruga forceps
Cottle caliper
Cottle chisel
Cottle clamp
Cottle elevator
Cottle forceps
Cottle guide
Cottle hook
Cottle incision
Cottle-Jansen forceps
Cottle-Joseph hook

Cottle-Kazanjian forceps
Cottle knife
Cottle-MacKenty elevator
Cottle mallet
Cottle-Neivert retractor
Cottle operation
Cottle osteotome
Cottle rasp
Cottle retractor
Cottle saw
Cottle scissors
Cottle speculum
Cottle suction tube
Cottle tenaculum
Cottle-Walsham forceps
Cottle-Walsham straightener
cotton applicator
cotton balls
cotton carrier
cotton elastic bandage
cotton pledgets
Cotton procedure
cotton-roll rubber-dam clamp
cotton sutures
cotton-tipped applicator
cotton wadding
cotton-wool bandage
Cottonoid strip
couching needle
coudé catheter
coudé electrode
coudé hemostatic bag
coudé-tip catheter
cough fracture
Coumadin
Councill catheter
Councill dilator
Councill stone basket

Councill stone dislodger
Councill stone extractor
Councilman chisel
counter rotating saw
counterbore
    cloverleaf
      Curry hip nail
    round
counterincision
countershock
countertraction
countertraction splint
coup de sabre deformity
Coupland elevator
Coupland suction tube
Cournand catheter
Cournand-Grino needle
Cournand needle
coursing
Courvoisier gallbladder
Courvoisier incision
Cowper's glands
Cowper's ligament
coxa vara
Coxeter catheter
CPI Maxilith pacemaker
CPI Minilith pacemaker
Crabtree dissector
Crafoord clamp
Crafoord-Cooley tunneler
Crafoord forceps
Crafoord operation
Crafoord retractor
Crafoord scissors
Craig forceps
Craig needle
Craig pin
Craig scissors

Craig-Sheehan retractor
Craig splint
Cramer splint
Crane chisel
Crane gouge
Crane mallet
Crane osteotome
cranial bur
cranial drill
cranial forceps
cranial fossa
cranial nerve
cranial nerve I (olfactory)
cranial nerve II (optic)
cranial nerve III (oculomotor)
cranial nerve IV (trochlear)
cranial nerve V (trigeminal)
cranial nerve VI (abducens)
cranial nerve VII (facial)
cranial nerve VIII (vestibulo-
    cochlear)
cranial nerve IX (glossopharyngeal)
cranial nerve X (vagus)
cranial nerve XI (accessory)
cranial nerve XII (hypoglossal)
cranial perforator
cranial puncture
cranial retractor
cranial rongeur
cranial trephine
craniales nerves
craniectomy
cranioclasis
cranioclast
    Auvard
    Braun
    DeLee-Zweifel
    Zweifel-DeLee

craniofacial fracture appliance
cranioplasty
craniotome
craniotomy
craniotomy scissors
Crapeau snare
crater
craterization
cravat bandage
Credo operation
Creevy dilator
Creevy evacuator
Creevy stone dislodger
cremaster fascia
cremaster muscle
cremasteric artery
cremasterica artery
Crenshaw forceps
crepe bandage
crepitus
crescendo
crescent incision
crescent-shaped incision
cretinism
cribriform fascia
cribriform process
cricoarytenoid ligament
cricoarytenoid muscle
cricoarytenoideus lateralis muscle
cricoarytenoideus posterior muscle
cricoesophageal tendon
cricoid cartilage
cricoidectomy
cricothyreotomy
cricothyroarytenoid ligament
cricothyroid ligament
cricothyroid muscle

cricothyroid trocar
cricothyroidectomy
cricothyroideus muscle
cricothyroidotomy
cricothyrostomy
cricothyrotomy
cricothyrotomy cannula
cricotomy
cricotracheal ligament
cricotracheotomy
Crigler evacuator
Crile blade
Crile clamp
Crile-Crutchfield clamp
Crile forceps
Crile head traction
Crile hemostat
Crile hook
Crile knife
Crile-Murray needle holder
Crile needle holder
Crile retractor
Crile spatula
Crile stripper
Crile-Wood needle holder
crimped dacron prosthesis
crimped wire
crimped woven prosthesis
crimper
crimper forceps
Cripps obturator
Cripps operation
Critchett excision of anterior
    eyeball
crocodile forceps
Cronin implant
Cronin operation

Crosby-Cooney operation for ascites
Crosby knife
cross-action clamp
cross-action forceps
cross bar
cross-cut bur
crossclamp
crossclamping
crosscut saw
crosshatch incision
crosspiece
Crotti retractor
Crowel-Beard ptosis procedure
crown-crimping pliers
crown debridement
crown drill
crown saw
crown stitch
crucial anastomosis
crucial bandage
crucial incision
cruciate head screw
cruciate incision
cruciate ligaments
cruciform screw
cruciform screwdriver
Cruickshank clamp
crura (*sing.* crus)
crura hook
crural canal
crural fascia
crural hernia
crural ligament
crurotomy
crurotomy chisel
crurotomy saw
crus (*pl.* crura)

crush vasectomy technique
crusher (see *spur crusher*)
crushing
crushing and removal of calculi
crushing clamp
crushing of calculus
crushing of nasal septum
crushing of nerve
crushing of vas deferens
crust
crusting
crutch
Crutchfield clamp
Crutchfield drill
Crutchfield operation
Crutchfield-Raney tongs
Crutchfield tongs
Cruveilhier's joint
Cruveilhier tumor
Cruveilhier ulcer
Cryer elevator
cryocautery
cryoconization
cryodestruction
cryoextraction
cryoextraction of cataract
cryoextractor (see also *extractor*)
    Amoils
    Bellows
    Frigitronics
    Krwawicz
    Thomas
cryogenic probe
cryogenic surgery
cryohypophysectomy
cryoleucotomy
cryo-ophthalmic unit
cryopexy

cryophake
    Alcon
    Keeler
cryoprobe (see *probe*)
cryopter
cryostat
cryostylet
cryosurgery
cryosurgery apparatus
cryothalamectomy
cryotherapy
crypt
crypt hook
crypt knife
cryptic tonsils
cryptitis
cryptorchidectomy
cryptorchidism
cryptotome
cryptotomy
crypts of Lieberkuhn
crypts of Luschka
Csapo abortion
Csapody operation
Cu-7 intrauterine device (IUD)
Cubbins operation
Cubbins screw
Cubbins screwdriver
cubital nerve
cubital vein
cuboid bone
cuff electrode
cuff resection
cuffed tube
cuffless tube
cul-de-sac
culdocentesis
culdoplasty

culdoscope
    Decker
    fiberoptic
    photoculdoscope
culdoscopy
culdotomy
Culley splint
Cullom-Mueller adenotome
Culp pyeloplasty
culture
culture and sensitivity
Cummings catheter
Cummings-Pezzer catheter
cuneiform
cuneiform bone
cuneiform ligament
Cunningham clamp
cup and ball osteotomy
cup arthroplasty
cup biopsy forceps
cup-biting forceps
cup-biting punch
cup forceps
cup impactor
cup pessary
cup positioner
cup-shaped electrode
cupped forceps
cupula (*pl.* cupulae)
Curad plastic bandage
curare
Curdy knife
Curdy sclerotome
curet
    adenoid
    Alvis
    Anderson
    Angell

curet *(continued)*
- angled
- antrum
- aortic
- Ballenger
- Bardic
- Barnhill
- Beaver
- Billeau
- biopsy
- Blake
- bone
- Brun
- Buck
- Bumm
- Carlens
- Carmack
- Carter
- cervical
- cervical biopsy
- chalazion
- Cloward
- Coakley
- Cobb
- Cone
- Converse
- corneal
- c. evacuation
- DeLee
- DePuy
- Derlacki
- dermal
- double-ended
- double-lumen
- down-biting
- Duncan
- ear
- embolectomy

curet *(continued)*
- endaural
- endocervical
- endometrial
- endotracheal
- Epstein
- ethmoid
- Faulkner
- Ferguson
- fine
- Fink
- foreign-body
- Fox
- Franklin-Silverman
- Freimuth
- Gifford
- Goldman
- Goldstein
- Govons
- Gracey
- Green
- Gross
- Gusberg
- Halle
- Hannon
- Harrison
- Harrison-Shea
- Hartmann
- Hayden
- Heaney
- Heath
- Hibbs
- Hibbs-Spratt
- Holden
- Holtz
- hook
- Hotz
- House

curet *(continued)*

- House-Paparella
- Houtz
- Hunter
- Ingersoll
- intervertebral
- Jones
- Kelly
- Kelly-Gray
- Kevorkian
- Kevorkian-Young
- Kezerian
- knife
- Kushner-Tandatnick
- Lempert
- long-handle
- Lounsbury
- Luer
- Luongo
- Lynch
- Magielski
- mastoid
- Mayfield
- McCaskey
- McElroy
- Meigs
- Meyerding
- Meyhoeffer
- Middleton
- Miller
- Molt
- Mosher
- Moult
- Mueller
- Myles
- nasal
- Nolan-Budd
- Novak

curet *(continued)*

- Paparella
- Piffard
- pituitary
- placenta
- plastic
- polyvinyl
- Pratt
- punch
- Randall
- Raney
- Ray
- Recamier
- rectal
- Reich-Nechtow
- Reiner
- reverse angle skid
- Rheinstaedter
- Richards
- Ridpath
- right-angle
- ring
- Rosen
- Rosenmueller
- ruptured disk
- salpingeal
- scarifying
- Schaeffer
- Schede
- Schroeder
- Schwartz
- Scoville
- serrated
- Shapleigh
- sharp
- Shea
- Simpson
- Sims

curet *(continued)*
  sinus
  Skeele
  skid
  Skillern
  Smith-Petersen
  soft rubber
  spinal fusion
  Spratt
  St. Clair-Thompson
  stapes
  stirrup-loop
  Strully
  Stubbs
  submucous
  suction
  suction tip
  Tabb
  Taylor
  Thomas
  Thompson
  Thorpe
  uterine
  uterine suction
  Vacurette
  vacuum
  Vogel
  Volkmann
  Walker
  Walsh
  Walton
  Weisman
  Whiting
  Wullstein
  Yankauer
curettage
curette (see *curet*)
curetted

curettement
curetting bur
Curry hip nail
Curry hip nail counterbore
Curry needle
Curry splint
Curtis forceps
Curtis operation
curvature
curved awl
curved cannula
curved catheter
curved forceps
curved gouge
curved hemostat
curved hook
curved incision
curved knife
curved needle
curved needle holder
curved nerve hook
curved-on-flat scissors
curved periosteal elevator
curved scissors
curved suture needle
curved tractor
curved valvulotome
curved zonule separator
curvilinear
curvilinear incision
curving incision
Cusco speculum
Cushing bur
Cushing clamp
Cushing clip
Cushing drill
Cushing elevator
Cushing forceps

Cushing Gigli-saw guide
Cushing hook
Cushing-Hopkins periosteal
  elevator
Cushing knife
Cushing needle
Cushing operation
Cushing perforator
Cushing retractor
Cushing rongeur
Cushing spatula
Cushing spoon
Cushing sutures
Cushing's ulcer
cushioning sutures
Cushman drain
cusp
cuspid
Custodis implant
Custodis sponge
Custodis sutures
cut and sew technique
cutanea vein
cutaneous amputation
cutaneous nerve
cutaneous punch
cutaneous sutures
cutaneous vein
cutaneus antebrachii lateralis
  nerve
cutaneus antebrachii medialis
  nerve
cutaneus antebrachii posterior
  nerve
cutaneus brachii lateralis inferior
  nerve
cutaneus brachii lateralis superior
  nerve

cutaneus brachii medialis nerve
cutaneus brachii posterior nerve
cutaneus dorsalis intermedius
  nerve
cutaneus dorsalis lateralis nerve
cutaneus dorsalis medialis nerve
cutaneus femoris lateralis nerve
cutaneus femoris posterior nerve
cutaneus surae lateralis nerve
cutaneus surae medialis nerve
cutdown catheter
cutdown incision
cuticle
cuticular sutures
cutis graft
Cutler-Beard technique
Cutler eye implant
Cutler operation
cutter
    Berbecker wire
    bone
    cast
    Kuhlman cast
    Lempert malleus
    malleus
    Martin wire
    rectal
    right-angled bone
    ring
    wire
Cutter-SCDK prosthesis
Cutter-Smeloff cardiac valve
  prosthesis
Cutter-Smeloff disk valve
cutting Bovie knife
cutting bur
cutting current
cutting forceps

cutting loop electrode
cutting needle
CVP (central venous pressure)
cyanosis
Cyclaine
cyclectomy
cyclicotomy
cycloanemization
cyclocryotherapy
cyclodialysis
cyclodialysis cannula
cyclodialysis spatula
cyclodiathermy
cyclodiathermy needle
cycloelectrolysis
cyclomethycaine sulfate
cyclopentane
cyclophotocoagulation
cyclopropane
cyclotomy
cylinder cast
cylindrical
cylindrical bougie
cylindrical-object forceps
cylindrical zonule separator
cyst
cystectomy
cystic
cystic artery
cystic cataract
cystic duct
cystic duct forceps
cystic duct scoop
cystic goiter
cystic vein
cystica artery
cystica vein
cysticolithectomy

cysticolithotripsy
cysticorrhaphy
cysticotomy
cystis
cystis fellea
cystitis
cystitome
cystocele
cystocele repair
cystocolostomy
cystodiaphanoscopy
cystoduodenostomy
cystogastrostomy
cystogram
cystography
cystojejunostomy
Cystokon
cystolithectomy
cystolitholapaxy
cystolithotomy
cystometer
    Lewis
    water
cystometric studies
cystometrogram (CMG)
cystometrography
cystometry
cystopexy
cystoplasty
cystoproctostomy
cystopyelogram
cystopyelography
cystorrhaphy
cystosarcoma
cystosarcoma phylloides
cystoscope
    ACMI
    Braasch

cystoscope *(continued)*
  Brown-Buerger
  Butterfield
  convertible
  c. accessory
  direct catheterizing
  double catheterizing
  electrocystoscope
  fiberoptic
  French Brown-Buerger
  infant
  Kelly
  Kidd
  Laidley
  Leiter
  Lowsley-Peterson
  McCarthy
  McCarthy-Campbell
  McCarthy-Peterson
  McCrea
  miniature
  National
  Nesbit
  Otis-Brown
  Ravich
  sheath
  universal
  Wappler
  Young
cystoscopic snare

cystoscopic urography
cystoscopy
cystostomy
cystostomy tube
cystotome
  Beard
  Graefe
  Holth
  Knapp
  von Graefe
  Wheeler
  Wilder
cystotomy
cystoureterolithotomy
cystourethral suspension
cystourethrogram
cystourethrography
cystourethropexy
cystourethroplasty
cystourethroscope
cystourethroscopy
cytologic
cytology
Czermak keratome
Czermak operation
Czerny herniorrhaphy
Czerny incision
Czerny-Lembert sutures
Czerny operation
Czerny sutures

d

D&C (dilation and curettage; dilatation and curettage)
dacron graft
dacron patch
dacron prosthesis
dacron sutures
dacryoadenectomy
dacryoadenotomy
dacryocystectomy
dacryocystogram
dacryocystography
dacryocystorhinostomy
dacryocystorhinostomy needle
dacryocystorhinostomy retractor
dacryocystorhinostomy trephine
dacryocystostomy
dacryocystosyringotomy
dacryocystotomy
dacryostomy
dactylocostal rhinoplasty
Daems clamp
Dakin tube
Dakin tubing
Dalkon shield intrauterine device (IUD)
Dallas operation
dam
Dammann-Muller operation
Damshek needle
Damshek trephine
Dana rhizotomy
Danberg forceps

Dandy clip
Dandy forceps
Dandy hemostat
Dandy hook
Dandy needle
Dandy rhizotomy
Dandy scissors
Dandy ventriculostomy
Daniel clamp
Daniels operation
Daniels tonsillectome
darkfield microscope
Darling capsulotome
Darrach ulnar resection
Darrach wrist procedure
Davat operation for varicocele
David speculum
Davidoff knife
Davidoff retractor
Davidson bur
Davidson clamp
Davidson collector
Davidson forceps
Davidson periosteal elevator
Davidson retractor
Davidson syringe
Davidson trocar
Daviel cataract extraction
Daviel knife
Daviel loupe
Daviel scoop
Daviel spoon

Davies-Colley operation
Davis and Kitlowski operation
Davis bronchoscope
Davis clamp
Davis conductor
Davis-Crowe mouth gag
Davis electrode
Davis forceps
Davis-Geck incision
Davis graft
Davis hemostat
Davis hook
Davis mouth gag
Davis needle
Davis needle holder
Davis operation
Davis periosteal elevator
Davis pin
Davis raspatory
Davis retractor
Davis rib spreader
Davis separator
Davis skid
Davis sound
Davis spatula
Davis splint
Davis spud
Davis stone dislodger
Davis uterine suspension
Davol catheter
Davol dermatome
Davol forceps
Davol pillows
Davol-Simon dermatome
Davol suction tube
Davol tube
Day cannula
Day hook

Day knife
dead space
De Alvarez forceps
Dean applicator
Dean forceps
Dean hemostat
Dean knife
Dean-MacDonald clamp
Dean needle
Dean periosteotome
Dean rasp
Dean rongeur
Dean scissors
Dean trocar
Deaver clamp
Deaver incision
Deaver retractor
Deaver scissors
Deaver T-drain
Deaver T-tube
DeBakey-Bahnson clamp
DeBakey-Bahnson forceps
DeBakey-Bainbridge forceps
DeBakey-Balfour retractor
DeBakey blade
DeBakey clamp
DeBakey-Cooley dilator
DeBakey-Cooley forceps
DeBakey-Cooley retractor
DeBakey forceps
DeBakey graft
DeBakey implant
DeBakey-Metzenbaum scissors
DeBakey needle holder
DeBakey prosthesis
DeBakey rib spreader
DeBakey scissors
DeBakey stripper

DeBakey suction tube
DeBakey tunneler
DeBakey valve prosthesis
DeBakey vascular prosthesis
Debove tube
debride
debridement
debridement of wound
debridement needle
debrider
    corneal
    Sauer
debris
decamethonium bromide
decamethonium iodide
decannulation plug
decapitation
decapitation hook
decapitation scissors
decapsulation
decapsulation of kidney
decerebrate
decidua
Decker culdoscope
Decker retractor
declotting
decompression
decompression laminectomy
decompression of imperforate anus
decompression of orbit
decompression of spinal cord
decompression retractor
decortical position
decortication
decortication of heart
decortication of lung
DeCourcy clamp
decubitus

decubitus position
decubitus ulcer
Dedo laryngoscope
Dedo-Pilling laryngoscope
deep artery of clitoris
deep artery of penis
deep brachial artery
deep dissection
deep fascia
deep femoral artery
deep lingual artery
deep retractor
deep-surgery forceps
deep-surgery scissors
deep veins of clitoris
deep veins of penis
deepening reamer
Dees needle
Dees suture needle
defatting of skin
defecation
defect
deferential artery
deferentialis artery
defibrillation
definite
definition
deflection
deformed
deformity
Defourmental forceps
defunctionalized
degenerative changes
degloving technique
Degnon sutures
de Grandmont operation
dehiscence
dehydration

DeJager elevator
dekalon sutures
deknatel needle
deknatel sutures
Del Toro operation
Delaborde dilator
Delaney retractor
delayed closure of wound
delayed skin flap
delayed sutures
delayed union
DeLee-Breisky pelvimeter
DeLee catheter
DeLee curet
DeLee forceps
DeLee knife
DeLee maneuver
DeLee operation
DeLee pelvimeter
DeLee-Perce perforator
DeLee retractor
DeLee-Simpson forceps
DeLee speculum
DeLee tenaculum
DeLee-Zweifel cranioclast
Delgado electrode
delicate
delicate scissors
delicate skin hook
delimiting keratotomy
delineate
delivery
Delore method
Delorme operation
Delphian node
deltoid ligament
deltoid muscle
deltoideus muscle

deltopectoral groove
deltopectoral incision
demand pacemaker
Demarest forceps
DeMartel clamp
DeMartel forceps
DeMartel retractor
DeMartel scissors
DeMartel-Wolfson clamp
DeMartel-Wolfson forceps
Demel and Ruttin operation
Demel forceps
Demerol
demigauntlet bandage
Deming nephropexy
demyelinating
demyelination
demyelinization
Denans operation
denervation
Denhardt-Dingman mouth gag
Denhardt mouth gag
Denis Browne forceps
Denis Browne needle
Denis Browne operation
Denis Browne splint
Denker operation
Denker trocar
Denker tube
Denman spontaneous version
Dennis anastomosis
Dennis clamp
Dennis forceps
Denonvilliers operation
dense
dense adhesions
density
dental anesthesia

dental arch bar
dental artery
dental bur
dental caries
dental debridement
dental drill
dental elevator
dental excavator
dental extraction
dental forceps
dental implant
dental knife
dental plate
dental pliers
dental prosthesis
dental restorative surgery
dental splint
dental syringe
dentate fracture
dentate ligament
dentate line
dentinoma
denture brush
denture splint
dentures
denudation
denude
Denuse operation
Depage-Janeway gastrostomy
Depage position
DePalma hip prosthesis
DePalma knife
Depaul tube
dependency
dependent
de Pezzer catheter
depilation
Depo-Medrol

depolarizing electrode
depolarizing relaxants
depressed
depressed fracture
depression
depressor anguli oris muscle
depressor labii inferioris muscle
depressor muscle
depressor septi nasi muscle
depressor supercilii muscle
depth perception
depths
DePuy arthroplasty
DePuy awl
DePuy bolt
DePuy curet
DePuy drill
DePuy extractor
DePuy fracture frame
DePuy head halter
DePuy pin
DePuy plate
DePuy-Pott splint
DePuy prosthesis
DePuy reamer
DePuy retractor
DePuy rongeur
DePuy screwdriver
DePuy splint
DePuy-Weiss needle
de Quervain fracture
Derby operation
Derf needle holder
Derlacki chisel
Derlacki curet
Derlacki gouge
Derlacki knife
Derlacki mobilizer

Derlacki operation
Derlacki punch
Derlacki-Shambaugh chisel
Derlacki-Shambaugh microscope
dermabrader
    Iverson
    lid
    sandpaper
    Stryker
dermabrasion
dermagraft
dermal curet
dermal sutures
Dermalene sutures
Dermalon sutures
dermatome
    air
    Bard-Parker
    Barker Vacu-tome
    Brown
    Brown-Blair
    Brown electrodermatome
    Castroviejo
    Davol
    Davol-Simon
    electric
    electrodermatome
    Hall
    Hood
    manual
    Meek-Wall
    microdermatome
    Padgett
    Padgett-Hood electro-
      dermatome
    Reese
    Simon
    Stryker

dermatoplasty
Dermicel tape
dermis
dermoepidermal junction
Derra clamp
Derra dilator
Derra knife
Derra valvulotome
D'Errico-Adson retractor
D'Errico bur
D'Errico chisel
D'Errico drill
D'Errico forceps
D'Errico knife
D'Errico perforator
D'Errico periosteal elevator
D'Errico retractor
D'Errico spatula
D'Errico trephine
Desault bandage
Desault ligation
Descemet's membrane
descending
descending aorta
descending colon
descending urogram
descending urography
descensus
descensus uteri
descensus ventriculi
Deschamps carrier
Deschamps compressor
Deschamps-Navratil needle
Deschamps needle
desensitize
desensitization
Deseret angiocatheter
Deseret catheter

Deseret sump drain
desiccate
desiccation
desiccation-fulguration needle
desiccation needle
de Signeux dilator
Desilet catheter
Desjardin forceps
Desjardin probe
Desjardin scoop
Desmarres clamp
Desmarres dissector
Desmarres elevator
Desmarres forceps
Desmarres knife
Desmarres needle
Desmarres retractor
Desmarres scarifier
desmoid
desmotomy
desoxycorticosterone
desquamation
destruction
destruction of lesion
destruction of lesion by
    cauterization
destruction of lesion by curettage
destruction of lesion by
    fulguration
detachment
Detakats-McKenzie forceps
deterioration
determinant
detorsion
detrusor pattern
detrusor response
detrusor urinae muscle
Deutschman knife

devascularization
devascularize
DeVega anuloplasty
deviated nasal septum
deviation
DeVilbiss bottle
DeVilbiss compressor
DeVilbiss forceps
DeVilbiss irrigator
DeVilbiss rongeur
DeVilbiss speculum
DeVilbiss-Stacey speculum
DeVilbiss suction tube
DeVilbiss trephine
Devine tube
devitalized
Devonshire catheter
Devonshire knife
Dewar elevator
Dewar procedure
dewebbing
DeWecker cannula
DeWecker-Pritikin scissors
DeWecker scissors
DeWecker sclerotomy
Dewey forceps
Dexon sutures
dextran
Deyerle drill
Deyerle pin
Deyerle plate
Deyerle punch
diabetes mellitus
diabetic cataract
diaclastic amputation
diacondylar fracture
diagnostic curettage
diagnostic laparoscopy

diagnostic procedure
dialysis
dialysis shunt
diamond bur
diamond drill
diamond-edge scissors
diamond green marker
diamond-inlay bone graft
diamond nail
Diamond needle holder
diamond-point suture needle
Diamond tube
Diamox
diaphanoscopy
diaphragm
diaphragm pessary
diaphragma
diaphragmatic
diaphragmatic arteries
diaphragmatic hernia
diaphragmatic hernia repair
diaphragmatic herniorrhaphy
diaphyseal-epiphyseal fusion
diaphysectomy
diaphysis
diarrhea
diastalsis
diastasis
diastasis recti abdominis
diastatic skull fracture
diastole
diathermia knife
diathermy
diathermy forceps
diathermy needle
diazepam
dibucaine hydrochloride

DIC (diffuse intravascular coagu-
    lopathy)
Dick dilator
Dickson-Dively operation
Dickson operation
didelphic uterus
die plate
Dieffenbach amputation
Dieffenbach clamp
Dieffenbach-Duplay operation
Dieffenbach forceps
Dieffenbach operation
Dieffenbach plastic closure
Dieffenbach-Warren operation
dieresis
Diertz shears
Dieter forceps
Diethrich clamp
diethyl oxide
Dietrich apparatus
Dieulafoy aspirator
Dieulafoy erosion
Dieulafoy ulcer
differential spinal anesthesia
differentiated
differentiated carcinoma
diffuse
digastric fossa
digastric triangle
digastricus muscle
digital
digital arteries
digital block
digital examination
digital nerves
digital veins
digitales dorsales hallucis lateralis
    et digiti secundi medialis nerves

digitales dorsales manus arteries
digitales dorsales nervi radialis
  nerves
digitales dorsales nervi ulnaris
  nerves
digitales dorsales pedis arteries
digitales dorsales pedis nerves
digitales dorsales pedis veins
digitales palmares communes
  arteries
digitales palmares communes nervi
  mediani nerves
digitales palmares communes nervi
  ulnaris nerves
digitales palmares propriae arteries
digitales palmares proprii nervi
  mediani nerves
digitales palmares proprii nervi
  ulnaris nerves
digitales palmares veins
digitales plantares communes
  arteries
digitales plantares communes
  nervi plantaris lateralis nerves
digitales plantares communes
  nervi plantaris medialis nerves
digitales plantares propriae
  arteries
digitales plantares proprii nervi
  plantaris lateralis nerves
digitales plantares proprii nervi
  plantaris medialis nerves
digitales plantares veins
digitalis
digitalize
Dilantin
dilaprobe
dilaprobe dilator

dilatable bougie
dilatation
dilatation and curettage
dilatation of cervix
dilate
dilating bougie
dilating forceps
dilating probe
dilation
dilation and curettage
dilation of bladder neck
dilation of cervix
dilation of punctum
dilation of urethra
dilation with metal sound
dilator
    aortic
    Arnott
    Atlee
    Backhaus
    Bailey
    Bakes
    Bard
    Barnes
    Beardsley
    Berens
    Black-Wylie
    bladder
    Bossi
    Bowman
    Bransford-Lewis
    Brock
    bronchial
    Browne-McHardy
    Broyles
    cardiac
    cardiac valve
    cardiospasm

dilator *(continued)*

Castroviejo
cervical
Clark
Clerf
common duct
Cooley
Councill
Creevy
DeBakey-Cooley
Delaborde
Derra
de Signeux
Dick
dilaprobe
Einhorn
esophageal
esophagospasm
expansile
Ferris
French
Frommer
Galezowski
gall duct
Garrett
Gerbode
Glover
Gohrbrand
Goodell
Guyon
Hanks
Hanks-Bradley
Heath
Hegar
Hegar-Goodell
Hosford
Hurst
Hurtig

dilator *(continued)*

hydrostatic
infant
Jackson
Jackson-Mosher
Jackson-Plummer
Jackson-Trousseau
Johnston
Jolly
Jones
Kahn
Kearns
Kelly
Kollmann
Kron
Laborde
lacrimal
laryngeal
Leader-Kollmann
Mahoney
Maloney
Mantz
meatal
mitral
mitral valve
Mixter
Muldoon
Murphy
Nettleship-Wilder
olive
Ottenheimer
Palmer
Patton
Plummer
Plummer-Vinson
pneumatic
Potts
Potts-Riker

dilator *(continued)*
> Pratt
> punctum
> pyloric stenosis
> Ramstedt
> Rapaport
> Ravich
> rectal
> Reich-Nechtow
> Ritter
> Rolf
> Russell
> Sims
> Sippy
> sphincter
> Starck
> Starlinger
> Steele
> tracheal
> transventricular
> Trousseau
> Trousseau-Jackson
> Tubbs
> Tucker
> Turner
> two-bladed
> ureteral
> urethral
> uterine
> valve
> van Buren
> vascular
> vibrodilator
> Wales
> Walther
> Wilder
> Williams
> Wylie

dilator *(continued)*
> Young
> Ziegler

dilator pupillae muscle
Dilaudid
diminution
Dimitry-Bell erysiphake
Dimitry erysiphake
Dimitry-Thomas erysiphake
Dimitry trephine
dimness
dimpling
Dingman abrader
Dingman clamp
Dingman-Denhardt mouth gag
Dingman elevator
Dingman forceps
Dingman mouth gag
Dingman needle
Dingman osteotome
Dingman periosteal elevator
Dingman retractor
Dingman-Senn retractor
Dingman wire passer
diopter
diploic vein
diploica frontalis vein
diploica occipitalis vein
diploica temporalis anterior vein
diploica temporalis posterior vein
diplopia
direct catheterizing cystoscope
direct forward-vision telescope
direct fracture
direct laryngoscope
direct ophthalmoscope
direct-vision adenotome
direct-vision telescope

director
    angled
    gorget
    grooved
    Larry
    Pratt
    probe
    Putti-Platt
    rectal
    Teale
disability
disarticulated
disarticulation
disarticulation chisel
disc (see also *disk*)
discission
discission knife
discission needle
discission of cataract
discission of lens
discogenic
discoid aortic prosthesis
discoid valve prosthesis
discomfort
discrete
disease
disembowelment
dish-pan fracture
disimpaction forceps
disinfectant
disk
disk electrode
disk endoscope
disk explorer
disk forceps
disk valve
disk valve prosthesis
diskogram

diskography
dislocation
dislocation fracture
dislocation operation
dispersing electrode
displacement
disposable
disposable airway
disposable catheter
disposable forceps
disposable sigmoidoscope
disposable speculum
disposable stripper
disposable syringe
dissecting aneurysm
dissecting chisel
dissecting clamp
dissecting forceps
dissecting hook
dissecting knife
dissecting probe
dissecting scissors
dissection
dissection forceps
dissection hook
dissector
    Allis
    aspirating
    attic
    Aufranc
    Beaver
    blunt
    Brunner
    bunion
    Carpenter
    Cavitron
    Cheyne
    Collin

dissector *(continued)*
  Colver
  corneal
  Crabtree
  Desmarres
  endarterectomy
  Gannetta
  goiter
  Green
  Hajek-Ballenger
  Harris
  Heath
  Holinger
  Hood
  House
  Hurd
  hydrostatic
  Israel
  joker
  King-Hurd
  Kistner
  Kitner
  Kocher
  lamina
  Lane
  Lang
  laryngeal
  Lewin
  Lothrop
  Lynch
  MacAusland
  MacDonald
  Madden
  McWhinnie
  Moorehead
  Morrison-Hurd
  Neivert

dissector *(continued)*
  Oldberg
  Olivecrona
  Penfield
  Pierce
  pleura
  Potts
  prostatic
  Raney
  Rienhoff
  Rogers
  Rosen
  rotary
  Sheldon-Pudenz
  Sloan
  Smith
  Smithwick
  Stolte
  submucous
  suction
  tonsil
  vascular
  Walker
  Wangensteen
  Watson-Cheyne
  Yasargil
  Yoshida
  Young
disseminate
disseminated carcinoma
dissemination
distal
distal arteriotomy
distal endarterectomy
distant skin flap
distend
distention
distortion

distraction rod
Dittel operation
Dittel sound
Dittrich plug
diuresis
diuretics
divergent
diversion
diverticula (*sing.* diverticulum)
diverticular hernia
diverticulectomy
diverticulitis
diverticulogram
diverticulography
diverticulopexy
diverticulosis
diverticulum (*pl.* diverticula)
divided colostomy
divinyl ether
division
division of adhesions
Dix gouge
Dix needle
Dix spud
Dixon blade
Dixon-Thomas-Smith clamp
dizziness
Dobbie-Trout clamp
Docktor forceps
Docktor needle
Doctor Collins clamp
Doctor Long clamp
Doderlein-Kronig operation
Doderlein operation
dog-legged filiforms
Dogliotti-Guglielmini clamp
Dogliotti valvulotome
Doherty eye implant

Dohlman hook
Doleris operation
dome
Donald clamp
Donald-Fothergill operation
Donald operation
Donaldson tube
donor
Dooley nail
Doppler apparatus
Doppler-Cavin monitor
Doppler monitor
Doppler operation
Doppler sound device
Dopplergram
Dopplergraphy
Doptone fetal stethoscope
dormant
Dormia basket
Dormia stone basket
Dormia stone basket catheter
Dormia stone dislodger
Dorrance operation
dorsal artery of clitoris
dorsal artery of foot
dorsal artery of nose
dorsal artery of penis
dorsal decubitus position
dorsal elevated position
dorsal inertia position
dorsal lithotomy position
dorsal nerve of clitoris
dorsal nerve of penis
dorsal plaster spline
dorsal position
dorsal recumbent position
dorsal rigid position
dorsal scapular nerve

dorsal scissors
dorsal slit of prepuce
dorsal strut
dorsal supine incision
dorsal veins of clitoris
dorsal veins of penis
dorsal veins of tongue
dorsal vertebrae
dorsales clitoridis superficiales
    veins
dorsales linguae veins
dorsales penis superficiales veins
dorsalis clitoridis artery
dorsalis clitoridis nerve
dorsalis clitoridis profunda vein
dorsalis nasi artery
dorsalis pedis artery
dorsalis penis artery
dorsalis penis nerve
dorsalis penis profunda vein
dorsalis scapulae nerve
Dorsey cannula
Dorsey forceps
Dorsey leukotome
Dorsey needle
Dorsey punch
Dorsey retractor
Dorsey screwdriver
Dorsey separator
Dorsey spatula
Dorsey tongue depressor
dorsiflexion
dorsodecubitus position
dorsolateral incision
dorsolithotomy position
dorsorecumbent position
dorsosacral position
dorsosupine position

dorsum
Dos Santos needle
Dott mouth gag
Dott retractor
Doubilet sphincterotome
double-action bone cutter
double-action hump forceps
double-action rongeur
double-angle blade plate
double-angle blade
double-angle valve
double-armed retention sutures
double-armed sutures
double-ball separator
double-barrel colostomy
double-barreled loop colostomy
double-button sutures
double catheterizing cystoscope
double-channel irrigating
    bronchoscope
double-concave forceps
double concave rotating saw
double-cuffed tube
double-current catheter
double-edged knife
double elevator
double-ended curet
double-ended elevator
double-ended periosteal elevator
double-ended retractor
double-ended spatula
double fixation hook
double-flap amputation
double fracture
double-hook skin tenaculum
double-lumen breast implant
    material
double-lumen cannula

double-lumen catheter
double-lumen curet
double-lumen tube
double-needle cataract operation
double-pedicle skin flap
double-pronged hook
double spatula
double towel clamp
double vision
double-woven wire
double-Y incision
doubled black silk sutures
doubly armed sutures
douche
Dougherty irrigator
doughnut headrest
doughnut pessary
Douglas cul de sac
Douglas forceps
Douglas knife
Douglas operation
Douglas snare
Douglas speculum
Douglas trocar
Dourmashkin bougie
dovetail
Dow Corning cannula
Dow Corning implant
Dow Corning shunt
dowel
Dowell hernia repair
down-biting curet
Downes cautery
Downing clamp
Downing knife
Downing retractor
Doyen bur
Doyen clamp

Doyen elevator
Doyen forceps
Doyen-Jansen mouth gag
Doyen needle
Doyen operation
Doyen periosteal elevator
Doyen raspatory
Doyen retractor
Doyen rib shears
Doyen scissors
Doyen screw
Doyen speculum
Doyle operation
Doyle vein stripper
Dragstedt operation
drain
    accordion
    angle
    cigarette
    closed
    controlled
    Cushman
    Deaver T-drain
    Deseret sump
    d. tube
    four-wing
    Freyer
    Hemovac
    Hendrickson
    intercostal
    Jackson-Pratt
    Keith
    Lahey
    latex
    Malecot
    Mikulicz
    Morris
    Mosher

drain *(continued)*
    Penrose
    Pezzer
    Pharmaseal
    polyethylene
    polyvinyl
    Redivac
    Ritter
    rubber
    rubber-dam
    seton
    Silastic
    soft rubber
    stab
    stab-wound
    suction
    sump
    suprapubic
    suprapubic suction
    T-drain
    T-tube
    thyroid
    tissue
    tube
    two-wing
    Vacutainer
    whistle-tip
    Wylie
    Y-drain
drainage catheter
drainage gastroscopy
drainage of abscess
drainage of ascites
drainage of cisterna magna
drainage of cyst
drainage of gland
drainage of kidney
drainage of sinus

drainage of tissues
drainage pump
drainage tube
drape
    Steri-Drape
    Thompson
Drapier needle
drawer sign
dressed tube
dressing (see also *bandage*)
    ABD
    Adaptic
    Adaptic gauze
    adhesive
    adhesive absorbent
    Aeroplast
    anorectal
    antiseptic
    Band-Aid
    barrel
    Barton
    binocular
    bolus
    brassiere-type
    bulky
    bulky compressive
    bulky pressure
    butterfly
    cellophane
    Clevis
    Coban
    cocoon
    collar
    collodion
    compound
    compression
    Cornish wool
    d. forceps

dressing *(continued)*
 d. pliers
 dry
 dry pressure
 dry sterile
 Elastoplast
 felt
 fixed
 fluff
 fluffy compression
 foam rubber
 four-tailed
 Fricke
 Fuller rectal
 Furacin
 gauze
 Gelfilm
 Gelfoam
 Gelocast
 hip spica
 immobilizing
 impermeable
 iodoform
 Ivalon
 jelly
 Jobst
 Kerlix
 Kling
 Koch-Mason
 Larrey
 light
 Lister
 Lubafax
 many-tailed
 mastoid
 MMM (3M)
 moist
 monocular

dressing *(continued)*
 mustache
 Nu-gauze
 occlusive
 Orthoplast
 paraffin
 patch
 petrolatum gauze
 plaster
 plaster-of-Paris
 plastic
 postnasal
 pressure
 propylene
 protective
 Queen Anne
 Robert Jones
 roller
 Scultetus
 semicompressive
 semi-pressure
 sheepskin
 stent
 sterile
 sterile compression
 stockinette
 styrofoam
 surgical
 Surgicel
 T-binder pressure
 Telfa
 3M
 tie-over
 triangular
 tulle gras
 Vaseline
 Vaseline gauze
 Vaseline wick

dressing *(continued)*
    Velpeau
    Velroc
    Victorian collar
    Vioform
    Wangensteen
    water
    Xeroform
Drew-Smythe catheter
drill
    Adson
    air
    Amico
    automatic cranial
    Bjork
    bone
    Bosworth
    Bunnell
    bur
    cannulated
    Carmody
    centering
    cervical
    Charnley
    Cherry
    Cherry-Austin
    chuck
    Cloward
    Codman
    Collison
    cortical step
    cranial
    crown
    Crutchfield
    Cushing
    dental
    DePuy
    D'Errico

drill *(continued)*
    Deyerle
    diamond
    d. guide
    d. hole
    d. point
    d. vise
    flat
    Hall
    hand
    high-speed
    Hudson
    intramedullary
    Jacobs
    Jordan-Day
    Kirschner wire
    Lentulo
    Light-Veley
    Luck
    Lusskin
    McKenzie
    micro-air
    Moore
    Neurain
    Neurairtome
    orthopedic
    penetrating
    perforating
    perforator
    pilot
    Ralks
    Raney
    rib
    Shea
    Smedberg
    Smith
    spiral
    Spirec

drill *(continued)*
    step-down
    Stille
    Stryker
    tap
    Thornwald
    twist
    universal
    Vitallium
    Zimmer
drilling
drip pyelogram
drip pyelography
driver
    d. impactor
    Ken
    Küntscher
    McReynolds
    Moore
    Moore-Blount
    Neufeld
    prostatic
    Rush
drooping
drop-foot brace
drop-foot procedure
drop-foot splint
dropper
drug-induced hypothermia
drum elevator
drum elevator knife
drum membrane
drum probe
Drummond-Morison operation
dry amputation
dry dressing
dry gangrene
dry needle holder

dry packing
dry packs
dry pressure dressing
dry sterile dressing (DSD)
dual distal lighted laryngoscope
dual-lead electrode
dual-pass pacemaker
Duane "U" clip
Dubois scissors
Dubois shears
Duchenne trocar
duckbill clamp
duckbill elevator
duckbill rongeur
duckbill speculum
duct
    alveolar
    bile
    biliary
    cochlear
    common bile
    cystic
    d. of Bartholin
    efferent
    ejaculatory
    endolymphatic
    excretory
    hepatic
    lacrimal
    lacrimonasal
    lactiferous
    lymphatic
    mammary
    mesonephric
    mullerian
    nasal
    nasolacrimal
    pancreatic

duct *(continued)*
    papillary
    paramesonephric
    paraurethral
    parotid
    prostatic
    salivary
    semicircular
    seminal
    sublingual
    submandibular
    submaxillary
    tear
    thoracic
ductal
ductal carcinoma
ductions
ductless glands
ductogram
ductography
ductus
ductus clamp
ductus deferentis artery
ductus spreader
Dudley hook
Dudley operation
Dudley-Smith speculum
Duffield scissors
Dufourmentel rongeur
Duhamel operation
Dührssen incision
Dührssen vaginofixation
Duke cannula
Duke-Elder operation
Duke level of carcinoma (A, B, C, or D)
Duke trocar
Duke tube

dull-pointed forceps
dull-pronged retractor
dull retractor
Dumont retractor
Dumont scissors
dumping
dumping syndrome
Duncan curet
Dunhill forceps
Dunhill hemostat
Dunlop stripper
Dunlop traction
Dunn-Brittain operation
Dunn operation
Dunn tongue depressor
Dunning elevator
Dunning periosteal elevator
Duo adhesive cement
duobiotic
duodenal
duodenal arteries
duodenal clamp
duodenal glands
duodenal pin
duodenal retractor
duodenal tube
duodenal ulcer
duodenectomy
duodenitis
duodenocholecystostomy
duodenocholedochostomy
duodenocholedochotomy
duodenocolic
duodenocystostomy
duodenoduodenostomy
duodenoenterostomy
duodenogram
duodenography

duodenoileostomy
duodenojejunal
duodenojejunal flexure
duodenojejunal hernia
duodenojejunostomy
duodenolysis
duodenopyloric
duodenopyloric constriction
duodenorrhaphy
duodenoscopy
duodenostomy
duodenotomy
duodenum
Duplay hook
Duplay-Lynch speculum
Duplay operation
Duplay I procedure
Duplay II procedure
Duplay speculum
Duplay tenaculum
Duplay tenaculum forceps
duplication
Dupuis cannula
Dupuy-Dutemps blepharoplasty
Dupuy-Dutemps operation
Dupuytren amputation
Dupuytren contracture
Dupuytren enterotome
Dupuytren fracture
Dupuytren knife
Dupuytren operation
Dupuytren splint
Dupuytren sutures
Dupuytren tourniquet
dura
dura elevator
dura forceps
dura hook

dura hook knife
dura mater
dura scissors
dura separator
dural elevator
dural incision
dural knife
dural plate
dural retractor
dural scissors
dural separator
Duranest
duraplasty
Durham needle
Durham operation
Durham trocar
Durham tube
durotomy
Duroziez sign
Durr operation
Duval-Allis forceps
Duval-Coryllos rib shears
Duval-Crile forceps
Duval forceps
Duverger and Velter operation
Duvergier sutures
Duverney fracture
Duvol bag
DuVries hammer toe repair
Dwyer instrumentation
Dyclone
dyclonine hydrochloride
dye
dynamic ileus
dynamic splint
dynamometer
dyscrasic fracture
dysesthesia

dysfunction

dysfunctional

dysfunctional uterine bleeding

dyskinesia

dyspareunia

dysphagia

dysphasia

dysplasia

dyspnea

dyssynergia

dystonia

dysuria

e

ear
ear bougie
ear curet
ear forceps
ear hook
ear knife
ear loupe
ear mobilizer
ear pinna
ear pinna prosthesis
ear piston prosthesis
ear probe
ear punch
ear punch forceps
ear rongeur
ear setback
ear snare
ear speculum
eardrum
eardrum elevator
Earle clamp
Earle probe
East-West retractor
Eastman clamp
Eastman forceps
Eastman retractor
Easy catheter
Eaton speculum
Eber forceps
Ebner's glands
ebonation
eburnation

eccentric amputation
ecchymosis (*pl.* ecchymoses)
eccrine gland
echinococcosis
echinococcotomy
Echinococcus
echinococcus cyst
echocardiogram
echocardiography
echoencephalogram
echoencephalography
ECG (electrocardiogram)
Eckstein-Kleinschmidt operation
écraseur
ectocolostomy
Ectocor pacemaker
ectokelostomy
ectopia
ectopic
ectopic beats
ectopic pregnancy
ectropion
Edebohls clamp
Edebohls incision
Edebohls operation
Edebohls position
Edelmann-Galton whistle
edema
edematous
Eden-Hybbinette operation
Eder-Chamberlin gastroscope
Eder forceps

Eder gastroscope
Eder-Hufford esophagoscope
Eder-Hufford gastroscope
Eder laparoscope
Eder-Palmer gastroscope
Eder tongs
edge-to-edge sutures
Edinburgh retractor
Edinburgh sutures
edrophonium chloride
Edwards-Carpentier aortic valve
    brush
Edwards catheter
Edwards clamp
Edwards clip
Edwards graft
Edwards hook
Edwards patch
Edwards prosthesis
Edwards Teflon intracardiac
    implant
Edwards Teflon intracardiac
    prosthesis
Edwards Ventrac pulse generator
EEA (end-to-end anastomosis)
EEA autosuture instrument
EEA stapler
EEG (electroencephalogram)
efferent
efferent duct
efficacious
Effler operation
Effler tack
effleurage
effusion
Eggers operation
Eggers plate
Eggers screw

Eggers splint
eggshell nails
Ehrhardt forceps
Eicher chisel
Eicher hip prosthesis
Eicher rasp
eikonometer
Einhorn dilator
Einhorn tube
Eisenmenger complex
Eitner operation
ejaculatory duct
Ekehorn operation
EKG (electrocardiogram)
elastic
elastic adhesive bandage
elastic bandage
elastic bougie
elastic hosiery
elastic ligature
elastic rubber bands
elastic sutures
elastic traction
Elasticon bandage
Elastoplast bandage
elbow joint
elbowed bougie
elbowed catheter
elective
elective surgery
electric anesthesia
electric aspirator
electric bur
electric caliper
electric cardiac pacemaker
electric cautery
electric dermatome
electric knife

electric meatotome
electric probe
electric retinoscope
electric saw
electric trephine
electrical implant
electrically driven bur
electricator
electricity-induced anesthesia
electroanesthesia
electrocardiogram (ECG, EKG)
electrocardiography
electrocautery
electrocautery unit
electrocholecystectomy
electrocholecystocausis
electrocoagulation
electrocoagulator
electrocochleogram
electrocochleography
electroconization
electrocystoscope
electrode
    ACMI
    angular
    angulated blade
    atrial
    ball
    ball tip
    Ballenger
    Bard
    Beaver
    Berens
    biopsy loop
    bipolar
    bipolar catheter
    Birtcher
    blade

electrode *(continued)*
    Bovie
    Bugbee
    Buie
    central terminal
    coagulating
    coagulation
    Collings
    conical tip
    conization
    coudé
    cuff
    cup-shaped
    cutting loop
    Davis
    Delgado
    depolarizing
    disk
    dispersing
    dual-lead
    EMG
    ENT
    epicardial
    equipotential
    exploring
    external
    fine needle
    fine-wire
    follicle
    flat-tip
    fulgurating
    fulguration
    Gradle
    Grantham
    Hamm
    Hubbard
    Hurd
    Iglesias

electrode *(continued)*
    impedance
    implanted
    inactive
    indifferent
    knife
    Kronfeld
    large loop
    lobotomy
    loop
    Lynch
    McCarthy
    McWhinnie
    meatotomy
    Moersch
    multi-lead
    multiple-point
    Myerson
    myocardial
    needle
    Nesbitt
    neutral
    New's
    pacemaker
    pacing wire
    pad
    panendoscope
    Pischel
    platinum blade
    point
    pointed-tip
    punctate
    reference
    retinal detachment
    retrograde
    Ringenberg
    rod
    small loop

electrode *(continued)*
        Smith
        Stern-McCarthy
        straight-blade
        straight-tip
        terminal
        therapeutic
        tonsil
        turbinate
        ultrasonic
        unipolar
        ureteral meatotomy
        Wappler
        Weve
        wire
    electrodermatome
    electrodesiccation
    electrodiaphake
    Electrodyne pacemaker
    electroencephalogram (EEG)
    electroencephalography
    electroenterostomy
    electrogastroenterostomy
    electrogastrogram
    electrogastrography
    electrogoniometer
    electrokeratotomy
    electrolysis
    electromagnet
    electromyogram (EMG)
    electromyography
    electron microscope
    electronarcosis agents
    electronic tonometer
    electronystagmogram (ENG)
    electronystagmography
    electroresection
    electroretinogram (ERG)

electroretinography
electroscope
    Bruening
    Haslinger
electroshock
electrosurgery
electrosurgery pencil
electrosurgical knife
electrosurgical unit
electrotome
    infant
    McCarthy
    Nesbit
    punctate
    Stern-McCarthy
elephant-ear clavicle splint
elephantiasis operation
elevating forceps
elevation
elevator
    Abbott
    Abraham
    Adson
    Alexander-Farabeuf
    Antole-Condale
    Aufricht
    Ballenger
    Ballenger-Hajek
    Baron
    Barsky
    Bennett
    Bethune
    Blair
    Boies
    bone
    Brophy
    Brown
    Cameron-Haight

elevator *(continued)*
    Campbell
    Cannon-Rochester
    Carter
    Chandler
    chisel
    cleft palate
    Cobb
    Cohen
    Converse-MacKenty
    Cooper
    Cordes-New
    costal
    Cottle
    Cottle-MacKenty
    Coupland
    Crawford
    Cryer
    Cushing
    DeJager
    dental
    Desmarres
    Dewar
    Dingman
    double
    double-ended
    Doyen
    drum
    duckbill
    Dunning
    dura
    dural
    eardrum
    elevator-dissector
    ethmoidal
    Farabeuf
    Ferris-Smith
    flap

elevator *(continued)*

Fomon
Frazier
Freer
Friedrich
Gillies
Gimmick
Graham
Hajek-Ballenger
Halle
Hamrick
hawk's beak
Hayden
heavy
Hedblom
Henner
Hibbs
Hoen
Horsley
House
Howorth
Hurd
inclined-plane
Jackson
Jannetta
joker
Joseph
Joseph-Killian
Key
Killian
Kinsella
Kirmisson
knife
Kocher
L-shaped
Ladd
lamina
Lamont

elevator *(continued)*

Lane
Langenbeck
Lee-Cohen
Lempert
lid
Love-Adson
Luongo
MacKenty
Magielski
malar
Matson
McIndoe
McKenty
Moore
Moorehead
mucosa
narrow
nasal
nostril
Overholt
palate
Paparella
Penfield
Pennington
perichondrial
periosteal
periosteum
Phemister
Pierce
Pischel
pituitary
Poppen
Potts
pressure
Proctor
Ralks
raspatory

elevator *(continued)*
    Ray-Parsons-Sunday
    rib
    Rochester
    Rosen
    Sachs
    Sayre
    scalene
    Schuknecht
    screw
    Sedillot
    septal
    septum
    Sewall
    Shambaugh
    Shambaugh-Derlacki
    sharp
    Smith-Petersen
    skin
    spinal
    spinal fusion
    stapes
    staphylorrhaphy
    straight
    submucous
    suction
    Sunday
    Tabb
    tonsil
    tooth
    Turner
    uterine
    Veau
    Walker
    Woodson
    zygoma
Ellik evacuator
Ellik meatotome

Ellik sound
Ellik stone basket
Elliot forceps
Elliot operation
Elliot position
Elliot trephination
Elliot trephine
ellipse
elliptic amputation
elliptical amputation
elliptical excision
elliptical incision
Ellis-Jones operation
Ellis needle holder
Ellis operation
Ellis spud
Ellsner gastroscope
Elmslie-Cholmeley operation
Eloesser flap
Eloesser operation
elongation
Elsberg cannula
Elsberg incision
Elschnig forceps
Elschnig knife
Elschnig-O'Brien forceps
Elschnig-O'Connor forceps
Elschnig operation
Elschnig retractor
Elschnig scoop
Elschnig spatula
Elschnig spoon
Ely operation
embarrassment
embolectomy
embolectomy catheter
embolectomy curet
emboli (*sing.* embolus)

embolic aneurysm
embolism
embolization
embolus (*pl.* emboli)
embryo
embryotomy
embryotomy knife
Emerson bronchoscope
Emerson pump
Emerson suction
Emerson suction tube
Emerson vein stripper
Emesco handpiece
EMG (electromyogram)
EMG electrode
EMI scan
EMI scanner
eminence
emissaria condylaris vein
emissaria mastoidea vein
emissaria occipitalis vein
emissaria parietalis vein
emissary vein
Emmert-Gellhorn pessary
Emmet forceps
Emmet needle
Emmet operation
Emmet probe
Emmet retractor
Emmet scissors
Emmet sutures
Emmet tenaculum
Emmet trocar
Empirin
empyema
empyema trocar
empyema tube
en bloc

en bloc resection
en coin fracture
en masse
en rave fracture
enamel
enamel rod
encapsulated
encephalocentesis
encephalogram
encephalography
encephalopuncture
Encerin soap
encircling procedure
encircling tube
encroach
encroachment
encrustation
encysted
encysted hernia
end colostomy
end-on mattress sutures
end-point
end-to-end anastomosis
end-to-side anastomosis
end tube
endarterectomized
endarterectomy
endarterectomy dissector
endarterectomy loop
endarterectomy scissors
endarterectomy spatula
endarterectomy stripper
endarteritis
endaural
endaural approach
endaural curet
endaural incision
endaural retractor

endaural rongeur
endaural speculum
endoaneurysmorrhaphy
endobronchial anesthesia
endobronchial tube
endocardial bipolar pacemaker
endocervical biopsy
endocervical biopsy punch
endocervical curet
endocervical os
endocervicitis
endocervix
endocholedochal
endocrine
endocrine fracture
endocrine glands
endodontia
endodontitis
endoesophageal prosthesis
endolymphatic duct
endolymphatic subarachnoid
    shunt
endolymphatic tube
endometrectomy
endometrial biopsy
endometrial curet
endometrial forceps
endometrial implants
endometrial polyp
endometriosis
endometritis
endometrium
endo-osseous implant
endophlebitis
endoplastic amputation
endoscope
    disk
    Kelly

endoscope *(continued)*
    Rockey
endoscopic bladder litholapaxy
endoscopic magnet
endoscopic retrograde cholangio-
    pancreatography (ERCP)
endoscopic tube
endoscopy
endospeculum
endospeculum forceps
endothelium
endotherm knife
endothermy
endothoracic fascia
endothyropexy
endotracheal
endotracheal anesthesia
endotracheal curet
endotracheal general anesthesia
endotracheal insufflation
    anesthesia
endotracheal stripper
endotracheal tube
enema
ENG (electronystagmogram)
Engel-Lysholm maneuver
Engel-May nail
Engel saw
engine reamer
Englemann splint
English forceps
English position
English rhinoplasty
engorgement
engraftment
enlargement
enlarging bur
Ennis forceps

ensiform
ensiform appendix
ensiform process
ENT (ear, nose, throat)
ENT electrode
enterauxe
enterectasis
enterectomy
enterelcosis
enteric
enteritis
enteroanastomosis
enteroapokleisis
enterocele
enterocelectomy
enterocentesis
enterochirurgia
enterocholecystostomy
enterocholecystotomy
enterocleisis
enteroclysis
enterocolectomy
enterocolitis
enterocolostomy
enteroenterostomy
enteroepiplocele
enterogastritis
enterohepatopexy
enterolith
enterolithiasis
enterolithotomy
enterolysis
enteromesenteric
enteropancreatostomy
enteropexy
enteroplasty
enteroplexy
enteroptosis

enterorrhaphy
enteroscope
enterostomy
enterostomy clamp
enterotome
    Abraham
    Dupuytren
    Lukens
enterotomy
enterotomy incision
entropion clamp
entropion forceps
entropion operation
enucleation
enucleation compressor
enucleation neurotome
enucleation of cyst
enucleation of eyeball
enucleation scissors
enucleation scoop
enucleation snare
enucleation spoon
enucleator
    Meding tonsil
    prostatic
    tonsil
    Young prostatic
epaulet shoulder pad
epic microscope
epicanthus
epicanthus repair
epicardial electrode
epicardiectomy
epicardiolysis
epicardium
epicranial muscle
epicranius muscle
epidermis

epidermoid
epididymectomy
epididymis (*pl.* epididymides)
epididymitis
epididymogram
eipdidymography
epididymoplasty
epididymorrhaphy
epididymotomy
epididymovasectomy
epididymovasostomy
epidural anesthesia
epidural space
epigastric
epigastric artery
epigastric fossa
epigastric hernia
epigastric herniorrhaphy
epigastric puncture
epigastric vein
epigastrica inferior artery
epigastrica inferior vein
epigastrica superficialis artery
epigastrica superficialis vein
epigastrica superior artery
epigastricae superiores veins
epigastrium
epigastrocele
epigastrorrhaphy
epiglottectomy
epiglottidectomy
epiglottis
epiglottis retractor
epilating forceps
epilation
epilation forceps
epilation needle
epimicroscope

epinephrine
epipharynx
epiphyseal arrest
epiphyseal-diaphyseal fusion
epiphyseal fracture
epiphyseal line
epiphysiodesis
epiphysiolysis
epiplocele
epiploectomy
epiploenterocele
epiploic
epiploitis
epiplomerocele
epiplomphalocele
epiploon
epiplopexy
epiploplasty
epiplorrhaphy
epiplosarcomphalocele
epiploscheocele
episclera
episcleral arteries
episcleral forceps
episcleral veins
episclerales arteries
episclerales veins
episioperineoplasty
episioperineorrhaphy
episioplasty
episioproctotomy
episiorrhaphy
episiotomy
episiotomy scissors
epispadias
epistaxis
epistaxis balloon
epistropheus

epithelial inlay operation
epithelial outlay operation
epithelialization
epithelialize
epithelialized
epithelium
epitrochlea
epitympanic
epitympanum
épluchage
eponychium
Epstein blade
Epstein curet
Epstein hammer
Epstein needle
Epstein osteotome
Epstein rasp
equalization
equator
Equen magnet
Equen-Neuffer knife
equilibrating
equilibration
equinovarus
equinus
equinus deformity
equipotential electrode
Equisetene sutures
ERCP (endoscopic retrograde cholangiopancreatography)
erector muscle
erector spinae muscle
erector spinae retractor
ERG (electroretinogram)
Ergotrate
Erhardt clamp
Erhardt forceps
Erhardt speculum

Erich arch bar
Erich forceps
Erich operation
Erich splint
erisiphake (see *erysiphake*)
Ernst applicator
Ernst radium application
erosion
erysiphake
    Barraquer
    Bell
    Dimitry
    Dimitry-Bell
    Dimitry-Thomas
    Harrington
    Kara
    L'Esperance
    Maumenee
    Nugent-Green-Dimitry
    Post-Harrington
    right-angled
    Sakler
    Searcy
    Viers
erythema
erythematous
eschar
escharectomy
escharotomy
eserine
ESI laryngoscope
ESI sigmoidoscope
Esmarch bandage
Esmarch operation
Esmarch probe
Esmarch scissors
Esmarch shears
Esmarch tourniquet

esogastritis
esophagalgia
esophageae veins
esophageal
esophageal anastomosis
esophageal biopsy
esophageal bougie
esophageal dilatation
esophageal dilator
esophageal diverticulectomy
esophageal fistula
esophageal fistula closure
esophageal forceps
esophageal repair
esophageal scissors
esophageal shears
esophageal speculum
esophageal stricture
esophageal tube
esophageal varices
esophageal veins
esophagectomy
esophagocardiomyotomy
esophagocologastrostomy
esophagocolostomy
esophagoduodenostomy
esophagoenterostomy
esophagoesophagostomy
esophagofundopexy
esophagogastrectomy
esophagogastric
esophagogastroanastomosis
esophagogastroduodenoscopy
esophagogastromyotomy
esophagogastropexy
esophagogastroplasty
esophagogastroscopy
esophagogastrostomy

esophagoileostomy
esophagojejunogastrostomosis
esophagojejunoplasty
esophagojejunostomy
esophagomyotomy
esophagopharynx
esophagoplasty
esophagoplication
esophagorrhaphy
esophagoscope
    Boros
    Broyles
    Bruening
    Chevalier Jackson
    Eder-Hufford
    e. obturator
    fiberoptic
    folding
    full-lumen
    Haslinger
    Haslinger tracheobroncho-
      esophagoscope
    Holinger
    Jackson
    Jesberg
    Lell
    Moersch
    Mosher
    Moure
    optical
    oval
    Roberts
    Sam Roberts
    Schindler
    Tucker
    Yankauer
esophagoscopic cannula
esophagoscopic catheter

esophagoscopic tube
esophagoscopy
esophagospasm
esophagospasm dilator
esophagostomy
esophagotomy
esophagus
esotropia
Esser operation
Esser skin graft
Essex-Lopresti maneuver
Essex-Lopresti method
Essex-Lopresti reduction tech-
    nique
Essig-type splint
Essrig forceps
Essrig scissors
Estes operation
estimated blood loss
Estlander cheiloplasty
Estlander operation
estrogen
ether
ether in oil
Ethibond sutures
Ethicon clip
Ethicon silk sutures
Ethicon sutures
Ethiflex sutures
Ethilon nylon sutures
Ethilon sutures
ethmoid
ethmoid bone
ethmoid curet
ethmoid-cutting forceps
ethmoid forceps
ethmoid fossa
ethmoid process

ethmoid sinus
ethmoidal artery
ethmoidal chisel
ethmoidal elevator
ethmoidal nerve
ethmoidal veins
ethmoidalis anterior artery
ethmoidalis anterior nerve
ethmoidalis posterior artery
ethmoidalis posterior nerve
ethmoidectomy
ethmoidotomy
ethocaine
Ethrane
Ethridge forceps
ethyl chloride
ethyl ether
ethyl oxide
ethyl vinyl ether
ethylene
etidocaine hydrochloride
eustachian bougie
eustachian bur
eustachian catheter
eustachian probe
eustachian tube
euthyroid
evacuation
evacuator
    bladder
    clot
    Creevy
    Crigler
    Ellik
    Ewald
    Hutch
    ice clot
    McCarthy

evacuator *(continued)*
    suction
    Timberlake
    Toomey
evagination
Evans forceps
Evans operation
eventration
Everett forceps
Everett-TeLinde operation
Eversbusch operation
eversion
everted
everting interrupted sutures
everting sutures
Eves snare
Evipal
evisceration
evisceration knife
evisceration of eyeball
evisceration of orbital contents
evisceration spoon
evulsion
Ewald evacuator
Ewald forceps
Ewald tube
exam
examination
examination retractor
examine
examining gastroscope
examining hook
examining telescope
exarticulation
excavation
excavator
    dental
    e. spoon

excavator *(continued)*
    House
    Lempert
    Schuknecht
    spoon
excentric amputation
excess
exchange transfusion
excision
excision and cautery
excision and fulguration
excochleation
excoriated
excoriation
excrement
excretion cystogram
excretion cystography
excretion pyelogram
excretion pyelography
excretion urogram
excretion urography
excretory duct
excretory urogram
excretory urography
excruciating pain
exenterated
exenteration
exenteration of orbital contents
exenteration of pelvic organs
exenteration spoon
exenteritis
exercise tolerance
exertion
exfoliation
Exner plexus
exocervix
exocrine glands
exodontia

exophthalmic
exophthalmic goiter
exophthalmometer
    Hertel
    Luedde
exophthalmos
exophytic
exophytic lesion
exostectomy
exostosectomy
exostosis
exotropia
expanding reamer
expansile
expansile dilator
expansile knife
expansile valvulotome
expiratory flow rate
exploration
exploratory
exploratory bougie
exploratory incision
exploratory laparotomy
exploratory operation
exploratory pneumonotomy
exploratory procedure
exploratory suction tip
exploratory thoracotomy
exploratory trephine
explorer
    disk
    Hoen
exploring cannula
exploring electrode
exploring needle
exposure
expressed skull fracture
expression

expressive
expressor (see also *lens expressor*)
    Arruga
    Heath
    Hess
    lens (see separate listing)
    Smith
    tonsil
exquisite pain
exquisite tenderness
exsanguinate
exsanguination
exsanguination transfusion
exsanguinotransfusion
exstrophy of bladder
extension
extension splint
extension tractor
extensive
extensor carpi radialis brevis
    muscle
extensor carpi radialis longus
    muscle
extensor carpi ulnaris muscle
extensor digiti minimi muscle
extensor digitorum brevis muscle
extensor digitorum longus muscle
extensor digitorum muscle
extensor hallucis brevis muscle
extensor hallucis longus muscle
extensor indicis muscle
extensor muscle
extensor pollicis brevis muscle
extensor pollicis longus muscle
exteriorization
exteriorize
external
external asynchronous pacemaker

external canthotomy
external capsule
external carotid artery
external demand pacemaker
external electrode
external ethmoidectomy
external frontal sinusotomy
external genitalia
external hemorrhoid
external hemorrhoidectomy
external-internal pacemaker
external nasal splint
external oblique fascia
external oblique muscle
external os
external osteotomy
external pacemaker
external rectus sheath
external rotation
external rotators
external sinusotomy
external splint
external stripper
external table
external traction
external version
externo-frontal retractor
extirpation
extirpation of cornea
extra-articular
extra-articular arthrodesis
extracapsular cataract extraction
extracapsular fracture
extracapsular lens extraction
extracorporeal
extracorporeal circulation
extracorporeal exchange hypo-
    thermia

extracting forceps
extraction
extraction of calculus
extraction of kidney stones
extraction of lens
extraction of tooth
extraction of ureteral stones
extractor (see also *cryoextractor*)
    Amico
    Austin Moore
    bone
    cataract
    Cherry
    Cilco
    cloverleaf pin
    comedo
    Councill stone
    DePuy
    femoral head
    Grieshaber
    hatchet
    head
    hoe
    hooked
    Jewett bone
    Kelman
    Krwawicz
    McLaughlin
    McReynolds
    Moore
    Moore-Blount
    nail
    Rush
    Saalfield
    Schamberg
    Smith-Petersen
    stone
    Unna

extractor *(continued)*
    ureteral stone
    Walton
extradural
extradural anesthesia
extrafascial apicolysis
Extrafil breast implant
extrahepatic
extraluminal
extraluminal stripper
extraneous
extraoral incision
extraperiosteal pneumonolysis
extraperitoneal
extraperitoneal approach
extraperitoneal cesarean section
extrapetrosal drainage
extrapleural apicolysis
extrapleural fascia
extrapleural pneumonolysis
extrapleural pneumothorax
extrapleural resection of ribs
extrapyramidal
extrasaccular
extrasaccular hernia
extrasystole
extrauterine pregnancy
extravasation
extrinsic
extrinsic pressure
extrusion
extubate
extubated
extubation
exudate
exudative
eye and ear cannula
eye bandage

eye caliper
eye drops
eye evisceration spoon
eye forceps
eye implant (see also *implant*)
    acorn-shaped
    acrylic
    acrylic ball
    Allen
    Arruga
    Berens
    Berens-Rosa
    Binkhorst
    Brown-Dohlman
    build-up
    Choyce
    Choyce Mark VIII
    conical
    conventional reform
    conventional shell-type
    corneal
    Cutler
    Doherty
    e.i. conformer
    Federov
    Fox
    Frey
    glass sphere
    gold sphere
    Guist
    Haik
    hemisphere
    hollow sphere
    Hughes
    Ivalon
    Levitt
    Lincoff
    lucite

eye implant *(continued)*
    magnetic
    McGhan
    Mules
    plastic sphere
    Plexiglas
    polyethylene
    pyramidal
    Rayner-Choyce
    reverse-shape
    scleral
    scleral buckler
    semishell
    shelf-type
    shell
    Silastic
    silicone
    Snellen
    sphere
    spherical
    sponge
    Stone
    surface
    tantalum
    tire
    Troutman

eye implant *(continued)*
    tunneled
    Vitalium
    Wheeler
    wire mesh
eye loupe
eye magnet
eye pad
eye retractor
eye scissors
eye shield
eye speculum
eye spoon
eye spud
eyed probe
eyed suture needle
eyeless atraumatic suture needle
eyeless suture needle
eyelet lag screw
eyelid
eyelid forceps
eyelid ptosis operation
eyelid retractor
eyelid speculum
Eyler operation

f

F. R. Thompson hip prosthesis
F. R. Thompson rasp
fabella
fabere sign
face-down position
face lift
facet
facet rasp
facetectomy
faceted
facial
facial artery
facial fracture appliance
facial nerve (cranial nerve VII)
facial nerve knife
facial triangle
facial vein
facialis artery
facialis nerve
facialis vein
faciei profunda vein
facilitation
facility
facioplasty
Fahey operation
Fahey pin
falces (*sing.* falx)
falciform
falciform ligament
Falk clamp
Falk forceps
Falk operation

Falk retractor
Falk-Shukuris operation
Falk spoon
fallopian
fallopian artery
fallopian cannula
fallopian catheter
fallopian tube
Falope ring
false aneurysm
false cord
false joint
false membrane
falx (*pl.* falces)
    aponeurotic
    f. aponeurotica
    f. cerebelli
    f. cerebri
    f. inguinalis
    f. ligamentosa
    f. of cerebellum
    f. of cerebrum
    f. septi
    inguinal
    ligamentous
familial
Fansler anoscope
Fansler proctoscope
Fansler speculum
far-and-near sutures
far sutures
Farabeuf amputation

Farabeuf elevator
Farabeuf forceps
Farabeuf-Lambotte clamp
Farabeuf-Lambotte forceps
Farabeuf operation
Farabeuf periosteal elevator
Farabeuf raspatory
Farabeuf retractor
Farabeuf saw
faradic electric stimulation
Farill operation
Farlow-Boettcher snare
Farlow snare
Farlow tongue depressor
Farnham forceps
Farr retractor
Farrington forceps
Farrior forceps
Farrior speculum
Farris forceps
Fasanella operation
Fasanella-Servat operation
fascia (*pl.* fasciae)
    aponeurotic
    Camper's
    Cloquet's
    cremaster
    crural
    deep
    endothoracic
    external oblique
    extrapleural
    f. cribrosa
    f. forceps
    f. graft
    f. lata
    f. lata femoris
    f. lata graft

fascia *(continued)*
    f. lata prosthesis
    f. needle
    f. punch
    f. sling operation
    f. stripper
    f. transversalis
    infundibuloform
    pectineal
    prepubic
    Scarpa's
    superficial
    thyrolaryngeal
    transverse
fascial
fascial graft
fasciaplasty
fasciatome
fasciculation
fasciectomy
fasciodesis
fascioplasty
fasciorrhaphy
fasciotomy
fat graft
fat transplant
fatigability
fatigue fracture
fatty tissue
faucial and lingual tonsillectomy
faucial catheter
faucial eustachian catheter
faucial tonsillectomy
faucial tonsils
Faulkner-Browne chisel
Faulkner chisel
Faulkner curet
Faulkner trocar

Fauvel forceps
Favoloro retractor
Favoloro tunneler
FB (fingersbreadth)
fecal
fecal fistula
fecal impaction
fecal incontinence
fecalith
feces
fecopurulent
Federoff operation
Federoff splenectomy
Federov eye implant
feeble
feeding tube
Fehland clamp
Feilchenfeld forceps
Fein needle
Fein trocar
Feldman retractor
Fell-O'Dwyer apparatus
felon
felt collar splint
felt dressing
felt foam padding
felt pads
felt patch
female catheter
femoral
femoral arteriotomy
femoral artery
femoral artery cannula
femoral broach
femoral canal
femoral clamp
femoral component
femoral condyle

femoral condyle plate
femoral head
femoral head extractor
femoral head prosthesis
femoral head reamer
femoral hernia
femoral hernia repair
femoral herniorrhaphy
femoral-inguinal herniorrhaphy
femoral neck reamer
femoral neck retractor
femoral nerve
femoral prosthesis
femoral prosthesis broach
femoral prosthesis pusher
femoral pusher
femoral shaft rasp
femoral splint
femoral triangle
femoral vein
femoralis artery
femoralis nerve
femoralis vein
femorocele
femoropopliteal bypass
femur
fence splint
fenestra (*pl.* fenestrae)
fenestrated catheter
fenestrated forceps
fenestrated lens scoop
fenestrated membrane
fenestrater
fenestration
fenestration bur
fenestration hook
fenestration of semicircular canals
fenestrometer

Fenger forceps
Fenger probe
Fenton bolt
Fergus operation
Ferguson angiotribe
Ferguson-Coley operation
Ferguson curet
Ferguson forceps
Ferguson inguinal herniorrhaphy
Ferguson-Metzenbaum scissors
Ferguson-Moon retractor
Ferguson needle
Ferguson operation
Ferguson probang
Ferguson retractor
Ferguson scissors
Ferguson scoop
Ferguson stone basket
Fergusson excision of maxilla
Fergusson incision
Fergusson speculum
fern test
Ferris dilator
Ferris forceps
Ferris-Robb knife
Ferris scoop
Ferris Smith elevator
Ferris Smith forceps
Ferris Smith-Gruenwald rongeur
Ferris Smith-Halle bur
Ferris Smith-Kerrison forceps
Ferris Smith-Kerrison rongeur
Ferris Smith knife
Ferris Smith retractor
Ferris Smith rongeur
Ferris Smith-Sewall retractor
Ferris Smith-Takahashi rongeur
ferrule

ferrule clamp
fetal basiotripsy
fetal cleidotomy
fetal cranioclasis
fetal craniotomy
fetal heart tones
fetal ischiopubiotomy
fetal membranes
fetal position
fetogram
fetography
fetoscopy
fetus
fiber
fiberglass
fiberglass graft
fiberglass sleeve trocar
fiberoptic culdoscope
fiberoptic cystoscope
fiberoptic esophagoscope
fiberoptic gastroscope
fiberoptic laryngoscope
fiberoptic probe
fiberoptic proctosigmoidoscope
fiberoptic sigmoidoscope
fiberoptic telescope
fiberscope
    gastroduodenal
    Hirschowitz
fibrillate
fibrillation
fibrin
fibrinopurulent
fibrinous
fibroadenoma
fibroadenosis
fibrocalcific

fibrocartilage
fibrocartilaginous
fibrocartilaginous joint
fibrocaseous
fibrocystic
fibroid
fibroid hook
fibroidectomy
fibroma
fibromatosis
fibromectomy
fibromuscular
fibromuscular junction
fibromyoma (*pl.* fibromyomata)
fibromyomata uteri
fibromyomectomy
fibromyotomy
fibrosis
fibrotic
fibrous
fibrous goiter
fibrous renal capsule
fibula
fibular
fibular artery
fibular head
fibular muscle
fibular nerve
fibular veins
fibulares veins
fibularis nerve
Fick operation
field
field block
figure-of-eight bandage
figure-of-eight sutures
fil d'Arion tube
Filatov-Marzinkowsky operation

Filatov operation
file
filiform bougie
filiform catheter
filiform-tipped catheter
filiforms and followers
filipuncture
Fillauer splint
fillet
filleting
filling of pulp canal
filmy adhesions
filter
fimbria (*pl.* fimbriae)
fimbriated
fimbriectomy
fine artery forceps
fine cautery
fine chromic sutures
fine curet
fine dissecting forceps
fine dissecting scissors
fine forceps
fine mesh gauze
fine needle electrode
fine-pointed hemostat
fine scissors
fine silk sutures
fine suture scissors
fine-toothed clamp
fine-toothed forceps
fine-wire electrode
finger cot splint
finger dissection
finger goniometer
finger plate
finger retractor
finger splint

fingerbreadth (*pl.* fingersbreadth)
finishing ball reamer
finishing cup reamer
Fink curet
Fink forceps
Fink hook
Fink-Jameson forceps
Fink laryngoscope
Fink retractor
Fink tendon tucker
Finney pyloroplasty
Finney operation
Finnoff transilluminator
Finochietto-Billroth I operation
Finochietto clamp
Finochietto forceps
Finochietto needle holder
Finochietto operation
Finochietto retractor
Finochietto rib spreader
Finochietto scissors
Finsterer-Hofmeister operation
Finsterer operation
Finsterer sutures
first-degree burn (1st degree burn)
first-stage procedure
Fischer needle
Fish forceps
fish-hook needle
Fisher-Arlt forceps
Fisher cannula
Fisher forceps
Fisher guide
Fisher knife
Fisher-Nugent retractor
Fisher operation
Fisher rasp
Fisher retractor

Fisher spoon
Fisher spud
fisherman pliers
fishmouth incision
fissure
fissure bur
fissure fracture
fissurectomy
fissured fracture
fistula (*pl.* fistulas or fistulae)
fistula closure
fistula hook
fistula knife
fistula needle
fistula probe
fistulectomy
fistulization
fistuloenterostomy
fistulogram
fistulography
fistulotome
fistulotome knife
fistulotomy
fistulous
fistulous tract
Fitzgerald forceps
Fitzpatrick suction tube
Fitzwater forceps
Fitzwater ligature carrier
fixation
fixation anchor
fixation bandage
fixation forceps
fixation graft
fixation hook
fixation pin
fixation ring
fixation sutures

fixed dressing
fixed-rate pacemaker
fixing screw
Flagg laryngoscope
flail
flail joint
Flajani operation
flaking
Flanagan gouge
flange
flank
flank incision
Flannery speculum
flap
flap amputation
flap elevator
flap knife
flap operation
flap scissors
flapless amputation
flapping of conjunctiva
flask
flat drill
flat spatula
flat-tip electrode
flat zonule separator
flatfoot
flattening
flatulent
flatus
flaval ligament
Flaxedil sutures
Fleischer ring
Fleming conization instrument
Fleming conization of cervix
Fletcher afterloading tandem
Fletcher AL tandem
Fletcher knife

Fletcher loading applicator
Fletcher tandem
Fletcher-Van Doren forceps
flexed incision
flexible catheter
flexible gastroscope
flexible metal catheter
flexible probe
flexible retractor
flexible rubber tube
flexible shaft retractor
flexible suction tube
flexible tourniquet
flexion
flexion crease
Flexitone sutures
Flexon sutures
flexor carpi radialis muscle
flexor carpi ulnaris muscle
flexor digiti minimi brevis manus
    muscle
flexor digiti minimi brevis pedis
    muscle
flexor digitorum brevis pedis
    muscle
flexor digitorum longus pedis
    muscle
flexor digitorum profundus
    muscle
flexor digitorum superficialis
    muscle
flexor hallucis brevis muscle
flexor hallucis longus muscle
flexor muscle
flexor pollicis brevis muscle
flexor pollicis longus muscle
flexorplasty
Flexsteel retractor

flexure
Flieringa scleral ring
floating catheter
floppy valve syndrome
floriform cataract
flow-directed catheter
flow rate
flow-regulator clamp
flowmeter
flowmetry
Floyd needle
fluctuant
fluctuating
fluctuation
fluff dressing
fluffed gauze
fluffs
fluffy compression dressing
fluorescein
fluorescein angioscopy
fluorescence microscope
fluorescent microscope
Fluoroma
fluoroscopic control
fluoroscopic foreign-body forceps
fluoroscopy
Fluothane
flush
flush tube
flutter
Flynt needle
foam rubber dressing
Foerster (see Förster)
Fogarty catheter
Fogarty clamp
Fogarty probe
foil carrier
folding esophagoscope

folding laryngoscope
Foley-Alcock catheter
Foley-Alcock hemostatic bag
Foley bag
Foley catheter
Foley forceps
Foley hemostatic bag
Foley plate
Foley pyeloplasty
Foley Y-plasty
follicle electrode
follicle stimulating hormone (FSH)
follicular
folliculi (*sing.* folliculus)
folliculi lymphatici aggregati
folliculi lymphatici aggregati
    appendicis vermiformis
folliculi lymphatici gastrici
folliculi lymphatici lienales
folliculi lymphatici recti
folliculi lymphatici solitarii
    intestini crassi
folliculi lymphatici solitarii
    intestini tenuis
folliculus (*pl.* folliculi)
Fomon chisel
Fomon elevator
Fomon knife
Fomon operation
Fomon periosteal elevator
Fomon periosteotome
Fomon rasp
Fomon retractor
Fomon scissors
Fontan operation
foot bones
footling breech
footpiece

footplate
footplate chisel
footplate hook
foramen (*pl.* foramina)
foramen of Bochdalek
foramen of Morgagni
foramen of Winslow
foramen ovale
foramen-plugging forceps
foramina (*sing.* foramen)
foraminal
foraminal hernia
foraminal punch
foraminotomy
Forane
Forbe amputation
forced duction tests
forced ductions
forceps
    ACMI
    Adair
    Adair-Allis
    adenoid
    Adler
    Adson
    Adson-Brown
    advancement
    Allen
    alligator
    alligator grasping
    Allis
    Allis-Adair
    Allis-Coakley
    Allis-Duval
    Allis-Ochsner
    anastomosis
    Andrews
    Andrews-Hartmann

forceps *(continued)*
    aneurysm
    angiotribe
    angled stone
    angular
    angulated
    anterior
    anterior segment
    aorta
    aortic aneurysm
    aortic occlusion
    applicator
    approximation
    Archer
    Arruga
    Arruga-Gill
    artery
    Asch
    Ashby
    atraumatic
    atraumatic tissue
    aural
    axis-traction
    Ayer
    Babcock
    Backhaus
    Bacon
    Bailey
    Bailey-Williamson
    Bainbridge
    Baird
    Baker
    Ballenger
    Ballenger-Förster
    Ballentine
    Ballentine-Peterson
    Bane
    Bard-Parker

forceps *(continued)*
  Barkan
  Barlow
  Barnes-Simpson
  Barraquer
  Barraya
  Barrett
  Barrett-Allen
  Barrett-Murphy
  Barton
  basket
  Bauer
  bayonet
  bean
  Beardsley
  Beaupre
  Beck
  Beebe
  Beer
  Benaron
  Bengolea
  Bennett
  Berens
  Berke
  Berne
  Berry
  Best
  Bevan
  Beyer
  Billroth
  biopsy
  biopsy punch
  biopsy specimen
  bipolar
  bipolar coagulation
  Birkett
  Bishop-Harmon
  biting

forceps *(continued)*
  bladder
  bladder specimen
  Blake
  Blakesley
  Blalock
  Blanchard
  Bloodwell
  Boettcher
  Boies
  Bonaccolto
  Bond
  bone
  bone-biting
  bone-breaking
  bone-cutting
  bone-grasping
  bone-holding
  bone septum
  bone-splitting
  Bonn
  Bonney
  Boston Lying-In cervical
  Botvin
  box-joint
  Boys-Allis
  Bozeman
  Braasch
  Bracken
  Bradford
  brain
  brain tumor
  Braun
  Brenner
  Bridge
  Brigham
  broad-blade
  bronchial biopsy

forceps *(continued)*
    bronchoscopic
    bronchus
    Brophy
    Brown
    Brown-Adson
    Brown-Buerger
    Broyles
    Bruening
    Brunner
    Brunschwig
    Buerger-McCarthy
    Buie
    bulldog
    bullet
    Bumpus
    Bunim
    Burch
    Burnham
    Cairns
    Calibri
    Callahan
    Campbell
    Cane
    cannulated
    capsule
    capsule fragment
    capsule grasping
    cardiovascular
    Carlens
    Carmalt
    Carmody
    Carmody-Brophy
    cartilage
    caruncle
    Cassidy-Brophy
    Castroviejo
    Castroviejo-Arruga

forceps *(continued)*
    cervical
    cervical punch
    cervical traction
    cervix-holding
    cesarean
    chalazion
    Chamberlen
    Chandler
    Charnley
    Cheatle
    Cheron
    Cherry-Adson
    Cherry-Kerrison
    Chevalier Jackson
    chicken-bill rongeur
    Child
    Child-Phillips
    Children's Hospital
    Cicherelli
    cilia
    Citelli
    clamp
    Clark
    Clark-Guyton
    Clark-Verhoeff
    cleft palate
    Clerf
    clip
    clip-applying
    clip-removing
    closing
    coagulating
    coagulation
    Coakley
    coarctation
    Cohen
    Colibri

forceps *(continued)*
    Coller
    Collin
    Collin-Duvall
    Colver
    Colver-Coakley
    compression
    Cone
    conjunctival
    Cooley
    Coppridge
    Corbett
    Cordes
    Cordes-New
    Corey
    corneal transplant
    corneoscleral
    Cornet
    Corwin
    Cottle
    Cottle-Arruga
    Cottle-Jansen
    Cottle-Kazanjian
    Cottle-Walsham
    Crafoord
    Craig
    cranial
    Crenshaw
    Crile
    crimper
    crocodile
    cross-action
    cup
    cup biopsy
    cup-biting
    cupped
    Curtis
    curved

forceps *(continued)*
    Cushing
    cutting
    cylindrical object
    cystic duct forceps
    Danberg
    Dandy
    Davidson
    Davis
    Davol
    De Alvarez
    Dean
    DeBakey
    DeBakey-Bahnson
    DeBakey-Bainbridge
    DeBakey-Cooley
    deep-surgery
    Defourmental
    DeLee
    DeLee-Simpson
    Demarest
    DeMartel
    DeMartel-Wolfson
    Demel
    Denis Browne
    Dennis
    dental
    D'Errico
    Desjardin
    Desmarres
    Detakats-McKenzie
    DeVilbiss
    Dewey
    diathermy
    Dieffenbach
    Dieter
    dilating
    Dingman

forceps *(continued)*
   disimpaction
   disk
   disposable
   dissecting
   dissection
   Docktor
   Dorsey
   double-action hump
   double-concave
   Douglas
   Doyen
   dressing
   dull-pointed
   Dunhill
   Duplay
   dura
   Duval
   Duval-Allis
   Duval-Crile
   ear
   ear punch
   Eastman
   Eber
   Eder
   Ehrhardt
   elevating
   Elliot
   Elschnig
   Elschnig-O'Brien
   Elschnig-O'Connor
   Emmet
   endometrial
   endospeculum
   English
   Ennis
   entropion
   epilating

forceps *(continued)*
   epilation
   episcleral
   Erhardt
   Erich
   esophageal
   Essrig
   ethmoid
   ethmoid-cutting
   Ethridge
   Evans
   Everett
   Ewald
   extracting
   eye
   eyelid
   Falk
   Farabeuf
   Farabeuf-Lambotte
   Farnham
   Farrington
   Farrior
   Farris
   fascia
   Fauvel
   Feilchenfeld
   fenestrated
   Fenger
   Ferguson
   Ferris
   Ferris Smith
   Ferris Smith-Kerrison
   fine
   fine artery
   fine dissecting
   fine-toothed
   Fink
   Fink-Jameson

forceps *(continued)*

Finochietto
Fish
Fisher
Fisher-Arlt
Fitzgerald
Fitzwater
fixation
Fletcher-Van Doren
fluoroscopic foreign-body
Foley
foramen-plugging
f. delivery
f. extraction
foreign-body
Förster
forward-grasping
Foss
fragment
Francis
Frangenheim
Fränkel
Frankfeldt
Fraser
Freer-Gruenwald
Fuchs
Furniss
Gabriel Tucker
galea
gall duct
gallbladder
gallstone
Garland
Garrigue
Garrison
gastrointestinal
Gavin-Miller
Gaylor

forceps *(continued)*

Gellhorn
Gelpi
Gelpi-Lowrie
Gemini
Gerald
GI
Gifford
Gilbert
Gill
Gill-Fuchs
Gill-Hess
Gill-Safar
Gillies
Ginsberg
Girard
Glassman
Glassman-Allis
Glenner
globular object
Glover
goiter
Gold
Goldman-Kazanjian
Gomco
Good
Goodhill
Goodyear-Gruenwald
Gordon
Gradle
Graefe
grasping
grasping and cutting
Gray
Grayton
Green
Green-Armytage
Greenwood

forceps *(continued)*

- Grieshaber
- Gross
- Gruenwald
- Gruenwald-Bryant
- Guggenheim
- Guist
- Gutglass
- Guyton-Noyes
- Haig Ferguson
- Hajek
- Hajek-Koffler
- Hale
- hallux
- Halsted
- Hamby
- Hamilton
- harelip
- Harken
- Harrington
- Harrington-Mayo
- Harrington-Mixter
- Harris
- Hartmann
- Hartmann-Citelli
- Hartmann-Gruenwald
- Hawkins
- Hawks-Dennen
- Hayes-Olivecrona
- Hayton-Williams
- Healy
- Heaney
- Heaney-Ballentine
- Heaney-Kanter
- Heaney-Rezek
- Heath
- Hegenbarth
- Heise

forceps *(continued)*

- hemorrhoid
- hemorrhoidal
- hemostasis
- hemostatic
- Hendren
- Henke
- Henrotin
- Hess
- Hess-Barraquer
- Hess-Gill
- Hess-Horwitz
- Heyman
- Hibbs
- high
- Hirschman
- Hirst
- Hirst-Emmet
- Hodge
- Hoen
- Hoffman
- Holinger
- hollow object
- Holmes
- Holth
- hook
- Hopkins
- Horsley
- Hosford-Hicks
- Hough
- House
- House-Wullstein
- Howard
- Hoxworth
- Hoyt
- Hubbard
- Hudson
- Hufnagel

forceps *(continued)*
    hump
    Hunt
    Hurd
    hyoid-cutting
    hysterectomy
    Imperatori
    inlet
    intestinal
    Iowa
    iris
    isolation
    IV disk
    Jackson
    Jacobs
    Jacobson
    Jameson
    Jansen
    Jansen-Gruenwald
    Jansen-Middleton
    Jansen-Struycken
    Jarcho
    Jesberg
    jeweler
    Johns Hopkins
    Johnson
    Jones
    Joplin
    Judd
    Judd-Allis
    Judd-DeMartel
    Juers
    Juers-Lempert
    Julian
    Jurasz
    Kahler
    Kalt
    Kantor

forceps *(continued)*
    Kantrowicz
    Katzin-Barraquer
    Kaufman
    Kazanjian
    Kazanjian-Cottle
    Kelly
    Kelly-Murphy
    Kelman
    Kennedy
    Kent
    keratotomy
    Kern
    Kerrison
    Kevorkian
    Kevorkian-Young
    kidney-elevating
    kidney-stone
    Kielland
    Kielland-Luikart
    Killian
    King-Prince
    Kingsley
    Kirby
    Kirkpatrick
    Kitner
    Kleenspec
    Knapp
    Knight
    Knight-Sluder
    Kocher
    Koeberle
    Koffler
    Koffler-Lillie
    Kolb
    Kolodny
    Krause
    Krause universal

forceps *(continued)*

Kronfeld
Kuhnt
Kulvin-Kalt
Laborde
Lahey
Lahey-Babcock
Lahey-Péan
Lambert
Lambotte
Lane
Langenbeck
Laplace
laryngeal
laryngeal biopsy
laryngeal punch
laryngofissure
Laufe
Laufe-Barton-Kielland
Laufe-Piper
Lawrence
Lawton
Leader
Lebsche
Lejeune
Leksell
Leland-Jones
Lemmon-Russian
Lempert
lens
Leonard
Leriche
Levret
Lewin
Lewis
Lewkowitz
Leyro-Diaz
lid

forceps *(continued)*

ligamenta flava
ligamentum-grasping
ligature
ligature-carrying
Lillie
Lillie-Killian
lingual
Linnartz
lion-jaw
Lister
Liston
Liston-Stille
lithotomy
Littauer
Littauer-Liston
Livingston
lobe-grasping
lobe-holding
lobectomy
Lockwood
Lockwood-Allis
Lombard-Beyer
London
Long
Long Island
Lordan
Lore
Lothrop
Love-Gruenwald
Love-Kerrison
Lovelace
low
Löwenberg
Lower
lower gall duct
Lowsley
Luc

forceps *(continued)*

- Lucae
- Luer
- Luer-Whiting
- Luikart
- Luikart-Kielland
- Luikart-McLane
- Luikart-Simpson
- lung
- lung-grasping
- Lutz
- Lynch
- Lyon
- MacKenty
- Magielski
- Magill
- Maier
- Malis
- malleus
- Mann
- marginal chalazion
- Marshik
- Martin
- Maryan
- mastoid rongeur
- Mathieu
- Maumenee
- Max Fine
- Mayfield
- Mayo
- Mayo-Blake
- Mayo-Harrington
- Mayo-Ochsner
- Mayo-Péan
- Mayo-Robson
- Mayo-Russian
- McCarthy
- McCarthy-Alcock

forceps *(continued)*

- McCoy
- McCullough
- McGannon
- McGee
- McGill
- McGuire
- McHenry
- McIndoe
- McIntosh
- McKay
- McKenzie
- McLane
- McLane-Tucker
- McLane-Tucker-Luikart
- McNealy-Glassman-Babcock
- McNealy-Glassman-Mixter
- McPherson
- meat
- meat-grasping
- medium
- Meeker
- meibomian
- membrane-puncturing
- Metzenbaum
- Metzenbaum-Tydings
- MGH
- Michel
- Michigan
- micro-forceps
- micro-pin
- mid
- Mikulicz
- Milex
- Miller
- Millin
- Mills
- miniature

forceps *(continued)*

Mitchell-Diamond
mitral
mitral valve-holding
Mixter
Mixter-McQuigg
Moehle
Moersch
Moore
Moritz-Schmidt
Morson
Mosher
mosquito
Mount
Mount-Mayfield
Mount-Olivecrona
mouse-tooth
Moynihan
Moynihan-Navratil
Muck
mucous
Mueller
multipurpose
Mundie
Murphy
muscle
muscle-recession
Museholdt
Myers
Myerson
Myles
nasal
nasal-cutting
nasal dressing
nasal-grasping
nasal hump-cutting
nasal-packing
nasal-polyp

forceps *(continued)*

Nelson
nephrolithotomy
New Orleans Eye and Ear
New's
Newman
Neidner
Nissen
Noble
nonfenestrated
nonslipping
nontoothed
Norwood
Noyes
Nugent
OB
O'Brien
obstetric
obstetrical
occluding
occlusion
Ochsner
Ochsner-Dixon
O'Connor
O'Hanlon
O'Hara
Oldberg
Olivecrona
oral
O'Shaughnessy
ossicle-holding
Overholt
Overstreet
ovum
Page
Palmer
Pang
papilloma

forceps *(continued)*
    parametrium
    Parker-Kerr
    partial occlusion
    patent ductus
    Paterson
    Paton
    Patterson
    Payne-Ochsner
    Payne-Péan
    Payne-Rankin
    Péan
    peanut
    peanut-grasping
    pediatric
    Pemberton
    Penfield
    Pennington
    Percy
    perforating
    peripheral iridectomy
    peripheral vascular
    Perritt
    Pfau
    Phaneuf
    phimosis
    phrenicectomy
    Pierce
    Pierce-Hoskins
    pile
    pillar
    pin-bending
    Piper
    Pischel
    Pitha
    pituitary
    placenta
    placenta previa

forceps *(continued)*
    placental
    plain
    plain tissue
    pleurectomy
    Pley
    point
    polyp
    polypus
    Poppen
    Porter
    posterior
    Potts
    Potts-Smith
    Poutasse
    Pratt
    Pratt-Smith
    prepuce
    pressure
    Price-Thomas
    Prince
    prostatic
    prostatic lobe-holding
    Providence
    Providence Hospital
    ptosis
    pulmonary artery
    pulmonary vessel
    punch
    Quervain
    Quevedo
    Ralks
    Randall
    Raney
    Rankin
    Rankin-Crile
    rat-tooth
    Ratliff-Blake

forceps *(continued)*

    Ratliff-Mayo
    Ray
    reach-and-pin
    recession
    rectal biopsy
    Reese advancement
    Reich-Nechtow
    Reiner-Knight
    Reisinger
    Rezek
    Richard
    Richard-Andrews
    Richter
    Rienhoff
    ring
    ring-end
    ring rotation
    Ritter
    Robb
    Roberts
    Robertson
    Rochester
    Rochester-Carmalt
    Rochester-Ewald
    Rochester-Harrington
    Rochester-Mixter
    Rochester-Ochsner
    Rochester-Péan
    Rochester-Rankin
    Rochester-Russian
    Rockey
    Roeder
    Rolf
    roller
    rongeur
    rotating
    rotation

forceps *(continued)*

    round punch
    Rowland
    rubber-dam clamp
    Rugby
    Rumel
    Ruskin
    Ruskin-Liston
    Russell
    Russian
    Russian-Péan
    Sachs
    Sam Roberts
    Sanders
    Santy
    Sarot
    Satinsky
    Sauer
    Sauerbruch
    Sawtell
    Sawtell-Davis
    scalp
    Scheinmann
    Schlesinger
    Schnidt
    Schoenberg
    Schroeder
    Schroeder-Braun
    Schubert
    Schutz
    Schwartz
    Schweigger
    Schweizer
    Scobee-Allis
    Scoville
    Scoville-Greenwood
    screw-holding
    Scudder

forceps *(continued)*
  Searcy
  secondary membrane
  Segond
  Seiffert
  Seletz
  Selman
  Semb
  Semken
  Senn
  Senturia
  septal compression
  septal ridge
  septum
  septum compression
  septum-cutting
  septum-straightening
  sequestrum
  serrated
  serrefine
  Sewall
  Shaaf
  Shallcross
  sharp-pointed
  Shearer
  Sheehy
  Shuster
  shuttle
  side-curved
  side-grasping
  Simpson
  Simpson-Luikart
  Singley
  Skene
  Skillern
  Skillman
  skin
  sliding capsule

forceps *(continued)*
  Smart
  Smith
  Smith-Petersen
  Smithwick
  Smithwick-Hartmann
  smooth tissue
  Snellen
  Snyder
  Somers
  specimen
  speculum
  Spence
  Spence-Adson
  Spencer
  Spencer Wells
  Spero
  sphenoid punch
  spicule
  spinal perforating
  spiral
  splinter
  sponge
  sponge-holding
  sponging
  spoon-shaped
  Spurling
  Spurling-Kerrison
  square specimen
  St. Clair
  St. Clair-Thompson
  St. Martin
  stapes
  staple
  Staude
  Staude-Moore
  sternum punch
  Stevens
  Stevenson

forceps *(continued)*

Stille
Stille-Adson
Stille-Bjork
Stille-Horsley
Stille-Liston
Stille-Luer
Stone
stone-grasping
Stoneman
Storey
strabismus
straight
Stratte
Struempel
strut
Struyken
subglottic
suction
suction-tube
suture
suture-holding
suture-tying
suturing
Sweet
T-shaped
tack-and-pin
Takahashi
tangential
Tarnier
Teale
tenaculum
tendon
tendon-pulling
Terson
Thoms
Thoms-Allis
Thoms-Gaylor

forceps *(continued)*

thoracic
Thorek-Mixter
Thorpe
throat
thumb
thyroid
thyroid traction
Tischler
tissue
tissue-grasping
Tivnen
Tobold
Tobold-Fauvel
Tomac
tongue
tongue-seizing
tonsil
tonsil artery
tonsil-holding
tonsil-ligating
tonsil-seizing
tonsil-suturing
tooth-extracting
toothed
torsion
towel
Tower
Townley
tracheal
trachoma
traction
transfer
transplant-grafting
triangular punch
Trousseau
Troutman
tube

forceps *(continued)*
- tubular
- Tucker
- Tucker-McLane
- tumor
- turbinate
- Turell
- Tuttle
- Tydings
- Tydings-Lakeside
- U-shaped
- universal
- upbiting biopsy
- ureter isolation
- urethral
- uterine
- uterine artery
- uterine biopsy
- uterine-dressing
- uterine-elevating
- uterine-packing
- uterine polyp
- uterine tenaculum
- uterine vulsellum
- utility
- vaginal hysterectomy
- van Buren
- Van Doren
- Van Struycken
- Vanderbilt
- Varco
- vas isolation
- vascular
- vascular tissue
- vasectomy
- vectis
- Verhoeff
- vessel

forceps *(continued)*
- Virtus
- viscera
- vise
- vomer
- von Graefe
- von Mondak
- vulsellum
- Wachtenfeldt
- Waldeau
- Walker
- Walsham
- Walter
- Walther
- Walton
- Walton-Schubert
- Wangensteen
- Watson
- Watson-Williams
- Weil
- Weingartner
- Weis
- Weisenbach
- Weisman
- Welch Allyn
- Wells
- Wertheim
- Wertheim-Cullen
- White
- White-Lillie
- White-Oslay
- White-Smith
- Wilde
- Wilde-Blakesley
- Willett
- Williams
- wire
- wire-closure

forceps *(continued)*
    wire-crimping
    wire-tightening
    Wittner
    Wolfe
    Woodward
    Worth
    wound clip
    Wullstein
    Wullstein-House
    Wylie
    Yankauer
    Yankauer-Little
    Yasargil
    Yeomans
    Young
    Ziegler
forearm and metacarpal splint
forearm splint
Foregger bronchoscope
Foregger laryngoscope
foreign body
foreign-body curet
foreign-body forceps
foreign-body spud
forequarter amputation
foreskin
fork
forked T-tube
formaldehyde
formation of fistula
formocresol
formocresol pulpotomy
fornix *(pl.* fornices)
fornix-based conjunctival flap
Foroblique cystourethroscope
Foroblique lens
Foroblique panendoscope

Foroblique telescope
Forrester brace
Forrester-Brown head halter
Forrester clamp
Forrester head halter
Forrester splint
Förster forceps
Förster operation
Förster-Penfield operation
Förster snare
Fort bougie
forward-grasping forceps
Fosler splint
Foss clamp
Foss forceps
Foss retractor
fossa *(pl.* fossae)
    amygdaloid
    cerebral
    condylar
    condyloid
    coronoid
    cranial
    digastric
    epigastric
    ethmoid
    f. ovalis
    f. ovalis cordis
    glenoid
    hyaloid
    hypophyseal
    iliac
    incisive
    infratemporal
    interpeduncular
    ischiorectal
    mandibular
    mastoid

fossa *(continued)*
- nasal
- navicular
- ovarian
- pituitary
- subarcuate
- subpyramidal
- subsigmoid
- supraspinous
- temporal
- tibiofemoral
- urachal

Foster-Ballenger speculum
Foster fracture frame
Fothergill-Donald operation
Fothergill operation
Fothergill-Shaw operation
fountain syringe
4-A Magovern prosthesis
four by fours (4 x 4s)
four-flanged nail
four-point biopsy
four-point cervical brace
four-poster cervical brace
four-prong retractor
four-quadrant biopsy
four-tailed bandage
four-tailed dressing
four-wing drain
four-wing Malecot retention catheter
fourchette
Fowler incision
Fowler operation
Fowler position
Fowler sound
Fowler-Weir incision
Fox balloon

Fox blepharoplasty
Fox conformer
Fox curet
Fox eye implant
Fox eye shield
Fox implant
Fox irrigator
Fox operation
Fox scissors
Fox speculum
Fox splint
Frackelton needle
fractional anesthesia
fractional biopsy
fractional curettage
fractional D&C (dilatation and curettage)
fractional epidural anesthesia
fractional spinal anesthesia
fracture
- agenetic
- apophyseal
- articular
- atrophic
- avulsion
- Barton
- basal skull
- bending
- Bennett
- bent
- blow-out
- boxer
- bucket-handle
- bumper
- bursting
- butterfly
- buttonhole
- capillary

fracture *(continued)*
- cementum
- chisel
- cleavage
- closed
- closed skull
- Colles
- comminuted
- complete
- complex simple
- complicated
- composite
- compound
- compound skull
- compression
- condylar
- congenital
- contrecoup
- cough
- de Quervain
- dentate
- depressed
- diacondylar
- diastatic skull
- direct
- dish-pan
- dislocation
- double
- Dupuytren
- Duverney
- dyscrasic
- en coin
- en rave
- endocrine
- epiphyseal
- expressed skull
- extracapsular
- fatigue

fracture *(continued)*
- fissure
- fissured
- f. appliance (See separate listing)
- f. by contrecoup
- f. clamp
- fracture-dislocation
- f. frame (See separate listing)
- f. nail
- f. plate
- f. rod
- f. splint
- f. table
- Galeazzi
- Gosselin
- greenstick
- grenade-thrower
- Guerin
- gutter
- hickory-stick
- horizontal
- horizontal maxillary
- impacted
- incomplete
- indirect
- inflammatory
- interperiosteal
- intra-articular
- intracapsular
- intraperiosteal
- intrauterine
- joint
- lead pipe
- LeFort (I, II, or III)
- linear
- linear skull
- longitudinal
- loose

fracture *(continued)*
- malunited
- march
- Monteggia
- Moore
- multiple
- neoplastic
- neurogenic
- oblique
- occult
- open
- paratrooper
- parry
- pathologic
- perforating
- periarticular
- pertrochanteric
- pillion
- ping-pong
- pond
- Pott
- pressure
- pyramidal
- Quervain
- resecting
- secondary
- segmental
- Shepherd
- silver-fork
- simple
- simple skull
- Skillern
- skull
- Smith
- spiral
- splintered
- spontaneous
- sprain

fracture *(continued)*
- sprinter's
- stellate
- Stieda
- strain
- stress
- subcapital
- subcutaneous
- subperiosteal
- supracondylar
- teardrop
- torsion
- torus
- transcervical
- transcondylar
- transverse
- transverse facial
- transverse maxillary
- trimalleolar
- trophic
- tuft
- ununited
- Wagstaffe
- willow

fracture appliance
- Cameron
- craniofacial
- facial
- Roger Anderson facial

fracture frame
- Balkan
- Böhler
- Bradford
- Cole
- DePuy
- Foster
- Goldthwait
- head

fracture frame *(continued)*
    Hibbs
    hyperextension
    occluding
    overhead
    rainbow
    reducing
    Stryker
    Thomson
    trial
    turning
    Whitman
fragility
fragment forceps
fragmentation
fragmentation probe
Frahur clamp
Frahur scissors
frame
Franceschetti operation
Franceschetti trephine
Francis forceps
Francis spud
Francke needle
Franco operation
Frangenheim forceps
Frangenheim-Goebell-Stoeckel
   operation
frank breech
Frank gastrostomy
Franke tabes operation
Fränkel forceps
Fränkel sinus probe
Fränkel speculum
Frankfeldt forceps
Frankfeldt needle
Frankfeldt sigmoidoscope
Frankfeldt snare

Franklin retractor
Franklin-Silverman curet
Franklin-Silverman needle
Franz retractor
Fraser forceps
Frater retractor
Frazier-Adson clamp
Frazier cannula
Frazier elevator
Frazier hook
Frazier knife
Frazier needle
Frazier operation
Frazier osteotome
Frazier-Paparella suction tube
Frazier retractor
Frazier-Sachs clamp
Frazier scissors
Frazier separator
Frazier-Spiller operation
Frazier suction tip
Frazier suction tube
Frazier trocar
Frazier tube
Frederick needle
Fredet-Ramstedt operation
Fredet-Ramstedt pyloromyotomy
free graft
free ligature
free tenotomy
free-tie sutures
free ties
freeing of adhesions
freely movable joint
freely movable mass
Freeman clamp
Freeman leukotome
Freeman-Swanson prosthesis

Freer chisel
Freer elevator
Freer gouge
Freer-Gruenwald forceps
Freer hook
Freer knife
Freer periosteal elevator
Freer periosteotome
Freer retractor
Freer spatula
freezing
Freiberg knife
Freiberg retractor
Freiberg traction
Freimuth curet
Frejka splint
frena (*sing.* frenum)
French bougie
French Brown-Buerger cystoscope
French catheter
French dilator
French-eye needle
French-eye needle holder
French Foley catheter
French-following metal sound
French-Iglesias resectoscope
French-McCarthy panendoscope
French retractor
French-Robinson catheter
French skin flap operation
French sound
French-Stern-McCarthy retractor
French sutures
frenectomy
frenotomy
frenulum (*pl.* frenula)
frenum (*pl.* frena)
frequency

Freund chondrectomy
Freund hysterectomy
Freund operation
Frey eye implant
Frey-Freer bur
Freyer drain
Freyer operation
friable
Fricke bandage
Fricke dressing
Fricke operation
Frickman operation
Friede operation
Friedenwald-Guyton operation
Friedenwald operation
Friedenwald ophthalmoscope
Friedenwald operation
Friedman clip
Friedman-Otis bougie
Friedman retractor
Friedman vein stripper
Friedrich clamp
Friedrich operation
Friedrich-Petz clamp
Friedrich raspatory
Friedrich rib elevator
Friend catheter
Friesner knife
Frigitronics cryoextractor
Frigitronics cryoprobe
Fritsch catheter
Fritsch operation
Fritsch retractor
Fritz aspirator
Fritz-Lange operation
frog-legged position
Frommel operation
Frommer dilator

frontal
frontal artery
frontal bone
frontal lobotomy
frontal nerve
frontal process
frontal sinus
frontal sinus cannula
frontal sinus chisel
frontal sinus operation
frontal sinus probe
frontal sinus rasp
frontal sinusotomy
frontal suture
frontalis nerve
frontoethmoidal suture
frontolacrimal suture
frontomaxillary suture
frontonasal suture
frontonasal process
frontotemporal craniotomy
    incision
frontozygomatic suture
frost anesthesia
Frost-Lang operation
Frost sutures
frozen section
FSH (follicle stimulating hormone)
Fuchs forceps
Fuchs operation
Fuchs position
Fukala operation
fulcrum
fulgurate
fulgurating electrode
fulguration
fulguration electrode
full-curve sound

full-curved clamp
full-lumen esophagoscope
full-thickness
full-thickness skin graft
full-view lumen finder
Fuller operation
Fuller rectal dressing
Fuller tube
fullness
fulminant
fulminate
fulminating
fulminating appendicitis
fulmination
Fulton retractor
Fulton rongeur
Fulton scissors
function study
functional
functional splint
fundectomy of stomach
fundectomy of uterus
fundi (*sing.* fundus)
fundic glands
fundoplication
fundus (*pl.* fundi)
fundus angioscopy
fundus glands
fundus photography
funduscope
funduscopy
fundusectomy
fungating
funicular
funicular artery
funicular hernia
funiculi (*sing.* funiculus)
funiculopexy

funiculus (*pl.* funiculi)
funiculus spermaticus
funnel
Furacin dressing
Furacin gauze
Furadantin
Furniss anastomosis
Furniss catheter
Furniss clamp
Furniss-Clute clamp
Furniss-Clute pin
Furniss forceps
Furniss incision
Furniss-McClure-Hinton clamp
furrier's sutures

furuncle
furuncular
furunculosis
fused hips
fusiform
fusiform aneurysm
fusiform bougie
fusiform cataract
fusion
fusion of bone
fusion of joint
fusion of spine
fusion operation
fusion tube

g

Gabarro operation
Gabriel proctoscope
Gabriel Tucker bougie
Gabriel Tucker forceps
Gabriel Tucker tube
Gaillard-Arlt sutures
Gaillard operation
gait
gaiter brace
galactocele
Galbiati bilateral fetal
    ischiopubiotomy
galea
galea forceps
galeaplasty
Galeazzi fracture
Galen anastomosis
Galen bandage
Galezowski dilator
gall duct
gall duct dilator
gall duct forceps
gall duct probe
gall duct scoop
gall duct spoon
gallamine
gallbladder
gallbladder aspirator
gallbladder bed
gallbladder cannula
gallbladder forceps
gallbladder operation

gallbladder retractor
gallbladder scissors
gallbladder spoon
gallbladder trocar
gallbladder tube
Gallie herniorrhaphy
Gallie needle
Gallie operation
Gallie tendon passer
Gallie transplant
gallop
gallstone
gallstone forceps
gallstone probe
gallstone scoop
Galt trephine
Galton whistle
galvanic cautery
galvanocaustic
galvanocaustic snare
galvanoionization
Gambee sutures
Gamgee tissue
Gamna-Gandy nodules
Gamna nodules
Gandhi knife
Gandy clamp
Gandy-Gamna nodules
ganglion (*pl.* ganglia or ganglions)
ganglion hook
ganglion knife
ganglionectomy

ganglionostomy
gangliosympathectomy
gangrene
gangrenous
Gannetta dissector
Gant clamp
Gant operation
gap
gape
gaping
gaping wound
Garamycin
Garceau catheter
Garden hip fracture
Gardner chair
Gardner chisel
Gardner headrest
Gardner needle
Gardner needle holder
Gardner operation
Gardner-Wells tongs
Garfield-Holinger laryngoscope
Gariel pessary
Garland clamp
Garland forceps
Garretson bandage
Garrett dilator
Garrigue forceps
Garrigue speculum
Garrison forceps
Garrison rongeur
Gärtner tonometer
gas cautery
gas laser
gaseous agents
Gaskell clamp
gasserectomy
gasserian ganglion

gasserian ganglion hook
gasserian ganglionectomy
gastrectomy
gastric
gastric arteries
gastric clamp
gastric freezing
gastric gavage
gastric glands
gastric neurectomy
gastric resection
gastric resection retractor
gastric tube
gastric ulcer
gastric veins
gastrica dextra artery
gastrica dextra vein
gastrica sinistra artery
gastrica sinistra vein
gastricae breves arteries
gastricae breves veins
gastritis
gastrocele
gastrocnemius muscle
gastrocolic
gastrocolic omentum
gastrocolitis
gastrocolostomy
gastrocolotomy
gastrocolpotomy
gastrodiaphany
gastroduodenal
gastroduodenal anastomosis
gastroduodenal artery
gastroduodenal fiberscope
gastroduodenal tube
gastroduodenal ulcer
gastroduodenalis artery

gastroduodenectomy
gastroduodenitis
gastroduodenoscopy
gastroduodenostomy
gastroenteric
gastroenteritis
gastroenteroanastomosis
gastroenterocolostomy
gastroenteroplasty
gastroenterostomy
gastroenterostomy catheter
gastroenterostomy clamp
gastroenterostomy tube
gastroenterotomy
gastroepiploic
gastroepiploic artery
gastroepiploic vein
gastroepiploica dextra artery
gastroepiploica dextra vein
gastroepiploica sinistra artery
gastroepiploica sinistra vein
gastroesophageal
gastroesophageal hernia
gastroesophagostomy
gastrogalvanization
gastrogastrostomy
gastrogavage
gastrohepatic
gastrohepatic ligament
gastrohepatic omentum
gastroileal anastomosis
gastroileitis
gastroileostomy
gastrointestinal
gastrointestinal clamp
gastrointestinal forceps
gastrointestinal needle
gastrointestinal surgical gut sutures

gastrointestinal surgical linen
    sutures
gastrointestinal surgical silk sutures
gastrointestinal tube
gastrojejunal
gastrojejunal anastomosis
gastrojejunal ulcer
gastrojejunocolic
gastrojejunostomy
gastrolysis
gastromegaly
gastromyotomy
gastronesteostomy
gastropexy
gastrophrenic
gastrophrenic ligament
gastroplasty
gastroplication
gastroptosis
gastropylorectomy
gastropyloric
gastrorrhaphy
gastrorrhexis
gastroscope
    ACMI
    Benedict
    Bernstein
    Cameron
    Chevalier Jackson
    Eder
    Eder-Chamberlin
    Eder-Hufford
    Eder-Palmer
    Ellsner
    examining
    fiberoptic
    flexible
    Herman-Taylor

gastroscope *(continued)*
> Hirschowitz
> Housset-Debray
> Janeway
> Kelling
> operating
> Schindler
> Wolf-Schindler

gastroscopy
gastrosplenic
gastrosplenic omentum
gastrostomy
gastrostomy plug
gastrostomy pump
gastrostomy scoop
gastrostomy tube
gastrotome
gastrotomy
Gatch bed
Gatellier incision
Gaucher disease
gauntlet bandage
gauntlet flap procedure
Gauvain brace
gauze
> absorbable
> absorbent
> Adaptic
> Aureomycin
> fine mesh
> fluffed
> Furacin
> g. bandage
> g. dressing
> g. pack
> g. packer
> g. packing
> g. scissors

gauze *(continued)*
> g. wick
> Gelfoam
> impregnated
> iodoform
> Kerlix
> Mersilene
> petrolatum
> plain
> Raytec
> sterile absorbent
> Surgicel
> Vaseline
> Xeroform

gavage
gavage tube
Gavello operation
Gavin-Miller clamp
Gavin-Miller forceps
gavinofixation
Gay's glands
Gayet operation
Gaylor forceps
Gaylor punch
Gaza operation
Gehrung pessary
Geiger-Downes cautery
gel-filled implant
gel-filled prosthesis
Gelfilm dressing
Gelfoam
Gelfoam dressing
Gelfoam gauze
Gelfoam packing
Gelfoam-soaked pledgets
Gellhorn forceps
Gellhorn pessary
Gellhorn punch

Gelocast dressing
Gelpi forceps
Gelpi-Lowrie forceps
Gelpi retractor
Gély sutures
gemellus inferior muscle
gemellus muscle
gemellus superior muscle
Gemini clamp
Gemini forceps
genal glands
general anesthesia
general closure sutures
General Electric pacemaker
general endotracheal anesthesia
general inhalation anesthesia
general insufflation anesthesia
generalized
Genga bandage
genicular artery
genicular veins
genioglossus muscle
geniohyoid muscle
geniohyoideus muscle
genioplasty
genitalia
genitofemoral nerve
genitofemoralis nerve
genitoplasty
gentamicin
gentian violet
gentle traction
genu recurvatum
genu valgus
genu varus
genucubital position
genufacial position
genupectoral position

genus descendens artery
genus inferior lateralis artery
genus inferior medialis artery
genus media artery
genus superior lateralis artery
genus superior medialis artery
genus vein
genyplasty
Geomedic arthroplasty
Geomedic femoral pusher
Geomedic jig
Geomedic prosthesis
geometric prosthesis
Georgariou operation
Gerald forceps
Gerbode dilator
Gerbode rib spreader
Gerdy knee tubercle
Gerota's fascia
Gersuny operation
Gerzog knife
Gerzog mallet
Gerzog-Ralks knife
Gerzog speculum
gestation
gestational size
Ghormley operation
ghost ophthalmoscope
ghost vessels
GI (gastrointestinal)
GI clamp
GI forceps
GIA (gastrointestinal anastomosis)
GIA staple
giant cell tumor
Gibbon hernia
Gibney bandage
Gibson-Balfour retractor

Gibson bandage
Gibson incision
Gibson irrigator
Gibson splint
Gibson sutures
Giertz-Shoemaker rib shears
Gifford applicator
Gifford curet
Gifford forceps
Gifford keratotomy
Gifford maneuver
Gifford operation
Gifford retractor
Gigli pubiotomy
Gigli-saw guide
Gigli wire saw
Gilbert catheter
Gilbert forceps
Gilbert-Graves speculum
Giliberty prosthesis
Gill blade
Gill forceps
Gill-Fuchs forceps
Gill-Hess forceps
Gill knife
Gill-Manning decompression
    laminectomy
Gill operation
Gill-Safar forceps
Gill scissors
Gill-Stein operation
Gillespie wrist excision
Gilliam-Doleris operation
Gilliam uterine suspension
Gillies-Dingman hook
Gillies elevator
Gillies forceps
Gillies-Fry operation

Gillies graft
Gillies hook
Gillies incision
Gillies needle holder
Gillies operation
Gillies scissors
Gillmore needle
Gilman-Abrams tube
Gilmer intermaxillary fixation
Gilmer splint
Gilmore probe
Gilvernet retractor
Gimbernat's ligament
Gimmick elevator
gingiva (*pl.* gingivae)
gingival clamp
gingival incision
gingival line
gingivectomy
gingivitis
gingivoplasty
Ginsberg forceps
Giordano operation
Giralde operation
Girard forceps
Girard probe
Girdlestone operation
Girdlestone-Taylor operation
Girdner probe
gladiolus
gland(s)
    acinous
    adrenal
    apocrine
    areolar
    axillary
    Bartholin's
    Bowman's

gland(s) *(continued)*
    bronchial
    Brunner's
    buccal
    bulbocavernous
    bulbourethral
    cardiac
    celiac
    ceruminous
    cervical
    ciliary
    circumanal
    Cobelli's
    coccygeal
    conglobate
    Cowper's
    ductless
    duodenal
    Ebner's
    eccrine
    endocrine
    exocrine
    fundic
    gastric
    Gay's
    genal
    glands of Lieberkühn
    glossopalatine
    gonad
    haversian
    hematopoietic
    hemolymph
    holocrine
    intestinal
    jugular
    Krause's
    lacrimal
    lingual

gland(s) *(continued)*
    Littre's
    lymph
    mammary
    marrow-lymph
    meibomian
    merocrine
    mixed
    Moll's
    Montgomery's
    mucous
    olfactory
    parathyroid
    peptic
    pineal
    pituitary
    preputial
    prostate
    pyloric
    salivary
    sebaceous
    sentinel
    seromucous
    serous
    sex
    sexual
    Skene's
    splenolymph
    sublingual
    submandibular
    submaxillary
    sudoriferous
    suprarenal
    sweat
    thymus
    thyroid
    Tyson's
    urethral

gland(s) *(continued)*
    vulvovaginal
    Waldeyer's
    Weber's
glans
glans penis
Glaser retractor
glass rod
glass sphere eye implant
glassblower's cataract
glasses
Glassman-Allis clamp
Glassman-Allis forceps
Glassman basket
Glassman brush
Glassman clamp
Glassman forceps
glaucoma
glaucoma knife
glaucomatous cataract
Glenn anastomosis
Glenn operation
Glenner forceps
Glenner retractor
glenohumeral ligaments
glenoid fossa
glenoid punch
glenoplasty
gliding prosthesis
glioma
Glisson's capsule
globe
globular
globular object forceps
globus pallidus
glomectomy
glomerular capsule
glomerulus *(pl.* glomeruli)

glossectomy
glossitis
glossopalatine glands
glossopalatine muscle
glossopexy
glossopharyngeal nerve (cranial nerve IX)
glossopharyngeal neurotomy
glossopharyngeus nerve
glossoplasty
glossorrhaphy
glossotomy
glottis
Glover clamp
Glover dilator
Glover forceps
Glover rongeur
glover's sutures
Gluck rib shears
Gluck shears
glutea inferior artery
glutea superior artery
gluteae inferiores veins
gluteae superiores veins
gluteal
gluteal artery
gluteal bonnet
gluteal hernia
gluteal line
gluteal nerve
gluteal veins
gluteus
gluteus inferior nerve
gluteus maximus muscle
gluteus medius muscle
gluteus minimus muscle
gluteus superior nerve
glycerin

glycosuria
Goebel-Frangenheim-Stoeckel
  operation
Goebel-Stoeckel operation
Goelet retractor
Goffe colporrhaphy
Gohrbrand dilator
Gohrbrand valvulotome
goiter
goiter clamp
goiter dissector
goiter forceps
goiter retractor
goiter scissors
goiter tenaculum
Golaski graft
gold crown
gold eye implant
Gold forceps
gold implant
gold sphere eye implant
Goldbacher anoscope
Goldbacher needle
Goldbacher proctoscope
Goldbacher speculum
Goldblatt clamp
Goldman curet
Goldman-Fox knife
Goldman hook
Goldman-Kazanjian forceps
Goldman knife
Goldman punch
Goldmann-McNeill blepharostat
Goldmann tonometer
Goldstein cannula
Goldstein curet
Goldstein irrigator
Goldstein retractor

Goldstein speculum
Goldthwait fracture frame
Goldthwait operation
Gomco clamp
Gomco forceps
Gomco pump
Gomco suction tube
Gomez-Marquez operation
gonadectomy
gonadotropin
gonads
gonarthrotomy
Gonin-Amsler marker
Gonin-Amsler sclera marker
Gonin operation
goniometer
        Conzett
        electrogoniometer
        finger
        international standard
        Tomac
gonioprism
goniopuncture
gonioscope
gonioscopy
gonioscopy lens
goniotomy
goniotomy knife
Good forceps
Good rasp
Good retractor
Good scissors
Goodell dilator
Goodell-Power operation
Goodfellow cannula
Goodhill forceps
Goodhill retractor
Goodwin clamp

Goodyear-Gruenwald forceps
Goodyear knife
Goodyear retractor
gooseneck chisel
gooseneck rongeur
Gordon forceps
Gordon splint
Gordon stethoscope
Gordon-Taylor amputation
gorget
gorget director
Gore-Tex graft
Gore-Tex prosthesis
Gosselin fracture
Gosset retractor
Gott-Daggett valve
Gott prosthesis
Gott valve
Gottschalk aspirator
Gottschalk operation
Gottschalk saw
gouge
    Abbott
    Alexander
    Andrews
    antrum
    Army
    arthroplasty
    Aufranc
    Ballenger
    Bishop
    bone
    Bowen
    Campbell
    Cave
    Cobb
    Compere
    Cooper

gouge *(continued)*
    Crane
    curved
    Derlacki
    Dix
    Flanagan
    Freer
    Guy
    Heerman
    Hibbs
    hip
    Hoen
    Holmes
    Kelly
    Kezerian
    Kuhnt
    Lahey
    lamina
    Lillie
    Martin
    mastoid
    Meyerding
    Moore
    Murphy
    nasal
    Nicola
    Putti
    scaphoid
    Schuknecht
    Smith-Petersen
    spinal fusion
    Stille
    swan-neck
    Todd
    trough
    Troutman
    Turner

gouge *(continued)*
    Walton
    Watson-Jones
    West
Gould sutures
Gouley catheter
Gouley sound
gout
gouty tophus
Goutz catheter
Govons curet
Gowers maneuver
Goyrand hernia
graafian cyst
graafian follicle
Graber-Duvernay operation
Gracey curet
gracilis muscle
gradient
Gradle electrode
Gradle forceps
Gradle operation
Gradle retractor
Gradle trephine
graduated sound
Graefe cystotome
Graefe forceps
Graefe hook
Graefe incision
Graefe knife
Graefe needle
Graefe speculum
Gräfenberg ring
graft (See also *patch* and
    prosthesis.)
    accordion
    aortic aneurysm
    arterial

graft *(continued)*
    autograft
    bifurcation
    bone
    bovine
    bypass
    bypass vein
    cancellous bone
    chessboard
    Cooley
    Dacron
    Davis
    DeBakey
    Edwards
    fat
    fixation
    Golaski
    Gor-Tex
    H
    heterograft
    homograft
    iliac
    iliac autograft
    Impra vein
    Marlex
    Mersilene
    Milliknit
    Ollier-Thiersch
    onlay
    osteoperiosteal
    pinch
    porcine
    prop
    replacement
    Reverdin
    ring
    Sauvage
    seamless arterial

graft *(continued)*
    slice
    Teflon
    tubular
    Weavenit
grafting
Graham elevator
Graham hook
Graham-Kerrison punch
Graham rib contractor
Graham-Roscie operation
Graham scissors
gram negative
gram positive
Grant needle holder
Grant operation
Grant retractor
Grant separator
Grant-Ward operation
Grantham electrode
Grantham needle
granular
granulate
granulating wound
granulation
granulation tissue
granulation tube
granuloma
granulomatous
grasping and cutting forceps
grasping clamp
grasping forceps
grasping punch
grattage
grattage of conjunctiva
Graves speculum
gravida (1, 2, 3, etc)
Gravindex

gravity cystography
gravity drainage
Gray clamp
Gray forceps
gray matter
Gray resectoscope
Grayton forceps
greater curvature of stomach
greater multangular bone
greater omentum
greater trochanter
Green-Armytage forceps
Green-Armytage operation
Green caliper
Green clamp
Green curet
Green dissector
Green forceps
Green hook
Green knife
Green mouth gag
Green needle holder
Green resectoscope
Green retractor
Green scoop
Green-Sewall mouth gag
Green spatula
Green strabismus tucker
Green trephine
Greenhow incision
Greenhow-Rodman incision
Greenough microscope
greenstick fracture
greenstick fracture splint
Greenwood forceps
Greenwood trephine
Greiling tube
grenade-thrower fracture

Grice-Green operation
Grice operation
grid
gridiron incision
Grieshaber extractor
Grieshaber forceps
Grieshaber keratome
Grieshaber needle
Grieshaber needle holder
Grieshaber retractor
Grieshaber trephine
Grieshaber vitrectomy tip
Grimsdale operation
grind test
Gritti amputation
Gritti-Stokes amputation
grittiness
gritty
Groenholm retractor
groin incision
grommet
grommet drain tube
groove
groove sutures
grooved director
grooving reamer
Gross clamp
Gross curet
Gross forceps
Gross hook
Gross-Pomeranz-Watkins retractor
Gross retractor
Gross spatula
Gross spoon
Gross spreader
Gross spud
Grossman operation
Gruber bougie

Gruber hernia
Gruber speculum
Gruenwald-Bryant forceps
Gruenwald forceps
Gruenwald punch
Gruenwald retractor
Gruenwald rongeur
grumose
grumous
Grüning magnet
Grynfelt hernia
guarded chisel
guarding
Gudebrod sutures
Guedel airway
Guedel blade
Guedel laryngoscope
guerney (also gurney)
Guepar prosthesis
Guerin fracture
Guggenheim forceps
Guggenheim scissors
guide
  acetabular
  Adson saw
  Bailey Gigli-saw
  basal ganglia
  Blair saw
  cartilage
  Cloward
  Cone
  Cooper
  Cottle
  Cushing Gigli-saw
  drill
  Fisher
  Gigli-saw
  g. pin

guide *(continued)*
    guide-pin holder
    g. sutures
    g. wire
    House
    Joseph saw
    Mumford Gigli-saw
    Raney Gigli-saw
    saw
    scaphoid screw
    Schlesinger Gigli-saw
    Stille Gigli-saw
    strut
    telescoping
    wire
Guild-Pratt speculum
Guilford-Schuknecht scissors
Guilford stapedectomy
guillotine
    g. amputation
    g. incision
    g. knife
    g. scissors
    guillotine-type orchiectomy
    hemostatic tonsil
    Lilienthal
    Molt
    rib
    Sluder
    Sluder-Sauer
    tonsil
    Van Osdel
Guisez tube
Guist-Black speculum
Guist eye implant
Guist forceps
Guist scissors
Guist speculum

Guleke-Stookey operation
Gullstrand ophthalmoscope
gum line
gum scissors
gun-barrel enterostomy
Gundelach punch
Gunning splint
gunshot wound
gurney (also guerney)
Gusberg curet
Gusberg punch
Gussenbauer clamp
Gussenbauer operation
Gussenbauer sutures
gut chromic sutures
gut plain sutures
gut sutures
Gutglass forceps
gutter
gutter fracture
guttering of bone
Guttmann retractor
Guttmann speculum
Gutzeit operation
Guy gouge
Guy knife
Guyon amputation
Guyon-Benique sound
Guyon bougie
Guyon's canal
Guyon clamp
Guyon dilator
Guyon-Péan clamp
Guyon sound
Guyton-Friedenwald sutures
Guyton-Park speculum
Guyton-Lundsgaard sclerotome
Guyton-Maumenee speculum

Guyton-Noyes forceps
Guyton operation
Guyton scissors
Gwathmey hook
Gwathmey oil-ether anesthesia
Gwathmey suction tube

gynecomastia
Gynefold pessary
gynoplastics
gynoplasty
gyrectomy
gyrus (*pl.* gyri)

h

H graft
H incision
Haab magnet
Haas operation
Hacker hypospadias
Hagedorn-Lemesurier operation
Hagedorn needle
Hagedorn operation
Hagerty operation
Hagie pin
Hagner catheter
Hagner hemostatic bag
Hagner operation
Hague lamp
Hahn cannula
Hahn gastrotomy
Hahn operation
Haidinger brush
Haig Ferguson forceps
Haight periosteal elevator
Haight retractor
Haight rib spreader
Haik eye implant
hair ball
hair-bearing graft
hair follicle
hairline
hairy nevus
Hajek-Ballenger dissector
Hajek-Ballenger elevator
Hajek chisel
Hajek forceps

Hajek-Koffler forceps
Hajek-Koffler punch
Hajek mallet
Hajek needle
Hajek punch
Hajek retractor
Hajek rongeur
Hajek-Skillern punch
Hakim-Cordis pump
Hakion catheter
Hale forceps
half-moon retractor
half-ring leg splint
Hall band intrauterine device
   (IUD)
Hall dermatome
Hall drill
Hall neurotome
Halle bur
Halle chisel
Halle curet
Halle elevator
Halle needle
Halle speculum
Halle-Tieck speculum
Hallpike maneuver
hallux
hallux equinus
hallux forceps
hallux malleus
hallux valgus

hallux varus
halo-pelvic traction
halo-to-bale traction
halo traction
halogen ophthalmoscope
halogen otoscope
halogenated agents
halothane
Halpin operation
Halsey needle
Halsey needle holder
Halsted clamp
Halsted-Ferguson operation
Halsted forceps
Halsted hemostat
Halsted incision
Halsted inguinal herniorrhaphy
Halsted-Meyer incision
Halsted operation
Halsted sutures
Halsted-Willy Meyer incision
halter
    DePuy head
    Forrester-Brown head
    Forrester head
    head
    Zimfoam head
hamartoma
hamate bone
Hamby forceps
Hamby-Hibbs retractor
Hamby retractor
Hamilton bandage
Hamilton forceps
Hamilton tongue depressor
Hamm electrode
hammer
    Cloward

hammer *(continued)*
    Epstein
    House
    intranasal
    Neef
    Quisling
    rotatory
    tack
    tapping
    vibratory
    Wagner
hammer toe
hammer toe correction
Hammersmith prosthesis
hammock bandage
hammock-method nephropexy
hammock pupil
Hammond operation
Hammond splint
Hampton operation
Hamrick elevator
Hamrick suction
hamstring tendons
hamstrings
Hanafee catheter
Hanafee catheter tip
Hancock amputation
Hancock valve replacement
hand cautery
hand cock-up splint
hand drill
hand pump
hand retractor
hand saw
hand splint
hand table
hand trephine
Handley incision

Handley operation
handpiece
hangnail
hanging-drop technique
hanging hip operation
Hanks-Bradley dilator
Hanks dilator
Hanna splint
Hannon curet
Hansen-Street nail
Hansen-Street pin
Hansen-Street plate
haptics
hard palate
Hardy speculum
harelip
harelip forceps
harelip needle
harelip operation
harelip suture
Hargin trocar
Hark operation
Harken clamp
Harken forceps
Harken needle
Harken prosthesis
Harken retractor
Harken rib spreader
Harken valve
Harken valvulotome
Harmon incision
Harmon operation
Harrington-Carmalt clamp
Harrington clamp
Harrington erysiphake
Harrington forceps
Harrington-Mayo forceps
Harrington-Mayo rib shears

Harrington-Mixter clamp
Harrington-Mixter forceps
Harrington-Pemberton retractor
Harrington retractor
Harrington rod
Harrington rod instrumentation
Harrington scissors
Harrington spinal fusion
Harrington strut
Harrington sutures
Harrington tonometer
Harris-Beath operation
Harris broach
Harris dissector
Harris forceps
Harris hip prosthesis
Harris operation
Harris segregator
Harris separator
Harris sutures
Harris trephine
Harris tube
Harris tube suction
Harrison curet
Harrison knife
Harrison prosthesis
Harrison retractor
Harrison scissors
Harrison-Shea curet
Harrison speculum
Harrison tucker
Hart splint
Hartley implant
Hartley-Krause operation
Hartmann catheter
Hartmann-Citelli forceps
Hartmann-Citelli punch
Hartmann curet

Hartmann-Dewaxer speculum
Hartmann forceps
Hartmann fossa
Hartmann-Gruenwald forceps
Hartmann-Herzfeld rongeur
Hartmann operation
Hartmann point
Hartmann pouch
Hartmann punch
Hartmann rongeur
Hartmann speculum
Hartmann tuning fork
Hartstein retractor
Harvard manometer
Harvard pump
Haseltine clamp
Hashimoto disease
Haslinger bronchoscope
Haslinger electroscope
Haslinger esophagoscope
Haslinger headrest
Haslinger laryngoscope
Haslinger retractor
Haslinger tracheobroncho-
    esophagoscope
Haslinger tracheoscope
Hasner operation
Hatch catheter
Hatcher pin
hatchet
hatchet extractor
Haultaim operation
Hauser operation
haustra (*sing.* haustrum)
haustra coli
haustration
haustrum (*pl.* haustra)
Haverfield cannula

Haverfield retractor
Haverfield-Scoville retractor
Haverhill clamp
haversian canal
haversian glands
hawk's beak elevator
Hawkins forceps
Hawkins fracture
Hawks-Dennen forceps
Hayden curet
Hayden elevator
Hayes clamp
Hayes-Olivecrona forceps
Hayes retractor
Haynes cannula
Haynes-Griffin splint
Haynes operation
Haynes pin
Hayton-Williams forceps
hazy
HEA (hemorrhages, exudates and
    aneurysms)
head dependent position
head extractor
head fracture frame
head halter (see *halter)*
head-low incision
head of pancreas
headgear
headrest
    Adson
    doughnut
    Gardner
    Haslinger
    Light
    Light-Veley
    Mayfield-Kees
    Multipoise

headrest *(continued)*
    neurosurgical
    Veley
healed per primam
healing
healing by first intention
healing by granulation
healing by second intention
healing by third intention
Healy forceps
Heaney-Ballentine forceps
Heaney clamp
Heaney curet
Heaney forceps
Heaney-Kantor forceps
Heaney needle holder
Heaney retractor
Heaney-Rezek forceps
Heaney-Simon retractor
Heaney sutures
Heaney vaginal hysterectomy
hearing whistle
heart block
heart catheterization
heart lung bypass
heart-lung machine
heart needle
heart prosthesis
heart transplant
heat cautery
heat-ray cataract
Heath curet
Heath dilator
Heath dissector
Heath expressor
Heath forceps
Heath operation
Heath scissors

Heaton inguinal herniorrhaphy
Heaton operation
heavy elevator
heavy silk retention sutures
heavy weighted speculum
hebosteotomy
Hedblom elevator
Hedblom raspatory
Hedblom retractor
heel bone
heel cords
heel pad
heel tendon
Heerman chisel
Heerman gouge
Heerman incision
Heffernan speculum
Hegar dilator
Hegar-Goodell dilator
Hegar needle holder
Hegar operation
Hegar perineorrhaphy
Hegenbarth forceps
Heidenhain rods
Heifitz clip
Heifitz operation
Heifitz retractor
Heile operation
Heimlich maneuver
Heimlich tube
Heine operation
Heineke colon resection
Heineke-Mikulicz gastro-
    enterostomy
Heineke-Mikulicz herniorrhaphy
Heineke-Mikulicz hypospadias
    operation
Heineke-Mikulicz operation

Heineke-Mikulicz pyloroplasty
Heineke operation
Heise forceps
Heisrath operation
Heitz-Boyer clamp
Helanca prosthesis
Helfrick retractor
helical sutures
helicinae penis arteries
helicine arteries of penis
helicis major muscle
helicis minor muscle
Heliodorus bandage
helium
helium-neon laser
helix
Heller cardiomyotomy
Heller myotomy
Heller operation
helminthiasis
helminthic appendicitis
hemangioma (*pl.* hemangiomas or
    hemangiomata)
hemangiosarcoma
hemarthrosis
hematemesis
hematoma
hematopoiesis
hematopoietic glands
hemiazygos accessoria vein
hemiazygos vein
hemiblock
hemicolectomy
hemicorporectomy
hemicraniectomy
hemicystectomy
hemidiaphragm
hemigastrectomy

hemiglossectomy
hemihepatectomy
hemilaminectomy
hemilaminectomy blade
hemilaminectomy prong
hemilaminectomy retractor
hemilaryngectomy
hemimastectomy
hemimaxillectomy
heminephrectomy
hemiparesis
hemipelvectomy
hemiplegia
hemipylorectomy
hemisect
hemisection
hemisphere
hemisphere eye implant
hemispherectomy
hemithyroidectomy
hemitransfixion incision
hemoclip
hemoclip clamp
hemoculture
hemocult negative
hemocult positive
hemocult slide
hemodialysis
hemodialysis tube
hemolymph glands
hemoptysis
hemorrhage
hemorrhagic
hemorrhoid
hemorrhoid forceps
hemorrhoidal
hemorrhoidal arteries
hemorrhoidal clamp

hemorrhoidal forceps
hemorrhoidal ligator
hemorrhoidal needle
hemorrhoidal nerves
hemorrhoidal tags
hemorrhoidal veins
hemorrhoidectomy
hemosiderin
hemospermia
hemostatis
hemostatis clip
hemostasis forceps
hemostat
    Adson
    Allis
    Boettcher
    Carmalt
    Coakley
    Corwin
    Crile
    curved
    Dandy
    Davis
    Dean
    Dunhill
    fine-pointed
    Halsted
    Jackson
    Kelly
    Kolodny
    Lewis
    Maingot
    Mayo-Péan
    McWhorter
    Sawtell-Davis
    scalp
    Schnidt
    Shallcross

hemostat *(continued)*
    Snyder
    straight
    tonsil
    tracheal
hemostatic bag
    Alcock
    Bardex
    Brodney
    coudé
    Foley
    Foley-Alcock
    Hagner
    Hendrickson
    Higgins
    Nesbit
    Owens
    Pilcher
    suprapubic
    two-way
hemostatic catheter
hemostatic clamp
hemostatic clip
hemostatic forceps
hemostatic ligatures
hemostatic sutures
hemostatic tonsil guillotine
hemostatic tonsillectome
Hemovac
Hemovac drain
Hemovac suction
Hemovac suction tube
Hemovac tube
Henderson chisel
Henderson operation
Henderson retractor
Hendren clamp
Hendren forceps

Hendrickson drain
Hendrickson hemostatic bag
Hendrickson lithotrite
Hendry operation
Henke forceps
Henke triangle
Henle's ligament
Henle's membrane
Henner elevator
Henner retractor
Henny rongeur
Henrotin forceps
Henrotin speculum
Henry femoral herniorrhaphy
Henry-Geist operation
Henry incision
Henry operation
Henry splenectomy
Henton hook
Henton needle
Henton suture needle
Hepacon cannula
Hepacon catheter
heparin
heparinized saline
hepatectomize
hepatectomy
hepatic
hepatic artery
hepatic cecum
hepatic duct
hepatic flexure
hepatic vein catheterization
hepatic veins
hepatica communis artery
hepatica propria artery
hepaticae veins
hepaticocholangiocholecyst-
    enterostomy
hepaticocholangiogastrostomy
hepaticocholangiojejunostomy
hepaticocystoduodenostomy
hepaticodochotomy
hepaticoduodenostomy
hepaticoenterostomy
hepaticogastrostomy
hepaticojejunostomy
hepaticolithectomy
hepaticolithotomy
hepaticolithotripsy
hepaticostomy
hepaticotomy
hepatitis
hepatobiliary
hepatocele
hepatocholangiocystoduoden-
    ostomy
hepatocholangioduodenostomy
hepatocholangioenterostomy
hepatocholangiostomy
hepatocholedochostomy
hepatocirrhosis
hepatoduodenal
hepatoduodenostomy
hepatoenterostomy
hepatogastric
hepatogastric ligament
hepatogastrostomy
hepatogenic
hepatojejunostomy
hepatolithectomy
hepatolithotomy
hepatomegaly
hepatopexy
hepatoptosis
hepatorenal
hepatorrhaphy

hepatosplenomegaly
hepatostomy
hepatotomy
Herbert Adams clamp
Herbert operation
Herbert prosthesis
Herff clamp
Herman-Taylor gastroscope
hernia
    abdominal
    acquired
    amniotic
    Barth
    Béclard
    Birkett
    cecal
    Cloquet
    Cooper
    crural
    diaphragmatic
    diverticular
    duodenojejunal
    encysted
    epigastric
    extrasaccular
    femoral
    foraminal
    funicular
    gastroesophageal
    Gibbon
    gluteal
    Goyrand
    Gruber
    Grynfelt
    h. adiposa
    h. in recto
    h. knife
    h. par glissement

hernia *(continued)*
    h. scissors
    Hesselbach
    Hey
    hiatal
    hiatus
    Holthouse
    incarcerated
    incisional
    indirect
    infantile
    inguinal
    inguinocrural
    inguinofemoral
    inguinoproperitoneal
    inguinosuperficial
    intermuscular
    interparietal
    intersigmoid
    interstitial
    irreducible
    ischiatic
    ischiorectal
    Kronlein
    Kuster
    labial
    Laugier
    levator
    linea alba
    Littre
    Littre-Richter
    lumbar
    Maydl
    mesenteric
    mesocolic
    mucosal
    oblique
    obturator

hernia *(continued)*
- omental
- ovarian
- pantaloon
- paraduodenal
- paraesophageal
- paraperitoneal
- parasaccular
- parietal
- parumbilical
- pectineal
- Petit
- properitoneal
- pudendal
- pulsion
- rectal
- reducible
- retrocecal
- retrograde
- retroperitoneal
- Richter
- Riex
- Rokitansky
- saddlebag
- sciatic
- scrotal
- sliding
- spigelian
- strangulated
- subpubic
- synovial
- thyroidal
- Treitz
- tunicary
- umbilical
- uterine
- vaginal
- vaginolabial

hernia *(continued)*
- Velpeau
- ventral
- vesical
- voluminous
- Von Bergmann
- w
- Wutzer

hernial sac
herniary
herniated
herniated disc
herniated nucleus pulposus
herniation
hernioappendectomy
hernioenterotomy
hernioid
herniolaparotomy
hernioplasty
herniopuncture
herniorrhaphy
herniotome
herniotome knife
herniotomy
herpes
herpes genitalis
herpes labialis
herpes progenitalis
herpes simplex
herpetic
Herrick clamp
hersage
Hertel exophthalmometer
hertz units (Hz)
Hess-Barraquer forceps
Hess expressor
Hess forceps
Hess-Gill forceps

Hess-Horwitz forceps
Hess operation
Hess scoop
Hess spoon
Hesselbach hernia
Hesselbach's ligament
Hesselbach's triangle
Hesseltine umbiliclip
heteroautoplasty
heterochromic cataract
heterocladic anastomosis
heterogenous graft
heterograft
heterologous graft
heterotransplant
heterotransplantation
Heuter operation
hexachlorophene
hexagonal wrench
hexamethylenamine
hexobarbital
hexylcaine hydrochloride
Hey amputation
Hey-Grooves operation
Hey hernia
Hey saw
Heyer-Schulte breast prosthesis
Heyman capsules
Heyman forceps
Heyman-Herndon operation
Heyman nasal scissors
Heyman operation
Heyman-Paparella scissors
hiatal
hiatal hernia
hiatopexy
hiatus
hiatus hernia

Hibbs chisel
Hibbs clamp
Hibbs curet
Hibbs elevator
Hibbs forceps
Hibbs fracture frame
Hibbs gouge
Hibbs mallet
Hibbs mouth gag
Hibbs operation
Hibbs osteotome
Hibbs periosteal elevator
Hibbs retractor
Hibbs spinal fusion
Hibbs-Spratt curet
hickory-stick fracture
Hicks version
hidradenitis
hidradenitis suppurativa
hidradenoma
Higbee speculum
Higgins catheter
Higgins hemostatic bag
Higgins incision
Higgins operation
high forceps
high-forceps delivery
high ligation
high lithotomy
high operation for femoral hernia
high-pressure anesthesia
high saphenous vein ligation
high-speed drill
hila (*sing.* hilum)
Hildreth cautery
Hildreth tip
Hilger nerve stimulator
Hilger tube

hili (*sing.* hilus)
Hill-Allison operation
Hill-Ferguson retractor
Hill hiatal herniorrhaphy
Hillis perforator
Hillis retractor
Hilsinger knife
hilum (*pl.* hila)
hilus (*pl.* hili)
Himmelstein retractor
Himmelstein valvulotome
Hinckle-James speculum
hindquarter amputation
Hines-Anderson pyelouretero-
    plasty
hinge joint
hinge position
hinged leaflet aortic valve
hinged leaflet vascular prosthesis
hinged skin hook
hingeless heart valve prosthesis
hinging
hip bone
hip flange
hip fusion
hip gouge
hip joint
hip nail
hip pin
hip prosthesis
hip retractor
hip ruler
hip screw
hip skid
hip spica dressing
Hippel operation
Hippel trephine
Hippocrates bandage

Hirschberg electromagnet
Hirschberg method
Hirschman anoscope
Hirschman clamp
Hirschman forceps
Hirschman-Martin proctoscope
Hirschman proctoscope
Hirschowitz fiberscope
Hirschowitz gastroscope
Hirschsprung disease
Hirschtick splint
Hirst-Emmet forceps
Hirst forceps
Hirst operation
His bundle
His bundle recording
His-Haas operation
Hiss bunionectomy
hoarseness
Hochenegg operation
hockey-stick incision
Hodge forceps
Hodge pessary
Hodgen splint
Hodgkin's disease
Hodgson hypospadias repair
hoe
    h. extractor
    Hough
    Joe's
    stapes
Hoen cannula
Hoen elevator
Hoen explorer
Hoen forceps
Hoen gouge
Hoen hook
Hoen needle

Hoen periosteal elevator
Hoen plate
Hoen raspatory
Hoen retractor
Hoen rongeur
Hoen scissors
Hoen separator
Hoffa-Lorenz operation
Hoffa operation
Hoffmann forceps
Hoffmann punch
Hofmeister-Billroth II gastrectomy
Hofmeister-Finsterer operation
Hofmeister gastrectomy
Hofmeister gastroenterostomy
Hofmeister-Polya operation
Hogan operation
Hoguet maneuver
Hohmann operation
Hohmann retractor
Hoke operation
Hoke osteotome
Hoke spoon
Hoke three-level incision
Holden curet
holder
     blade
     Juers-Derlacki
     needle (See separate listing.)
     speculum
     suture
hole saw
Holinger applicator
Holinger bougie
Holinger bronchoscope
Holinger cannula
Holinger dissector
Holinger esophagoscope

Holinger forceps
Holinger-Garfield laryngoscope
Holinger-Hurst bougie
Holinger-Jackson bronchoscope
Holinger laryngoscope
Holinger magnet
Holinger needle
Holinger scissors
Holinger telescope
Holinger tube
hollow
hollow cannula
hollow chisel
hollow-object forceps
hollow sphere eye implant
hollow sphere implant
hollow sphere prosthesis
Holman-Mathieu cannula
Holman retractor
Holmes forceps
Holmes gouge
Holmes nasopharyngoscope
Holmes operation
Holocaine
holocrine gland
Holter monitor
Holter shunt
Holter tube
Holter valve
Holth cystotome
Holth forceps
Holth operation
Holth punch
Holth sclerectomy
Holthouse hernia
Holtz curet
Homans' sign
homeograft

homocladic anastomosis
homogeneous
homograft
homograft implant
homokeratoplasty
homologous graft
homoplastic
homoplasty
homotransplant
homotransplantation
Honore-Smathers tube
Hood and Kirkland incision
Hood dermatome
Hood dissector
Hood-Graves speculum
hooded transilluminator
hook

    Adson
    Allport
    Aufranc
    ball-end
    Bane
    Barr
    bent
    Berens
    Bethune
    Blair
    blunt
    Boettcher
    bone
    Bose
    Boyes-Goodfellow
    brain
    Braun
    Braun-Jardine-DeLee
    Brown
    Buck
    calvarial

hook *(continued)*

    cautery
    Cloward
    Colver
    compression
    Converse
    cordotomy
    Cottle
    Cottle-Joseph
    Crile
    crura
    crypt
    curved
    curved nerve
    Cushing
    Dandy
    Davis
    Day
    decapitation
    delicate skin
    dissecting
    dissection
    Dohlman
    double-fixation
    double-pronged
    Dudley
    Duplay
    dura
    ear
    Edwards
    examining
    fenestration
    fibroid
    Fink
    fistula
    fixation
    footplate
    Frazier

hook *(continued)*
    Freer
    ganglion
    gasserian ganglion
    Gillies
    Goldman
    Graefe
    Graham
    Green
    Gross
    Gwathmey
    Henton
    hinged skin
    Hoen
    h. curet
    h. forceps
    hook-on bronchoscope
    hook-on laryngoscope
    hook-on loupe
    h. retractor
    h. scissors
    House
    incus
    intracapsular lens expression
    iris
    Jackson
    Jaeger
    Jameson
    jaw
    Johnson
    Joseph
    Kelly
    Kilner
    Kimball
    Kirby
    Klemme
    Knapp
    knot-tier

hook *(continued)*
    Kobyashi
    Lahey
    Leader
    lid
    lid-retracting
    ligature
    Lillie
    Linton
    long palate
    Lordan
    Loughnane
    Madden
    Magielski
    Malgaigne
    Martin
    Mayo
    McReynolds
    microscopic
    Murphy
    muscle
    muscle-splitting
    nasal polyp
    Neivert
    nephrostomy
    nerve
    New's
    Newman
    Nugent
    O'Connor
    oval-window
    Pajot
    palate
    palate pusher
    patellar
    posterior palate
    Pratt
    prostatic

hook *(continued)*

- Ramsbotham
- rectal
- rectus muscle
- Rosser
- rubber-shod
- Sachs
- Saunders-Paparella
- Schuknecht
- Schwartz
- scleral
- Scobee
- Scoville
- Searcy
- Selverstone
- Shambaugh
- sharp
- Shea
- skin
- skin graft
- Sluder
- Smellie
- Smith
- Smithwick
- squint
- stapes
- Stevens
- Stewart
- strabismus
- straight nerve
- Strully
- suture
- swivel
- sympathectomy
- Tauber
- tenaculum
- tenotomy
- tonsil

hook *(continued)*

- tonsil suture
- tracheal
- tracheostomy
- tracheotomy
- Tyrrell
- universal nerve
- Updegraff
- uterine tenaculum
- vas
- vein
- von Graefe
- Weary
- Welch Allyn
- Wiener
- Zoellner

hooked extractor
hooked nail
Hooper scissors
Hope resuscitator
Hopkins clamp
Hopkins forceps
Hopkins operation
Hopkins raspatory
Hopkins telescope
Hopp blade
Hopp laryngoscope
Horay operation
Horgan blade
horizontal
horizontal fracture
horizontal incision
horizontal mattress sutures
horizontal maxillary fracture
horizontal position
horizontal retractor
horizontal tube
hornpipe position

horsehair sutures
horseshoe magnet
horseshoe sutures
horseshoe tear
Horsley bone wax
Horsley elevator
Horsley forceps
Horsley operation
Horsley pyloroplasty
Horsley rongeur
Horsley separator
Horsley sutures
Horsley trephine
Horvath operation
Horwitz-Adams operation
Hosford dilator
Hosford-Hicks forceps
Hosford spud
hosiery
hot conization
hot knife
hot snare
Hotchkiss operation
Hotz-Anagnostakis procedure
Hotz curet
Hotz operation
Hotz probe
Houget operation
Hough bed
Hough forceps
Hough's hoe
Hough operation
Hough osteotome
hourglass anterior commissure
    laryngoscope
hourglass bladder
Hourin needle
House-Barbara needle

House-Bellucci scissors
House bur
House chisel
House curet
House-Dieter nipper
House dissector
House elevator
House excavator
House forceps
House guide
House hammer
House hook
House irrigator
House knife
House-Metzenbaum scissors
House needle
House-Paparella curet
House pick
House prosthesis
House retractor
House rod
House-Rosen needle
House scissors
House separator
House speculum
House stapedectomy
House suction tube
House tube
House-Urban retractor
House wire
House-Wullstein forceps
Housset-Debray gastroscope
Houston valve
Houtz curet
Howard abrader
Howard forceps
Howard stone basket
Howard stone dislodger

Howorth elevator
Howorth operation
Howorth osteotome
Howorth retractor
Hoxworth clip
Hoxworth forceps
Hoyt forceps
Hryntschak catheter
hub saw
Hubbard bolt
Hubbard electrode
Hubbard forceps
Hubbard plate
Hubbard tank
Hubell meatoscope
Hudgins cannula
Hudson brace
Hudson bur
Hudson clamp
Hudson drill
Hudson forceps
Hudson retractor
Hudson rongeur
Hueter bandage
Hueter-Mayo operation
Huey scissors
Huffman-Graves speculum
Huffman speculum
Huffman vaginoscope
Hufnagel clamp
Hufnagel forceps
Hufnagel knife
Hufnagel operation
Hufnagel valve
Hufnagel valve prosthesis
Huggins operation
Hughes eye implant
Hughes operation

Hughes-Young adrenalectomy
Hughes-Young incision
Humby knife
Humby operation
Hume clamp
humeroradial articulation
humeroulnar articulation
humerus
humerus splint
hump forceps
Humphries clamp
Hunt clamp
Hunt forceps
Hunt needle
Hunt operation
Hunt retractor
Hunt sound
Hunt trocar
Hunter's canal
Hunter curet
Hunter operation
Hunter separator
Huntington chorea
Hupp retractor
Hurd dissector
Hurd electrode
Hurd elevator
Hurd forceps
Hurd retractor
Hurst bougie
Hurst dilator
Hurtig dilator
Hurwitz clamp
Hurwitz trocar
Huschke canal
Huschke foramen
Huschke valve
Huse cannula

Husks rongeur
Hutch diverticulum
Hutch evacuator
Hutch operation
Hutchins needle
hyaline membrane
hyalinization
hyaloid artery
hyaloid fossa
hyaloidea artery
Hyams clamp
Hyams operation
Hybbinette-Eden operation
hybrid prosthesis
hydatidiform mole
hydraclip
hydraclip clamp
hydration
hydrocele
hydrocele repair
hydrocele trocar
hydrocelectomy
hydrochloride
hydrocollator packs
hydrocortisone
hydronephrosis
hydroperitoneum
hydrops
hydrops abdominis
hydrops fetalis
hydrostatic dilator
hydrostatic dissector
hydrostatic irrigator
hydrotherapy
hyfrecator
hyfrecator coagulator
hygroma
hymen

hymenectomy
hymenoplasty
hymenorrhaphy
hymenotomy
hyoepiglottic ligament
hyoglossal membrane
hyoglossus muscle
hyoid
hyoid bone
hyoid-cutting forceps
Hypaque
hyperalimentation
hyperbaric
hyperbaric anesthesia
hyperbaric spinal anesthesia
hyperemesis gravidarum
hyperemic
hyperextension
hyperextension brace
hyperextension fracture frame
hyperinsulinism
hyperkeratosis
hypermastia
hypermature cataract
hyperparathyroidism
hyperpituitarism
hyperplasia
hyperplastic
hypertelorism
hypertension
hyperthermia
hyperthyroid
hyperthyroidism
hypertonic
hypertrophic
hypertrophic gastritis
hypertrophy
hypertropia

hyperventilate
hyperventilation
hypnosis
hypnotic agents
hypobaric
hypobaric anesthesia
hypobaric spinal anestheisa
hypochondrium (*pl.* hypo-
   chondria)
hypocystotomy
hypodermatotomy
hypodermic microscope
hypodermic needle
hypodermic syringe
hypogastric artery
hypogastric nerve
hypogastric vein
hypogastric vessel
hypogastricus dexter nerve
hypogastricus sinister nerve
hypoglossal
hypoglossal canal
hypoglossal nerve (cranial nerve
   XII)
hypoglossus nerve
hypomastia
hypoparathyroidism
hypopharynx
hypophyseal fossa
hypophysection
hypophysectomy
hypophysis
hypopituitarism
hypoplasia
hypoplastic
hypopyon
hypopyon operation
hypospadias

hypospadias operation
hypotension
hypotensive
hypotensive agents
hypotensive anesthesia
hypothenar
hypothermia
hypothermia blankets
hypothermic
hypothermic anesthesia
hypothyroid ligament
hypothyroidism
hypotonic
hypotympanotomy
hypotympanum
hypoxia
Hyrtl anastomosis
Hyrtl loop
Hyrtl sphincter
hysterectomy
hysterectomy clamp
hysterectomy forceps
hysterectomy knife
hysterectomy retractor
hysterocolpectomy
hysterocolposcope
hysteroflator
hysterogram
hysterography
hysterolysis
hysteromyomectomy
hysteromyotomy
hystero-oophorectomy
hysteropexy
hysteroplasty
hysterorrhaphy
hysterosalpingectomy
hysterosalpingogram

hysterosalpingography
hysterosalpingo-oophorectomy
hysterosalpingorrhaphy
hysterosalpingostomy
hysteroscope
hysteroscopy

hysterotomy
hysterotrachelectomy
hysterotracheloplasty
hysterotrachelorrhaphy
hysterotrachelotomy
Hz (hertz units)

i

I & D (incision and drainage)
I-131 (radioactive iodine)
I-131 uptake
ICCE (intracapsular cataract extraction)
ice clot evacuator
ice-tong caliper
iced saline
ICLH apparatus (Imperial College, London Hospital)
icterus
ICU (intensive care unit)
ideal arch wire
Iglesias electrode
Iglesias resectoscope
IHSS (idiopathic hypertrophic subaortic stenosis)
ileac
ileal
ileal arteries
ileal conduit
ileal veins
ileectomy
ilei arteries
ileitis
ileo-ileal anastomosis
ileobladder cystoscopy
ileobladderoscopy
ileocecal
ileocecal valve
ileocecostomy
ileocecum

ileocolectomy
ileocolic
ileocolic artery
ileocolic vein
ileocolica artery
ileocolica vein
ileocolitis
ileocolitis ulcerosa chronica
ileocolostomy
ileocolotomy
ileocystoplasty
ileoduodenotomy
ileoentectropy
ileoesophagostomy
ileoileostomy
ileoloopogram
ileoneocystostomy
ileopancreatostomy
ileopexy
ileoproctostomy
ileorectal
ileorectostomy
ileorrhaphy
ileoscopy
ileosigmoid
ileosigmoidostomy
ileostogram
ileostomy
ileotomy
ileotransverse colostomy
ileotransverse colotomy
ileotransversostomy

ileoureterostomy
ileum
ileus
Ilfeld-Gustafson splint
iliac
iliac artery
iliac autograft
iliac colon
iliac crest
iliac flexure
iliac fossa
iliac graft
iliac muscle
iliac vein
iliac vessels
iliaca communis artery
iliaca communis vein
iliaca externa artery
iliaca externa vein
iliaca interna artery
iliaca interna vein
iliacus muscle
Iliff operation
Iliff trephine
iliococcygeus muscle
iliocostal muscle
iliocostalis cervicis muscle
iliocostalis lumborum muscle
iliocostalis muscle
iliocostalis thoracis muscle
iliofemoral ligament
iliohypogastric
iliohypogastric nerve
iliohypogastricus nerve
ilioinguinal
ilioinguinal nerve
ilioinguinalis nerve
iliolumbalis artery

iliolumbalis vein
iliolumbar artery
iliolumbar vein
iliolumbocostoabdominal
iliopectineal
iliopectineal line
iliopsoas muscle
iliopubic
ilium
Illinois needle
IMA (inferior mesenteric artery)
imbricate
imbricated sutures
imbricating sutures
imbrication
immature cataract
Immergut suction tube
Immergut tube
immobile
immobilization
immobilize
immobilizing bandage
immobilizing dressing
immovable bandage
immovable joint
immunization
impacted
impacted fracture
impaction
impactor
impedance
impedance electrode
Imperatori forceps
imperforate
imperforate anus
impermeable dressing
impinge
impingement

implant (See also *eye implant.*)
    acrylic
    adhesive silicone
    artificial joint
    Berens
    bone
    cartilage
    celluloid
    cochlear
    Cronin
    Custodis
    DeBakey
    dental
    double-lumen breast
    Dow Corning
    Edwards Teflon intracardiac
    electrical
    endo-osseous
    Extrafil breast
    eye (See separate listing.)
    Fox
    gel-filled
    gold
    Hartley
    hollow-sphere
    homograft
    i. fork
    interstitial
    iridium wire
    Ivalon
    Lash-Löffler
    lens
    magnetic
    Marlex mesh
    Mules
    paraffin
    penile
    permanent

implant *(continued)*
    pin
    plastic
    plastic sphere
    Plexiglas
    polyethylene
    polyurethane
    polyvinyl
    radium
    shell
    Silastic
    silicone
    silicone rod
    silicone sponge
    sphere
    sponge
    stainless steel
    subdermal
    submucosal
    subperiosteal
    Supramid
    Swanson
    tantalum mesh
    Teflon
    tendon
    Tensilon
    ureteral
    Usher Marlex mesh
    Vitallium
    Vivosil
    Weber
    Wheeler
    wire mesh
implantable pacemaker
implantation
implanted electrode
implanted pacemaker
implanted sutures

Impra vein graft
impregnated gauze
impression tonometer
Imre operation
in situ
in toto
in utero
inactive electrode
incarcerated
incarcerated hernia
incarceration
incipient cataract
incise
incision
    ab-externo
    abdominal
    abdominothoracic
    Agnew-Verhoeff
    alar
    Alexander
    angular
    anterior pillar
    aortotomy
    arcuate
    areolar
    arteriotomy
    Auvray
    backcut
    Bar
    Bardenheuer
    Battle
    Battle-Jalaguier-Kammerer
    bayonet
    Bergmann
    Bergmann-Israel
    Bevan
    bivalved elliptical
    Bosworth-Shawler

incision *(continued)*
    bowling-pin
    Boyd
    Brackin
    Brock
    Brunner
    Bruser
    bur-hole
    buttonhole
    Caldwell-Luc
    Cave
    celiotomy
    cervical
    Chamberlain
    Cheatle-Henry
    Cherney
    Chernez
    Chiene
    circular
    circular guillotine
    circumareolar
    circumcisional
    circumcorneal
    circumferential
    circumferentiating skin
    circumlimbar
    circumoral
    circumscribing
    classic
    classical
    clean and dry
    Clute
    Codman
    Coffey
    collar
    confirmatory
    conjunctival
    Connell

incision *(continued)*

corneoscleral
corollary
coronal
cortical
Cottle
counterincision
Courvoisier
crescent
crescent-shaped
crosshatch
crucial
cruciate
curved
curvilinear
curving
cut-down
Czerny
Davis-Geck
Deaver
deltopectoral
dorsal supine
dorsolateral
double-Y
Dührssen
dural
Edebohls
elliptical
Elsberg
endaural
enterotomy
exploratory
Fergusson
fishmouth
flank
flexed
Fowler
Fowler-Weir

incision *(continued)*

frontotemporal craniotomy
Furniss
Gatellier
Gibson
Gillies
gingival
Graefe
Greenhow
Greenhow-Rodman
gridiron
groin
guillotine
H-incision
Halsted
Halsted-Meyer
Halsted-Willy Meyer
Handley
Harmon
Heerman
hemitransfixion
Henry
Higgins
hockey-stick
Hoke three-level
Hood and Kirkland
horizontal
Hughes-Young
i. knife
inframammary
infraumbilical
inguinal
intercartilaginous
intracapsular
intranasal intercartilagenous
inverted-T
J-shaped

incision *(continued)*

- Jackson
- Jalaguier
- Kammerer
- Kehr
- keratome
- Killian
- Kocher
- Küstner
- lamellar
- Lamm
- Langenbeck
- lateral
- lateral flank
- lateral rectus
- lazy-S
- Lempert
- Lilienthal
- limbal
- line
- linear
- linear skin
- linear transverse
- Linton
- long oblique
- longitudinal
- longitudinal midline
- Longuet
- low
- low midline
- lower midline
- lumboiliac
- Lynch
- Mackenrodt
- malar
- Mason
- Maylard
- Mayo-Robson

incision *(continued)*

- McArthur
- McBurney
- McKissock
- McLaughlin
- McVay
- meatal
- medial
- median
- median parapatellar
- Meyer
- Meyer-Halsted
- Meyer hockey-stick
- midline
- midsternum splitting
- Mikulicz
- Monroe-Kerr
- Morison
- muscle
- muscle-splitting
- myringotomy
- Nagamatsu
- nasal
- oblique
- oblique relaxing
- Obwegeser
- Ollier
- operative
- orbicular
- Orr
- oval
- paracostal
- parainguinal
- parallel
- paramedian
- paramuscular
- parapatellar
- pararectal

incision *(continued)*

- pararectus
- parasagittal
- parascapular
- paraumbilical
- paravaginal
- Parker
- Péan
- perianal
- periareolar
- perilimbal
- periscapular
- peritoneal
- Perthes
- Pfannenstiel
- Phemister
- popliteal
- postauricular
- posterior
- posterior stab
- posterolateral
- Pringle
- proximal
- puncture
- pyelotomy
- racket
- radial
- rectus
- rectus muscle splitting
- relaxing
- relief
- retroauricular
- right rectus
- rim
- Risdon
- Rocky-Davis
- Rodman
- Rollet

incision *(continued)*

- Rosen
- Roux-en-Y
- Russe
- S-shaped
- saber-cut
- salmon backcut
- Sanders
- scalp
- Schobinger
- Schuchardt
- scratch
- scrotal
- semicircular
- semiflexed
- semilunar
- serpentine
- Shambaugh
- sharp
- Shea
- shelving
- shield
- Shoepinger
- shoulder-strap
- Simon
- Singleton
- skin
- skinfold
- skinline
- Sloan
- slot
- slot-type rim
- smile
- smiling
- Smith-Petersen
- Souttar skin
- spiral
- St. Marks

incision *(continued)*
- stab
- stab-wound
- stellate
- stepladder
- sternal-splitting
- Stewart
- stocking-seam
- straight
- Strombeck mammoplasty
- subcostal
- subcostal flank
- subinguinal
- submammary
- suboccipital
- subtrochanteric
- subumbilical
- supracervical
- suprapubic
- supraumbilical
- T-incision
- T-shaped
- temporal
- tennis-racket
- Thomas-Warren
- thoracoabdominal
- thoracotomy
- Timbrall-Fisher
- transection
- transmeatal
- transrectus
- transverse
- trap
- trap-door
- U-shaped
- Uchida
- upper abdominal midline
- upper midline

incision *(continued)*
- upward gaze
- uterine
- V-shaped
- vermis
- vertical
- vertical bur hole
- vertical elliptical
- vertical lateral parapatellar
- Vischer
- Vischer lumboiliac
- W-shaped
- Warren
- Watson-Jones
- Weber-Fergusson
- wedge
- Whipple
- Wilde
- Willy Meyer
- Y-incision
- Y-type
- Z-flap
- Z-incision
- Z-plasty
- Z-shaped

incision and drainage (I & D)
incision and packing
incision and packing of wound
incision and resuture of wound
incisional
incisional hernia
incisive fossa
incisive muscle
incisivi labii inferioris muscle
incisivi labii superioris muscle
incisor
incisura (*pl.* incisurae)
incisura angularis ventriculi

incisura cardiaca ventriculi
incisurae helicis muscle
inclined-plane elevator
inclusion
inclusion cyst
incompetence
incompetent
incompetent cervix
incompetent veins
incomplete
incomplete abortion
incomplete fracture
incontinence
incontinence clamp
increment
incubator
incudectomy
incudomalleolar articulation
incudopexy
incudostapedial
incudostapedial articulation
incudostapedial knife
incudostapediopexy
incus
incus hook
incus replacement prosthesis
indentation
index finger
Indian operation
Indian rhinoplasty
Indian skin flap operation
Indiana reamer
indicator
indifferent electrode
indigestion
indirect fracture
indirect hernia
indirect ophthalmoscope

indiscrete
Indocin
induction
indurated
induration
indwelling
indwelling catheter
infant abdominal retractor
infant abduction splint
infant bougie
infant bronchoscope
infant catheter
infant cystoscope
infant dilator
infant electrotome
infant feeding tube
infant female catheter
infant male catheter
infant rib shears
infant rib spreader
infant sound
infant vaginal speculum
infant vaginoscope
infant vascular clamp
infantile cataract
infantile hernia
infarct
infarction
infection
inferior
inferior carotid triangle
inferior laryngotomy
inferior maxilla
inferior mesenteric artery (IMA)
inferior nasal concha
inferior pole of thyroid
inferior tracheotomy
inferior turbinate

inferior vessels
inferotemporal
infiltrating
infiltrating carcinoma
infiltrating ductal cell carcinoma
infiltration
infiltration anesthesia
inflamed
inflammation
inflammatory fracture
inflatable
inflatable mammary prosthesis
inflatable splint
inflation
infolding
infraclavicular
infraclavicular triangle
infracted
infraction
infraction of turbinate
inframamillary
inframammary
inframammary incision
inframaxillary
infraoccipital nerve
infraorbital
infraorbital artery
infraorbital block
infraorbital canal
infraorbital nerve
infraorbitalis artery
infraorbitalis nerve
infrared microscope
infraspinatus muscle
infraspinous muscle
infratemporal fossa
infratrochlear nerve
infratrochlearis nerve

infraumbilical incision
infundibula (*sing.* infundibulum)
infundibular punch
infundibulectomy
infundibulectomy rongeur
infundibuliform
infundibuliform fascia
infundibulopelvic
infundibulopelvic ligament
infundibulum (*pl.* infundibula)
infusion
infusion pyelogram
infusion pyelography
infusion tube
Ingals cannula
Ingals speculum
Inge procedure
Ingersoll curet
Ingersoll needle
ingrown toenail
inguinal
inguinal adenopathy
inguinal canal
inguinal falx
inguinal hernia
inguinal hernia repair
inguinal herniorrhaphy
inguinal incision
inguinal ligament
inguinal ring
inguinal triangle
inguinoabdominal
inguinocrural
inguinocrural hernia
inguinofemoral
inguinofemoral hernia
inguinolabial
inguinoproperitoneal

inguinoproperitoneal hernia
inguinoscrotal
inguinosuperficial
inguinosuperficial hernia
inhalation anesthesia
inhibition
initial incision
injection
injection cannula
injection into nerve
injection needle
injection of air
injection of dye
injection of hemorrhoids
injection of varices
inlay graft
inlay inguinal herniorrhaphy
inlet
inlet forceps
inlet views
inner ear ablation
inner layer
innominate
innominate artery
innominate bone
innominate veins
Innovar
inoculation
inoperable
insemination
insertion
insertion of cannula
insertion of catheter
insertion of intrauterine radium
insertion of metal plate
insertion of nail
insertion of pacemaker
insertion of pack

insertion of pin
insertion of prosthesis
insertion of radioactive material
insertion of screw
insertion of tampon
insertion of traction device
insertion of tube
insertion of wire
instillation
instrument
instrumental dilation
insufflation
insufflation anesthesia
insufflation of fallopian tubes
insufflation of uterus
insufflator
    Buckstein
    colonic
    Kidde
    tubal
    Ventri
    Weber
insulin
intact
integrating microscope
intensive care unit (ICU)
intercapital veins
intercapitales veins
intercarpal articulation
intercartilaginous
intercartilaginous incision
interchondral articulation
intercostal
intercostal anesthesia
intercostal arteries
intercostal articulation
intercostal catheter
intercostal drain

intercostal muscle
intercostal trocar
intercostal vein
intercostales anteriores veins
intercostales externi muscles
intercostales interni muscles
intercostales muscles
intercostales posteriores arteries
intercostales posteriores veins
intercostalis superior dextra vein
intercostalis superior sinistra vein
intercostalis suprema artery
intercostalis suprema vein
intercostobrachial nerves
intercostobrachiales nerves
intercricothyroidotomy
intercricothyrotomy
interdental splint
interdental wire
interdigital
interdigitation
interference microscope
interilioabdominal amputation
interinnominoabdominal amputation
interlobar arteries of kidney
interlobar veins of kidney
interlobares renis arteries
interlobares renis veins
interlobular arteries of kidney
interlobular arteries of liver
interlobular veins of kidney
interlobular veins of liver
interlobulares hepatis arteries
interlobulares hepatis veins
interlobulares renis arteries
interlobulares renis veins
interlocked mesh prosthesis
interlocking sound
interlocking sutures
intermaxillary suture
intermaxillary traction
intermediary amputation
intermediate amputation
intermediate nerve
intermediate tendon of diaphragm
Intermedics pulse generator
Intermedics Thinlith II pacemaker
intermedius nerve
intermetacarpal articulation
intermetatarsal articulation
intermittent
intermittent claudication
intermittent positive pressure
  breathing (IPPB)
intermuscular
intermuscular hernia
internal
internal capsule
internal carotid artery
internal decompression trocar
internal fixating device
internal fixation
internal fixation device
internal hemorrhoidectomy
internal hemorrhoids
internal oblique muscle
internal os
internal sphincter
internal table
internal traction
internal urethrotomy
internal version
internasal suture
international standard goniometer
interossea anterior artery

interossea communis artery
interossea posterior artery
interossea recurrens artery
interossei dorsales manus muscles
interossei dorsales pedis muscles
interossei palmares muscles
interossei plantares muscles
interosseous anterior nerve
interosseous artery
interosseous cruris nerve
interosseous muscle
interosseous nerve
interosseous posterior nerve
interosseous veins
interpalpebral
interparietal
interparietal hernia
interpeduncular fossa
interpelviabdominal amputation
interperiosteal fracture
interphalangeal
interphalangeal articulation
interposition of uterus
interposition operation
interposition uterine suspension
interrupted sutures
interrupted vertical mattress
    sutures
interscapular amputation
interscapulothoracic amputation
intersigmoid
intersigmoid hernia
interspinal muscle
interspinales muscles
interstice
interstitial
interstitial hernia
interstitial implant

intertarsal articulation
interthoracoscapular amputation
intertransversarii muscles
intertransverse muscles
intertrochanteric line
intertrochanteric plate
interureteric ridge
interval
interval operation
intervertebral
intervertebral curet
intervertebral disk
intervertebral disk rongeur
intervertebral punch
intervertebral vein
intervertebralis vein
intestinal
intestinal anastomosis
intestinal arteries
intestinal clamp
intestinal decompression
intestinal decompression trocar
intestinal forceps
intestinal glands
intestinal infarction
intestinal needle
intestinal obstruction
intestinal occlusion clamp
intestinal occlusion retractor
intestinal plication needle
intestinal ring clamp
intestinal scissors
intestinal tube
intestine
intima
intimectomy
intra-abdominal
intra-abdominal exploration

intra-abdominal vasectomy
intra-amniotic saline injection
intra-articular fracture
intra-atrial baffle
intracapsular cataract extraction
   (ICCE)
intracapsular fracture
intracapsular incision
intracapsular lens expressor hook
intracapsular lens extraction
intracapsular lens loupe
intracapsular lens spoon
intracardiac catheter
intracardiac patch
intracardiac retractor
intracavitary radium insertion
intracervical bag
intracervical pack
intracondylar
intracranial aneurysm
intractable
intracystic
intradermal mattress sutures
intradermal nevus
intradermic sutures
intraductal
intrahepatic
intrahepatic cholangiojejunostomy
intraluminal
intraluminal stripper
intraluminal tube
intraluminal tube prosthesis
intramedullary
intramedullary anesthesia
intramedullary bar
intramedullary drill
intramedullary nail
intramedullary nailing

intramedullary pin
intramedullary rod
intramedullary wire
intramural
intranasal
intranasal anesthesia
intranasal antrum speculum
intranasal ethmoidectomy
intranasal hammer
intranasal intercartilaginous
   incision
intranasal packing
intranasal sinusotomy
intranasal splint
intranasal tube
intraocular
intraocular contents
intraocular lens (IOL)
intraoral anesthesia
intraoral wire
intraosseous anesthesia
intraperiosteal fracture
intraperitoneal injection
intrapleural pneumonolysis
intrapulpal anesthesia
intrapyretic
intraspinal anesthesia
intratracheal anesthesia
intratracheal tube
intrauterine cannula
intrauterine catheter
intrauterine curettage
intrauterine device (IUD)
   Bernberg bow
   bow
   coil
   CU-7
   Dalkon shield

intrauterine device *(continued)*
    Hall band
    Lippes loop
    loop
    Mazlin spring
intrauterine fracture
intrauterine pack
intrauterine pessary
intrauterine pregnancy
intrauterine probe
intrauterine radium application
intravascular
intravenous
intravenous anesthesia
intravenous catheter
intravenous pyelogram
intravenous pyelography
intravenous regional anesthesia
intravenous urogram
intravenous urography
intrinsic
introducer (see *sphere introducer*)
introduction
introduction of radiopaque substance
introduction of radium
introitus
intubation
intubation anesthesia
intubation laryngoscope
intubation tube
intumescence
intumescent cataract
intussusception
intussusceptum
intussuscipiens
invaginated
invaginated nipple

invaginated stump
invagination
invasive
invasive carcinoma
invasive procedure
inversion
inversion of tarsus
inversion operation
inverted
inverted cone bur
inverted jackknife position
inverted sutures
inverted-T incision
inverter
    appendix
    Barrett
    Mayo-Boldt
    Mayo-Kelly
inverting sutures
investing fascia
involution
involution cyst
iodized surgical gut sutures
iodoform dressing
iodoform gauze
iodoventriculogram
iodoventriculography
IOL (intraocular lens)
ion microscope
Ionescu method
Ionescu-Shiley valve
ionization
ionotherapy
iontophoresis
Iowa forceps
Iowa periosteal elevator
IPPB (intermittent positive pressure breathing)

iridectomesodialysis
iridectomize
iridectomy
iridencleisis
iridesis
iridium wire implant
iridocapsulectomy
iridocapsulotomy
iridocapsulotomy scissors
iridocorneosclerectomy
iridocyclectomy
iridocystectomy
iridodesis
iridodialysis
iridomesodialysis
iridoplasty
iridosclerectomy
iridosclerotomy
iridostasis
iridotomy
iris
iris forceps
iris hook
iris knife needle
iris needle
iris replacer
iris repositor
iris retractor
iris scissors
iris spatula
iris stretching
iritis
iritomy
irradiation
irradiation cataract
irreducible
irreducible hernia
irrigating bronchoscope

irrigating catheter
irrigating tip
irrigating valve
irrigation
irrigation of sinuses
irrigation syringe
irrigator
    anterior chamber
    antrum
    Bishop-Harmon
    Buie
    DeVilbiss
    Doss
    Dougherty
    eye
    Fox
    Gibson
    Goldstein
    House
    hydrostatic
    Moncrieff
    percolator
    Rollet
    Shambaugh
    Shea
    Sylva
    Thornwald
    Valentine
    Wells
irritable
irritable colon
irritant
Irvine scissors
Irving sterilization
Irving tubal ligation
Irwin operation
Isaacs aspiration syringe
ischemia

ischiadic nerve
ischiadicus nerve
ischial
ischial weightbearing brace
ischiatic
ischiatic hernia
ischiatic hernioplasty
ischiectomy
ischioanal
ischiocavernosus muscle
ischiocavernous muscle
ischiococcygeal
ischiofemoral arthrodesis
ischiohebotomy
ischiopubiotomy
ischiorectal
ischiorectal abscess
ischiorectal fossa
ischiorectal hernia
ischium
ischochymia
Ishihara plate
island
island flap
island of Reil
islands of Langerhans
islets of Langerhans
isobaric anesthesia
isobaric spinal anesthesia
isolate
isolation
isolation forceps
isoperistaltic
isoperistaltic anastomosis

isoperistaltic gastroenterostomy
isoperistaltic jejunostomy
isotonic
Israel dissector
Israel operation
Israel rasp
Israel retractor
isthmectomy
isthmorrhaphy
isthmus
Isuprel
Italian operation
Italian rhinoplasty
Itard catheter
IUD (See *intrauterine device.*)
IV (intervertebral, intravenous)
IV catheter (intravenous)
IV disk (intervertebral)
IV disk forceps
IV disk rongeur
IV pyelogram (intravenous)
IV pyelography
IVAC pump
Ivalon dressing
Ivalon eye implant
Ivalon implant
Ivalon patch
Ivalon sponge
Ivalon sutures
Iverson dermabrader
Ives anoscope
Ives speculum
Ivy rongeur
Ivy wire

j

J&J Band-Aid sterile drape
J-point treadmill test
J-shaped incision
Jaboulay amputation
Jaboulay button
Jaboulay operation
Jaboulay pyloroplasty
jacket
jackknife position
Jackson applicator
Jackson atomizer
Jackson bougie
Jackson bronchoscope
Jackson clamp
Jackson dilator
Jackson elevator
Jackson esophagoscope
Jackson forceps
Jackson hemostat
Jackson hook
Jackson incision
Jackson knife
Jackson laryngoscope
Jackson laryngostat
Jackson-Moore shears
Jackson-Mosher dilator
Jackson-Plummer dilator
Jackson-Pratt drain
Jackson probe
Jackson punch
Jackson retractor
Jackson scissors

Jackson shears
Jackson speculum
Jackson tenaculum
Jackson tracheoscope
Jackson-Trousseau dilator
Jackson tube
Jacobaeus operation
Jacobaeus thoracoscope
Jacobs clamp
Jacobs chuck and key
Jacobs chuck drill
Jacobs forceps
Jacobs-Palmer laparoscope
Jacobs tenaculum
Jacobson clamp
Jacobson forceps
Jacobson punch
Jacobson retractor
Jacobson scissors
Jacobson spatula
Jaeger hook
Jaeger keratome
Jaeger knife
Jaeger lid plate
Jaeger lid retractor
Jaeger-Whiteley catheter
Jaesche-Arlt operation
Jaesche operation
Jahnke-Cook-Seeley clamp
Jako knife
Jako laryngoscope
Jalaguier cleft lip repair

Jalaguier incision
Jamar dynamometer
Jameson caliper
Jameson forceps
Jameson hook
Jameson needle
Jameson operation
Jamshidi needle
Janeway gastroscope
Janeway gastrostomy
Jannetta elevator
Jannetta retractor
Jansen forceps
Jansen-Gifford retractor
Jansen-Gruenwald forceps
Jansen-Middleton forceps
Jansen-Newhart probe
Jansen operation
Jansen periosteotome
Jansen raspatory
Jansen retractor
Jansen rongeur
Jansen-Struycken forceps
Jansen-Wagner retractor
Jaquet apparatus
Jarcho cannula
Jarcho forceps
Jarcho tenaculum
Jarvis clamp
Jarvis operation
Jarvis snare
jaundice
Javal ophthalmometer
Javid catheter
Javid clamp
Javid shunt
Javid tube
jaw

jaw hook
jaw splint
Jefferson retractor
jejunal
jejunal and ileal veins
jejunal arteries
jejunal loop
jejunal ulcer
jejunal veins
jejunales arteries
jejunales et ilei veins
jejunectomy
jejunitis
jejunocecostomy
jejunocholecystostomy
jejunocolostomy
jejunoileitis
jejunoileostomy
jejunojejunostomy
jejunopexy
jejunorrhaphy
jejunostomy
jejunotomy
jejunum
Jelanko bar
Jelanko splint
Jelco catheter
Jelco needle
Jelks operation
jelly dressing
Jelm catheter
Jendrassik maneuver
Jennings mouth gag
Jennings-Skillern mouth gag
Jergesen I-beam
Jergesen tube
Jergeson reamer
Jesberg bronchoscope

Jesberg clamp
Jesberg esophagoscope
Jesberg forceps
Jesberg tube
Jesse-Stryker saw
jeweler forceps
Jewett bone extractor
Jewett brace
Jewett nail
Jewett plate
Jewett prosthesis
Jewett reamer
Jewett screw
Jewett sound
Jianu-Beck operation
jib
jig
Jobert de Lamballe operation
Jobert de Lamballe sutures
Jobert sutures
Jobst dressing
Jobst stockings
Joe's hoe
Joel-Baker anastomosis
Joel-Baker tube
Johansen urethroplasty
Johns Hopkins clamp
Johns Hopkins forceps
Johns Hopkins needle holder
Johns Hopkins retractor
Johns Hopkins stone basket
Johns Hopkins tube
Johnson basket
Johnson forceps
Johnson hook
Johnson-Kerrison punch
Johnson knife
Johnson needle holder

Johnson operation
Johnson retractor
Johnson screwdriver
Johnson splint
Johnson stone basket
Johnson stone dislodger
Johnson-Tooke knife
Johnson tube
Johnston clamp
Johnston dilator
Johnston plug
joint (See also *articulation.*)
    amphidiarthrodial
    ankle
    ball-and-socket
    biaxial
    bilocular
    cartilaginous
    Chopart's
    composite
    compound
    costochondral
    Cruveilhier's
    elbow
    false
    fibrocartilaginous
    flail
    freely movable
    hinge
    hip
    immovable
    j. capsule
    j. fracture
    j. instability
    j. line
    j. of Luschka
    j. stability
    knee

joint *(continued)*
    ligamentous
    Lisfranc's
    midcarpal
    mixed
    pivot
    shoulder
jointed vein stripper
joker (endarterectomy instrument)
joker dissector
joker elevator
Jolly dilator
Jonas-Graves speculum
Jonell splint
Jones clamp
Jones curet
Jones dilator
Jones forceps
Jones hammer toe operation
Jones operation
Jones pin
Jones position
Jones retractor
Jones scissors
Jones splint
Jones suspension traction
Jones sutures
Jones tube
Jonge position
Jonnesco operation
Joplin forceps
Joplin operation
Joplin stripper
Joplin tendon passer
Joplin toe prosthesis
Jordan bur
Jordan-Day bur

Jordan-Day drill
Jorgenson retractor
Jorgenson scissors
Joseph chisel
Joseph clamp
Joseph elevator
Joseph hook
Joseph-Killian elevator
Joseph knife
Joseph-Maltz knife
Joseph-Maltz saw
Joseph-Maltz scissors
Joseph operation
Joseph perforator
Joseph periosteal elevator
Joseph periosteotome
Joseph punch
Joseph rasp
Joseph raspatory
Joseph ruler
Joseph saw
Joseph saw guide
Joseph scissors
Joseph splint
joule units
Judd-Allis clamp
Judd-Allis forceps
Judd clamp
Judd-DeMartel forceps
Judd forceps
Judd-Masson retractor
Judd operation
Judd trocar
Judet dissector
Judet operation
Judet prosthesis
Juers crimper
Juers-Derlacki holder

Juers forceps
Juers-Lempert forceps
Juers-Lempert rongeur
Juevenelle clamp
jugular
jugular gland
jugular nerve
jugular vein
jugularis anterior vein
jugularis interna vein
jugularis nerve
Julian-Fildes clamp
Julian forceps
Julian needle holder
jump graft
jump skin flap

junction
    corneoscleral
    dermoepidermal
    fibromuscular
    manubriogladiolar
    mucogingival
    myoneural
    neuromuscular
    sclerocorneal
    ureteropelvic
    ureterovesical
junctional
junctional nevus
juncture
Jurasz forceps
Jutte tube
juvenile cataract

k

K-Gar clamp
K-nail
K-S adhesive needle holder
K-wire (Kirschner wire)
Kader needle
Kader operation
Kader-Senn operation
Kahler forceps
Kahn cannula
Kahn dilator
Kahn-Graves speculum
Kahn scissors
Kahn tenaculum
Kal-Dermic sutures
Kalt forceps
Kalt needle
Kalt needle holder
Kalt spoon
Kalt sutures
Kammerer incision
kanamycin
kanamycin solution
Kanavel cannula
Kanavel conductor
Kanavel splint
Kane clamp
kangaroo tendon sutures
Kantor clamp
Kantor forceps
Kantrex solution
Kantrowicz clamp
Kantrowicz forceps

Kapel operation
Kaplan needle
Kapp-Beck clamp
Kapp clamp
Kara erysiphake
Karras needle
Kasai operation
Kaslow tube
Katsch chisel
Katzin-Barraquer forceps
Katzin scissors
Kaufman forceps
Kaufman operation
Kaufman penile prosthesis
Kaufman syringe
Kaufman vitrector
Kaufman II vitrector
Kay-Shiley valve
Kay-Shiley valve prosthesis
Kay-Suzuki valve prosthesis
Kaye antihelix operation
Kayser-Fleischer ring
Kazanjian button
Kazanjian-Cottle forceps
Kazanjian forceps
Kazanjian operation
Kazanjian scissors
Kazanjian splint
Kazanjian T-bar
Kearns dilator
Keegan operation
Keel operation

Keeler cryophake
Keeler cryophake unit
Keeley vein stripper
Keen operation
Keflin
Kehr incision
Kehr operation
Kehr tube
Keidel tube
Keith drain
Keith needle
Keith scissors
Keith-Wagener retinopathy
Keitzer urethrotome
Keller-Blake splint
Keller bunionectomy
Keller operation
Kelling gastroscope
Kellogg-Speed operation
Kelly adenotome
Kelly clamp
Kelly curet
Kelly cystoscope
Kelly-Deming operation
Kelly dilator
Kelly endoscope
Kelly forceps
Kelly gouge
Kelly-Gray curet
Kelly hemostat
Kelly hook
Kelly-Kennedy operation
Kelly-Murphy forceps
Kelly needle
Kelly operation
Kelly proctoscope
Kelly retractor
Kelly scissors

Kelly sigmoidoscope
Kelly-Sims retractor
Kelly speculum
Kelly sphincteroscope
Kelly-Stoeckel operation
Kelly sutures
Kelly tube
Kelman cryostylet
Kelman cystotome
Kelman extractor
Kelman forceps
keloid
keloplasty
kelotomy
Kelsey clamp
Ken driver
Ken nail
Ken plate
Kenalog
Kennedy bar
Kennedy forceps
Kennedy operation
Kent forceps
keratectomy
keratocentesis
keratoleptynsis
keratome
    Agnew
    Beaver
    Berens
    Castroviejo
    Czermak
    Grieshaber
    Jaeger
    k. incision
    Kirby
    Lancaster
    Landolt

keratome *(continued)*
 Lichtenberg
 McReynolds
 pterygium
 Rowland
 Thomas
 Wiener
keratomileusis
keratoplasty
keratoplasty scissors
keratoprosthesis
keratosis
keratotomy
keratotomy forceps
keratotomy knife
Kerley B lines
Kerlix bandage
Kerlix dressing
Kerlix fluffs
Kerlix gauze
Kerlix rolls
Kern forceps
Kernan-Jackson bronchoscope
Kernig sign
Kerr cesarean section
Kerr rongeur
Kerr splint
Kerrison forceps
Kerrison punch
Kerrison retractor
Kerrison rongeur
Kessel plate
Kessler operation
Kessler sutures
Kestenbach-Anderson procedure
Ketaject
Ketalar
ketamine hydrochloride

Kevorkian curet
Kevorkian forceps
Kevorkian-Young curet
Kevorkian-Young forceps
Key elevator
key-in-lock maneuver
Key operation
Key periosteal elevator
Keyes chisel
Keyes lithotrite
Keyes punch
Kezerian chisel
Kezerian curet
Kezerian gouge
Kezerian osteotome
Kidd cystoscope
Kidd trocar
Kidd tube
Kidde insufflator
Kidde-Robbins tourniquet
Kidde tourniquet
Kidner operation
kidney
kidney clamp
kidney-elevating forceps
kidney pedicle clamp
kidney pelvectomy
kidney position
kidney retractor
kidney stone
kidney-stone forceps
kidney transplant
Kielland forceps
Kielland-Luikart forceps
Kielland operation
Killian bronchoscope
Killian cannula
Killian chisel

Killian-Eichen cannula
Killian elevator
Killian forceps
Killian incision
Killian-King retractor
Killian knife
Killian operation
Killian-Reinhard chisel
Killian rongeur
Killian speculum
Killian suspension apparatus
Killian tube
Kilner-Dott mouth gag
Kilner hook
Kilner operation
Kilner scissors
Kilner suture carrier
Kimball catheter
Kimball hook
Kimpton-Brown tube
Kimpton spreader
Kinematic prosthesis
kineplastic amputation
kineplasty
King brace
King-Hurd dissector
King-Hurd retractor
King needle
King operation
King-Prince forceps
King retractor
King-Richards operation
King-Steelquist amputation
King traction
Kingsley forceps
Kingsley splint
Kinsella-Buie clamp
Kinsella elevator
Kinsella periosteal elevator
Kirby forceps
Kirby hook
Kirby keratome
Kirby knife
Kirby lens expressor
Kirby operation
Kirby retractor
Kirby scissors
Kirby separator
Kirby sliding technique
Kirby spatula
Kirby spoon
Kirby sutures
Kirk amputation
Kirk mallet
Kirkaldy-Willis operation
Kirkland knife
Kirkland retractor
Kirkpatrick forceps
Kirmisson elevator
Kirmisson operation
Kirmisson periosteal elevator
Kirmisson raspatory
Kirschner operation
Kirschner sutures
Kirschner traction apparatus
Kirschner wire (K-wire)
Kirschner-wire drill
Kirschner-wire splint
Kirschner-wire spreader
Kirschner-wire tightener
Kirschner-wire tractor
Kistner button
Kistner dissector
Kistner probe
Kistner tube
Kitlowski operation

Kitner dissector
Kitner forceps
Kiwisch bandage
Klaff speculum
Klatskin needle
Kleenspec forceps
Kleenspec laryngoscope
Kleenspec sigmoidoscope
Kleenspec speculum
Klein punch
Kleinert operation
Kleinert sutures
Klemme hook
Klemme retractor
Kling bandage
Kling dressing
Kling elastic
Kling gauze
Knapp cystotome
Knapp forceps
Knapp hook
Knapp-Imre operation
Knapp iris repositor & probe
Knapp knife
Knapp needle
Knapp operation
Knapp retractor
Knapp scissors
Knapp scoop
Knapp spatula
Knapp speculum
Knapp spoon
knee bone
knee-chest position
knee-elbow position
knee joint
knee plate
knee retractor

knee splint
kneeling-squatting position
knife
    Abraham
    acetabular
    Adson
    Agnew
    Allen-Barkan
    amputating
    amputation
    angle
    angular
    appendotome
    Armour
    ASR
    Atkin
    Austin
    Ayerst
    Ayre
    Ayre-Scott
    Bailey-Glover-O'Neil
    Bailey-Morse
    Ballenger
    Bard-Parker
    Barkan
    Barker Vacu-tome
    Baron
    Barraquer
    Barrett
    Beard
    Beaver
    Beck
    Beer
    Berens
    bistoury
    Bizzari-Guiffrida
    bladebreaker
    Blair

knife *(continued)*
- Blair-Brown
- Bonta
- Bosher
- Bovie
- brain
- Brock
- Brophy
- Brown
- Buck
- Bucy
- button
- button-end
- Caltagirone
- canal
- canaliculus
- Canfield
- capsule
- Carpenter
- Carter
- cartilage
- Castroviejo
- cataract
- Catling amputation
- cautery
- Cave
- cervical
- cervical cordotomy
- chalazion
- cirsotome
- cleft palate
- coagulating
- Cobbett
- cold-cone
- Collings
- Colver
- commissurotomy
- cone

knife *(continued)*
- conization
- Converse
- cordotomy
- cornea
- Cottle
- Crile
- Crosby
- crypt
- Curdy
- curved
- Cushing
- cutting Bovie
- Davidoff
- Daviel
- Day
- Dean
- DeLee
- dental
- DePalma
- Derlacki
- Derra
- D'Errico
- Desmarres
- Deutschman
- Devonshire
- discission
- dissecting
- double-edged
- Douglas
- Downing
- drum elevator
- Dupuytren
- dura hook
- dural
- ear
- electric
- electrosurgical

knife *(continued)*
    Elschnig
    embryotomy
    endotherm
    Equen-Neuffer
    evisceration
    expansile
    facial nerve
    Ferris-Robb
    Ferris-Smith
    Fisher
    fistula
    fistulotome
    flap
    Fletcher
    Fomon
    Frazier
    Freer
    Freiberg
    Friesner
    Gandhi
    ganglion
    Gerzog
    Gerzog-Ralks
    Gill
    glaucoma
    Goldman
    Goldman-Fox
    goniotomy
    Goodyear
    Graefe
    Green
    guillotine
    Guy
    Haab
    Harris
    Harrison
    hernia

knife *(continued)*
    herniotome
    Hilsinger
    hot
    House
    Hufnagel
    Humby
    hysterectomy
    incision
    incudostapedial
    Jackson
    Jaeger
    Jako
    Johnson
    Johnson-Tooke
    Joseph
    Joseph-Maltz
    keratotomy
    Killian
    Kirby
    Kirkland
    Knapp
    k. biopsy
    k. curet
    k. electrode
    k. elevator
    k. handle
    k. needle
    k. retractor
    k. spud
    Kreissl
    Krull
    Kyle
    Ladd
    lamina
    Lancaster
    Lang
    Langenbeck

knife *(continued)*
laparotrachelotomy
laryngeal
Lebsche
Lee
Lee-Cohen
Leland
Lempert
lenticular
lid
Lillie
Liston
Lothrop
Lowe-Breck
Lowell
Lundsgaard
Lynch
MacKenty
Maltz
Marcks
mastectomy
Mayo
McHugh
McKeever
McMurray
McPherson-Wheeler
McPherson-Ziegler
McReynolds
meatotomy
meniscus
Merrifield
Metzenbaum
Meyhoeffer
Mitchell
mitral
mitral stenosis
Moebius
Moorehead

knife *(continued)*
mucosa
Murphy
myringoplasty
myringotome
myringotomy
nasal
Neivert
Newman
Niedner
Nunez-Nunez
obtuse angle
Oertli
O'Malley
ophthalmic
Pace
Page
Paparella
paracentesis
Parker
Paton
Paufique
pituitary capsulectomy
plaster
plaster cast
Politzer
Potts
Prince
pterygium
ptosis
pulmonary valve
Ralks
Ramsbotham
Reese
Reiner
reversible
Ridlon
Rish

knife *(continued)*

Robb
Robertson
Rochester
roller
Rosen
Royce
Sato
Scheie
Scholl
Schuknecht
Schultze
Schwartz
scimitar-blade
sclerotomy
Seiler
Sellor
semilunar cartilage
septum
serrated
Sexton
Shambaugh
Shambaugh-Lempert
Shea
Sheehy
Sichel
sickle-shaped
skin-graft
Sluder
Smillie
Smith
Smith-Fisher
Smith-Green
stapedius tendon
sternum
Stewart
Strayer
submucous

knife *(continued)*

suction
swivel
Tabb
tenotomy
Thiersch
Tobold
tonsil
Tooke
tracheal
Tubby
twin
Tydings
tympanoplastic
uterine
Vacu-tome
valvotomy
Vannas
Virchow
von Graefe
Walton
Weber
Webster
Wheeler
Wullstein
Yasargil
Ziegler
Knight brace
Knight forceps
Knight scissors
Knight-Sluder forceps
knitted vascular prosthesis
knock-knee
Knowles pin
Knowles pin nail
Knowles scissors
knuckle binder splint
knuckle of bowel

knuckle of tube
Kobak needle
Kobyashi hook
Koch-Mason dressing
Kocher approach
Kocher clamp
Kocher-Crotti retractor
Kocher dissector
Kocher elevator
Kocher forceps
Kocher incision
Kocher maneuver
Kocher operation
Kocher periosteal elevator
Kocher raspatory
Kocher retractor
Kocher sound
Kocher spoon
Kocher ulcer
kocherization
Kocks operation
Koeberle forceps
Koeberle operation
Koenig operation
Koenig-Wittek operation
Koeppe lens
Koffler forceps
Koffler-Lillie forceps
Koffler operation
Kogan endospeculum
Kohn needle
koilonychia
Kolb forceps
Kolb trocar
Kolle-Lexer operation
Kollmann dilator
Kolodny clamp
Kolodny forceps

Kolodny hemostat
Kolomnin operation
Kondoleon operation
König operation
Kono procedure
Kopetzky bur
Korotkoff method
Körte-Ballance operation
Kortzeborn operation
Kos cannula
Kowalzig operation
Kramer speculum
Kramer telescope
Kraske approach
Kraske position
Kraske retractor
Kraupa operation
Krause cannula
Krause forceps
Krause's gland
Krause punch
Krause snare
Krause universal forceps
Krause-Wolfe operation
Kreiker operation
Kreischer chisel
Kreiselman incubator
Kreiselman unit
Kreissl knife
Kreuscher operation
Kreuscher scissors
Kreutzmann cannula
Kreutzmann trocar
Kriebig operation
Krimer operation
Kristeller retractor
Kristeller speculum
Kristiansen screw

Kroener fimbriectomy
Kroener operation
Kron dilator
Kron probe
Kronecker needle
Kroner tubal ligation
Kronfeld electrode
Kronfeld forceps
Kronfeld retractor
Kronig cesarean section
Krönlein-Berke orbital decompression
Krönlein hernia
Krönlein operation
Krukenberg amputation
Krukenberg operation
Krull knife
Krwawicz cataract extractor
Krwawicz cryoextractor
Kryostik
krypton laser
KUB (kidneys, ureters, bladder)
KUB x-ray
Kuhlman brace
Kuhlman cast cutter
Kuhlman traction
Kuhn tube

Kuhnt forceps
Kuhnt gouge
Kuhnt operation
Kuhnt-Szymanowski operation
Kulenkampff anesthesia
Kulvin-Kalt forceps
Küntscher driver
Küntscher nail
Küntscher pin
Küntscher reamer
Küntscher rod
Kurten vein stripper
Kurten wire brush
Kushner-Tandatnick curet
Kussmaul respirations
Kuster hernia
Kuster operation
Küstner incision
Küstner operation
Kutler amputation
Kydex body jacket
Kyle applicator
Kyle knife
Kyle speculum
Kyoto-Barrett-Boyes perfusion technique
Kypher sutures

I

L-osteotomy
L-plate
L-shaped elevator
L-type nose-bridge prosthesis
Labbé operation
labia (*sing.* labium)
labia majora
labia minora
labial
labial arteries
labial bar
labial flange
labial hernia
labial nerves
labial splint
labial veins
labiales anteriores nerves
labiales anteriores veins
labiales inferiores veins
labiales posteriores nerves
labiales posteriores veins
labialis inferior artery
labialis superior artery
labialis superior vein
labiectomy
labium (*pl.* labia)
Laborde dilator
Laborde forceps
labyrinthectomy
labyrinthi arteries
labyrinthi veins
labyrinthine veins

labyrinthotomy
Lacarrere operation
lace sutures
lacerated
laceration
lacidem sutures
lacrimal artery
lacrimal bone
lacrimal canaliculi
lacrimal cannula
lacrimal dilator
lacrimal duct
lacrimal glands
lacrimal needle
lacrimal probe
lacrimal retractor
lacrimal sac
lacrimal sac retractor
lacrimal sound
lacrimal syringe
lacrimal trephine
lacrimal tube
lacrimal vein
lacrimalis artery
lacrimalis nerve
lacrimalis vein
lacrimoconchal suture
lacrimomaxillary suture
lacrimonasal duct
lactated Ringer's solution
lactation
lacteal

lacteal cataract
lactiferous duct
lacuna (*pl.* lacunae)
lacuna musculorum
lacuna vasorum
lacunar
lacunar ligament
Ladd caliper
Ladd clamp
Ladd elevator
Ladd knife
Ladd operation
Ladd raspatory
Laennec's cirrhosis
Laforce adenotome
Laforce-Grieshaber adenotome
Laforce spud
Laforce-Stevenson adenotome
Laforce tonsillectome
Laforce tonsillectomy
LAG (lymphangiogram)
lag screw
Lagleyze operation
Lagrange operation
Lagrange scissors
Lagrange sclerectomy
Lahey-Babcock forceps
Lahey carrier
Lahey clamp
Lahey Clinic instruments
Lahey drain
Lahey forceps
Lahey gouge
Lahey hook
Lahey ligature carrier
Lahey needle
Lahey operation
Lahey osteotome

Lahey-Péan forceps
Lahey retractor
Lahey scissors
Lahey tenaculum
Lahey trephine
Lahey tube
Laidley cystoscope
Laing plate
Lambda pacemaker
lambdoid suture
Lambert-Berry raspatory
Lambert forceps
Lambert-Lowman clamp
Lambotte chisel
Lambotte clamp
Lambotte forceps
Lambotte-Henderson osteotome
Lambotte osteotome
Lambrinudi operation
Lambrinudi splint
lamella (*pl.* lamellae)
lamellar cataract
lamellar incision
lamellar keratoplasty
lamina (*pl.* laminae)
lamina dissector
lamina elevator
lamina gouge
lamina knife
laminar
laminar air flow
laminaria
laminaria insertion
laminectomy
laminectomy chisel
laminectomy punch
laminectomy raspatory
laminectomy retractor

laminectomy rongeur
laminectomy scissors
laminectomy shears
laminogram
laminography
laminotomy
Lamm incision
Lamont elevator
Lamont rasp
Lamont saw
lamp
Lancaster keratome
Lancaster knife
Lancaster magnet
Lancaster-O'Connor speculum
Lancaster operation
Lancaster sclerotome
Lancaster speculum
lance
lancet
Landolt keratome
Landolt operation
Landzert fossa
Lane catheter
Lane clamp
Lane dissector
Lane elevator
Lane forceps
Lane-Lannelongue operation
Lane mouth gag
Lane needle
Lane operation
Lane periosteal elevator
Lane plate
Lane raspatory
Lane retractor
Lane screwdriver
Lane suture needle

Lang dissector
Lang knife
Lang scoop
Lang speculum
Lange operation
Lange position
Lange punch
Lange retractor
Lange speculum
Langenbeck amputation
Langenbeck elevator
Langenbeck forceps
Langenbeck incision
Langenbeck knife
Langenbeck-O'Brien raspatory
Langenbeck operation
Langenbeck periosteal elevator
Langenbeck raspatory
Langenbeck retractor
Langenbeck saw
Langerhans islands
Lannelongue operation
Lanz operation
Lanz tube
lap tapes
laparectomy
laparoaminoscopy
laparocholecystotomy
laparocolostomy
laparocolotomy
laparocystectomy
laparocystidotomy
laparoenterostomy
laparoenterotomy
laparogastroscopy
laparogastrostomy
laparogastrotomy
laparohepatotomy

laparoileotomy
laparomyomectomy
laparorrhaphy
laparoscope
    ACMI
    Eder
    Jacobs-Palmer
    Lent
laparoscopic cannula
laparoscopic trocar
laparoscopic tubal ligation
laparoscopic tubal sterilization
laparoscopy
laparosplenectomy
laparosplenotomy
laparotome
laparotomy
laparotomy pack
laparotomy pads
laparotrachelotomy
laparotrachelotomy knife
laparotyphlotomy
Lapides catheter
Lapides needle
Lapides needle holder
Lapides procedure
Laplace forceps
Laplace retractor
Lardennois button
large bowel
large intestine
large loop electrode
LaRocca tube
La Roque-Branson hernia repair
La Roque hernia repair
La Roque sutures
La Roque technique
Laroyenne operation

Larrey amputation
Larrey bandage
Larrey dressing
Larry director
Larry probe
laryngea inferior artery
laryngea inferior vein
laryngea superior artery
laryngea superior vein
laryngeal
laryngeal applicator
laryngeal artery
laryngeal biopsy forceps
laryngeal cannula
laryngeal dilator
laryngeal dissector
laryngeal enterotome
laryngeal forceps
laryngeal knife
laryngeal mirror
laryngeal nerve
laryngeal punch
laryngeal punch forceps
laryngeal retractor
laryngeal saw
laryngeal scissors
laryngeal snare
laryngeal speculum
laryngeal stridor
laryngeal syringe
laryngeal tube
laryngeal vein
laryngectomy
laryngectomy clamp
laryngectomy saw
laryngectomy tube
laryngeus inferior nerve
laryngeus recurrens nerve

laryngeus superior nerve
laryngocentesis
laryngoesophagectomy
laryngofissure
laryngofissure forceps
laryngofissure profilometer
laryngofissure retractor
laryngofissure saw
laryngofissure scissors
laryngofissure shears
laryngogram
laryngography
laryngopharyngectomy
laryngopharyngoesophagectomy
laryngoplasty
laryngorrhaphy
laryngoscope
    adult
    Albert-Andrews
    anterior commissure
    Atkins-Tucker
    Bizzarri-Giuffrida
    Broyles
    Chevalier Jackson
    Clerf
    Dedo
    Dedo-Pilling
    direct
    dual distal lighted
    ESI
    fiberoptic
    Fink
    Flagg
    folding
    Foregger
    Garfield-Holinger
    Guedel
    Haslinger

laryngoscope *(continued)*
    Holinger
    Holinger-Garfield
    hook-on
    Hopp
    hourglass anterior commissure
    intubation
    Jackson
    Jako
    Kleenspec
    Lewy
    Lundy
    Lynch
    MacIntosh
    Magill
    Miller
    mirror
    multipurpose
    optical
    polio
    reverse-bevel
    Roberts
    rotating
    Rusch
    Sam Roberts
    Sanders
    self-retaining
    shadow-free
    Siker
    slotted
    standard
    straight-blade
    suspension
    Tucker
    wasp-waist
    Welch Allyn
    Wis-Foregger

laryngoscope *(continued)*
   Wis-Hipple
   Yankauer
laryngoscopy
laryngospasm
laryngostat
laryngostomy
laryngotomy
laryngotracheobronchoscopy
laryngotracheoscopy
laryngotracheostomy
laryngotracheotomy
larynx
Lasègue sign
laser
   argon
   gas
   helium-neon
   krypton
   l. microscope
   neodymium
   ruby
LASH (left anterior superior
   hemiblock)
Lash operation
Lash-Löffler implant
Lasix
lateral
lateral condyle
lateral decubitus position
lateral flank incision
lateral gutter
lateral incision
lateral ligament
lateral malleolus
lateral meniscus
lateral osteotomy
lateral position

lateral prone position
lateral rectus incision
lateral recumbent position
lateral sinus
latex catheter
latex drain
latex tube
Lathbury applicator
latissimus dorsi muscle
Latrobe retractor
Latzko cesarean section
Latzko closure
Latzko colpocleisis
Latzko fistula repair
Latzko radical hysterectomy
Laufe-Barton-Kielland forceps
Laufe forceps
Laufe-Piper forceps
Laugier hernia
Lauren operation
lavage
Law position
Lawrence forceps
Lawson-Thornton plate
Lawton forceps
Lawton scissors
layer closure
layered
lazy-S incision
lead-pipe colon
lead-pipe fracture
Leadbetter operation
Leadbetter-Politano operation
Leadbetter-Politano uretero-
   neocystotomy
Leader forceps
Leader hook
Leader-Kollmann dilator

leads
leaflet
Leahey operation
leapfrog position
leaves of broad ligament
Leboyer delivery technique
Lebsche chisel
Lebsche forceps
Lebsche knife
Lebsche punch
Lebsche raspatory
Lebsche rongeur
Lebsche shears
lecithin/sphingomyelin ratio
    (L/S ratio)
Ledbetter maneuver
Le Dentu sutures
Le Dran sutures
Lee-Cohen elevator
Lee-Cohen knife
Lee knife
Lees clamp
LeFort amputation
LeFort bougie
LeFort catheter
LeFort follower
LeFort fracture (I, II, or III)
LeFort operation
LeFort osteotomy (I, II, or III)
LeFort sound
LeFort sutures
left coronary artery
left lateral position
left lower lobe (LLL)
left lower quadrant (LLQ)
left-to-right shunt
left upper lobe (LUL)
left upper quadrant (LUQ)

leg extension splint
leg roll
leg splint
Legg operation
Legg osteotome
Legueu retractor
Lehman catheter
Lehman syringe
Leinbach osteotome
Leinbach prosthesis
Leinbach screw
leiomyoma (*pl.* leiomyomata)
leiomyomata uteri
Leiter cystoscope
Leiter tube
Lejeune applicator
Lejeune forceps
Lejeune scissors
Leksell forceps
Leksell frame
Leksell rongeur
Leksell sternal approximator
Leksell sternal spreader
Leland-Jones forceps
Leland knife
Lell esophagoscope
Lell saw
Lell tube
Lem-Blay clamp
Lembert sutures
LeMesurier operation
Lemmon rib spreader
Lemmon-Russian forceps
Lemmon sternal approximator
Lemmon sternal retractor
Lemmon sternal spreader
Lempert bur
Lempert-Colver retractor

Lempert-Colver speculum
Lempert curet
Lempert elevator
Lempert excavator
Lempert forceps
Lempert incision
Lempert knife
Lempert malleus cutter
Lempert operation
Lempert perforator
Lempert punch
Lempert retractor
Lempert rongeur
Lempka vein stripper
lengthening of bone
lengthening of tendon
Lennander operation
Lennarson suction tube
Lennarson tube
lens
lens capsule
lens expressor (See also *expressor.*)
    Arruga
    Berens
    Kirby
    medallion
    Rizzuti
    Smith
    Verhoeff
lens extraction
lens forceps
lens implant
lens loupe
lens scoop
lens spoon
lenticular
lenticular cataract
lenticular knife

Lentulo drill
Leonard forceps
Leopold operation
Lepley-Ernst tube
L'Episcopo operation
Leriche forceps
Leriche operation
Lermoyez punch
lesion
L'Esperance erysiphake
Lespinasse sutures
lesser curvature of stomach
lesser multangular bone
lesser trochanter
lethargic
leucotomy (See *leukotomy.*)
leukoma
leukonychia
leukoplakia
leukotome
    Bailey
    Dorsey
    Freeman
    Lewis
    Love
    McKenzie
    transorbital
leukotomy
Levant stone dislodger
levator
levator anguli oris muscle
levator ani muscle
levator glandulae thyroideae
    muscle
levator hernia
levator labii superioris alaeque
    nasi muscle
levator labii superioris muscle

levator muscle
levator palpebrae superioris
   muscle
levator prostatae muscle
levator scapulae muscle
levator veli palatini muscle
levatores costarum muscles
LeVeen dialysis shunt
LeVeen peritoneal shunt
lever pessary
Levin tube
Levine operation
Levis splint
Levitt eye implant
Levret forceps
Lewin clamp
Lewin dissector
Lewin forceps
Lewin splint
Lewin-Stern splint
Lewis cystometer
Lewis forceps
Lewis hemostat
Lewis leukotome
Lewis loupe
Lewis mouth gag
Lewis rasp
Lewis raspatory
Lewis retractor
Lewis scoop
Lewis snare
Lewis tongue depressor
Lewis tube
Lewkowitz forceps
Lewy laryngoscope
Lewy-Rubin needle
Lewy suspension apparatus
Lexer chisel

Lexer operation
Lexer scissors
Leyro-Diaz forceps
Lichtenberg keratome
Lichtenberg trephine
Lichtwicz needle
Lichtwicz trocar
lid clamp
lid dermabrader
lid elevator
lid everter
   Berens
   Walker
lid forceps
lid-fracturing blepharoplasty
lid hook
lid knife
lid operation
lid plasty
lid plate
lid ptosis operation
lid-retracting hook
lid retractor
lid scalpel
lid speculum
lid suture operation
lidocaine hydrochloride
Lieberkühn crypts
Lieberkühn follicles
Lieberkühn glands
Lieberman abrader
Lieberman proctoscope
Lieberman sigmoidoscope
lien
lien accessorius
lien mobilis
lienal
lienalis artery

lienalis vein
lienculus
lienocolic
lienopancreatic
lienophrenic
lienorenal
lienorenal ligament
life-saving suction tube
Liga clip
ligament(s)
    accessory
    acromioclavicular
    acromiocoracoid
    adipose
    annular
    anterior
    arcuate
    brachioradial
    broad l. of uterus
    calcaneofibular
    calcaneonavicular
    capsular
    cardinal
    carpometacarpal
    caudal
    ciliary
    conoid
    Cooper's
    coracoacromial
    coracoclavicular
    coracohumeral
    costoclavicular
    costotransverse
    Cowper's
    cricoarytenoid
    cricothyroarytenoid
    cricothyroid
    cricotracheal

ligament(s) *(continued)*
    cruciate
    crural
    cuneiform
    deltoid
    dentate
    falciform
    flaval
    gastrohepatic
    gastrophrenic
    Gimbernat's
    glenohumeral
    Henle's
    hepatogastric
    Hesselbach's
    hyoepiglottic
    hyothyroid
    iliofemoral
    infundibulopelvic
    inguinal
    lacunar
    lateral
    lienorenal
    l. of Treitz
    Lisfranc's
    Lockwood's
    longitudinal
    medial
    medial collateral
    meniscofemoral
    nephrocolic
    nuchal
    ovarian
    pancreaticosplenic
    patellar
    pectinate
    pectineal
    periodontal

ligament(s) *(continued)*
    Petit's
    phrenicocolic
    phrenicolienal
    phrenicosplenic
    Poupart's
    pulmonary
    radiocarpal
    rectouterine
    rhomboid
    round l. of femur
    round l. of liver
    round l. of uterus
    sacrogenital
    sacrospinous
    sacrouterine
    splenocolic
    splenorenal
    suspensory l. of axilla
    suspensory l. of lens
    sutural
    tendinotrochanteric
    transverse humeral
    trapezoid
    umbilical
    uteropelvic
    uterosacral
    ventricular
    vesicouterine
    vestibular
    vocal
    Weitbrecht's
ligamenta (*sing.* ligamentum)
ligamenta flava
ligamenta flava forceps
ligamenti teretis uteri artery
ligamentous
ligamentous falx

ligamentous joint
ligamentum (*pl.* ligamenta)
ligamentum-grasping forceps
ligate
ligation
ligation and stripping
ligation of artery
ligation of fallopian tubes
ligation of vas deferens
ligation of vein
ligation sutures
ligator (See also *sutures.*)
    hemorrhoidal
    McGivney
ligature (See *sutures.*)
ligature carrier
ligature-carrying forceps
ligature forceps
ligature hook
ligature needle
ligature wire
light
    l. application
    l. coagulation
    l. coagulator
    l. dressing
    l. microscope
    l. treatment
    neurosurgical
    overhead
Light headrest
Light-Veley apparatus
Light-Veley drill
Light-Veley headrest
lighted retractor
lightning cataract
lignocaine
Lilienthal guillotine

Lilienthal incision
Lilienthal probe
Lilienthal rib spreader
Lilienthal-Sauerbruch retractor
Lilienthal-Sauerbruch rib spreader
Lillie cannula
Lillie forceps
Lillie gouge
Lillie hook
Lillie-Killian forceps
Lillie knife
Lillie probe
Lillie retractor
Lillie rongeur
Lillie scissors
Lillie speculum
Lillie trocar
limb
limb splint
limbal groove
limbal incision
limbal sutures
limbus (*pl.* limbi)
Lincoff eye implant
Lincoff sponge
Lincoln scissors
Linde walker
Lindeman cannula
Lindeman hysteroflator
Lindeman needle
Lindeman-Silverstein tube
Lindholm operation
Lindner operation
Lindner spatula
line
    epiphyseal
    gingival
    gluteal

line *(continued)*
    gum
    iliopectineal
    intertrochanteric
    l. incision
    l. of Douglas
    lip
    median
    mylohyoid
    nuchal
    pectinate
    semilunar
    temporal
    terminal
    visual
linea (*pl.* lineae)*
    l. alba
    l. alba hernia
    ll. albicantes
    l. aspera
    ll. atrophicae
    l. nigra
    l. semilunaris
linear
linear amputation
linear cautery
linear fracture
linear incision
linear polyethylene sutures
linear skin incision
linear skull fracture
linear transverse incision
linen sutures
linen thread sutures
lingual

*l. = linea [L.]
ll. = lineae [L., pl.]

lingual artery
lingual bar
lingual block
lingual flange
lingual forceps
lingual glands
lingual hemorrhoid
lingual nerve
lingual splint
lingual tonsillectome
lingual tonsillectomy
lingual vein
lingualis artery
lingualis nerve
lingualis vein
lingula (*pl.* lingulae)
lingulectomy
lining
linitis
linitis plastica
Linnartz clamp
Linnartz forceps
Linton-Blakemore needle
Linton clamp
Linton hook
Linton incision
Linton operation
Linton retractor
Linton-Talbott operation
Linton tourniquet
Linton tube
Linton vein stripper
lion-jaw clamp
lion-jaw forceps
lip clamp
lip line
lip retractor
lip shave

lip sutures
lipectomy
lipoma (*pl.* lipomas or lipomata)
lipomatous
Lippes loop intrauterine device
    (IUD)
Lippman hip prosthesis
liquefaction
liquid conductor Bovie
liquid nitrogen
Lisfranc amputation
Lisfranc's joint
Lisfranc's ligament
Lister-Burch speculum
Lister dressing
Lister forceps
Lister scissors
Liston forceps
Liston knife
Liston operation
Liston rongeur
Liston scissors
Liston shears
Liston splint
Liston-Stille forceps
lithiasis
lithium pacemaker
lithocystotomy
litholapaxy
lithonephrotomy
lithotome
lithotomy
lithotomy forceps
lithotomy position
lithotomy-Trendelenburg position
lithotresis
lithotripsy
lithotriptoscope

lithotriptoscopy
lithotrite
    Alcock
    Alcock-Hendrickson
    Bigelow
    Hendrickson
    Keyes
    Lowenstein
    Lowsley
    Reliquet
    Thompson
lithotrity
Littauer forceps
Littauer-Liston forceps
Littauer rongeur
Littauer scissors
Little retractor
Littler scissors
Littlewood amputation
Littlewood operation
Littre's glands
Littre hernia
Littre operation
Littre-Richter hernia
Littre sutures
Litwak scissors
Litwin scissors
live splint
liver
liver bed
liver biopsy needle
liver edge
liver retractor
Livermore trocar
Livingston bar
Livingston forceps
Lizar operation
LLL (left lower lobe)

Lloyd catheter
Lloyd-Davies operation
Lloyd tube
LLQ (left lower quadrant)
lobe
lobe-grasping forceps
lobe-holding forceps
lobe of lung
lobe of thyroid gland
lobectomy
lobectomy forceps
lobectomy of lung
lobectomy of prostate
lobectomy of thyroid
lobectomy scissors
lobectomy tourniquet
lobotomy
lobotomy electrode
lobotomy needle
lobotomy of brain
lobster-tail catheter
lobular
lobular carcinoma
lobulate
lobulated
lobule
lobulette
lobulus (*pl.* lobuli)
local anesthesia
local excision
local excision of lesion
local recurrence of carcinoma
localized
lochia
lock needle
lock-stitch sutures
locking clamp
locking sutures

Lockwood-Allis forceps
Lockwood clamp
Lockwood forceps
Lockwood's ligament
locomotor ataxia
loculate
Löffler sutures
Löhlein operation
loin
Lombard-Beyer forceps
Lombard-Beyer rongeur
Lombard-Boies rongeur
Lombard rongeur
Londermann operation
London forceps
London prosthesis
long-arm cast
long-armed cast
Long forceps
long-handle curet
Long Island forceps
long-leg brace
long-leg cast
long muscle
long needle
long oblique incision
long palate hook
long periosteal elevator
long scissors
Longdwel catheter
Longdwel needle
longissimus capitis muscle
longissimus cervicis muscle
longissimus muscle
longissimus thoracis muscle
longitudinal
longitudinal cystotomy
longitudinal fracture

longitudinal incision
longitudinal ligament
longitudinal midline incision
longitudinal muscle
longitudinalis superior linguae
    muscle
Longmire operation
Longmire valvulotome
Longuet incision
Longuet operation
longus capitis muscle
longus colli muscle
loop (See also *loupe.*)
    Beck
    Cannon endarterectomy
    endarterectomy
    Lippes
    l. colostomy
    l. electrode
    l. ileostomy
    l. intrauterine device (IUD)
    l. of bowel
    l. of intestine
    l. stripper
    l. sutures
    l. transverse colostomy
    l. wire
    P-loop
    snare
    twisted wire
    wire
loopogram
loose fracture
Lopez-Enriquez operation
Lord-Blakemore tube
Lord operation
Lordan forceps
Lordan hook

Lore forceps
Lore-Lawrence tube
Lore suction tube
Lorenz operation
Lorenz osteotomy
Lorenz tube
Lorenzo reamer
Lorenzo screw
Lorenzo SMO prosthesis
Lorfan anesthesia
Lorie retractor
Lorie trephine
Loring ophthalmoscope
Lossen operation
Lotheissen herniorrhaphy
Lotheissen-McVay operation
Lotheissen operation
Lothrop dissector
Lothrop forceps
Lothrop knife
Lothrop retractor
Lottes nail
Lottes operation
Lottes pin
Lottes reamer
Loughnane hook
Lounsbury curet
loupe (See also *loop.*)
    Arlt
    Berens
    binocular
    corneal
    Daviel
    ear
    eye
    hook-on
    intracapsular lens
    Lewis

loupe *(continued)*
    magnifying
    New Orleans
    Wilder
Love-Adson elevator
Love-Adson periosteal elevator
Love-Gruenwald forceps
Love-Gruenwald rongeur
Love-Kerrison forceps
Love-Kerrison rongeur
Love leukotome
Love retractor
Love splint
Lovelace forceps
Low-Beers projection
low cervical cesarean section
low cesarean section
low forceps
low forceps delivery
low-friction arthroplasty
low incision
low ligation
low midline incision
low profile valve prosthesis
low spinal anesthesia
Lowe-Breck knife
Lowe ring
Lowell knife
Löwenberg forceps
Lowenstein lithotrite
Lowenstein operation
Lower forceps
lower gall duct forceps
lower GI series
lower jaw
lower lobe of lung
lower midline incision
lower operation for femoral hernia

lower uterine segment cesarean section
Lowman clamp
Lowsley forceps
Lowsley lithotrite
Lowsley needle
Lowsley nephropexy
Lowsley operation
Lowsley-Peterson cystoscope
Lowsley retractor
Lowsley tractor
Lowsley urethroscope
L/S ratio (lecithin/sphingomyelin)
Lubafax dressing
Lubraseptic
Luc forceps
Luc operation
Lucae forceps
Lucae mallet
Lucae probe
Lucas-Cottrell operation
Lucas-Murray operation
lucite
lucite eye implant
lucite pessary
Luck drill
Luck fasciotome
Luck operation
Luck saw
Luckett operation
Ludloff incision
Ludloff operation
Ludloff osteotomy
Luedde exophthalmometer
Luer curet
Luer forceps
Luer-Hartmann rongeur
Luer-Korte scoop

Luer-Lok syringe
Luer needle
Luer retractor
Luer rongeur
Luer scoop
Luer speculum
Luer syringe
Luer tube
Luer-Whiting forceps
lugged plate
Lugol solution
Luikart-Bill traction handle
Luikart forceps
Luikart-Kielland forceps
Luikart-McLane forceps
Luikart-Simpson forceps
Lukens aspirator
Lukens cannula
Lukens catgut sutures
Lukens collector
Lukens enterotome
Lukens retractor
Lukens suction tube
LUL (left lower lobe)
Lulu clamp
lumbales arteries
lumbales nerves
lumbales veins
lumbalis ascendens vein
lumbalis ima artery
lumbar
lumbar aortogram
lumbar aortography
lumbar aortography needle
lumbar arteries
lumbar colotomy
lumbar epidural anesthesia
lumbar hernia

lumbar laminectomy
lumbar nephrectomy
lumbar nerve block
lumbar nerves
lumbar puncture
lumbar puncture needle
lumbar veins
lumbar vertebrae
lumbocostoabdominal triangle
lumbodorsal
lumboiliac incision
lumbosacral fusion
lumbosacral trunk
lumbrical muscles
lumbricales manus muscles
lumbricales pedis muscles
lumen (*pl.* lumina)
lumen finder
    Carabelli
    full-view
lumina (*sing.* lumen)
luminous ophthalmoscope
lunate bone
Lund operation
Lundsgaard blade
Lundsgaard-Burch knife
Lundsgaard-Burch rasp
Lundsgaard-Burch sclerotome
Lundsgaard knife
Lundsgaard rasp
Lundsgaard sclerotome
Lundy-Irving needle
Lundy laryngoscope
Lundy needle
lung clamp
lung exclusion clamp
lung forceps
lung-grasping forceps

lung retractor
lung scissors
lung tourniquet
lunula
Luongo cannula
Luongo curet
Luongo elevator
Luongo needle
Luongo retractor
LUQ (left upper quadrant)
Luschka crypts
Lusskin drill
Lutz forceps
luxation
Luys segregator
Luys separator
LVEDP (left ventricular end
    diastolic pressure)
Lyman-Smith brace
lymph
lymph gland
lymph node
lymphadenectomy
lymphadenitis
lymphadenopathy
lymphadenotomy
lymphangiectomy
lymphangiography
lymphangioplasty
lymphangiorrhaphy
lymphangiotomy
lymphangitis
lymphatic
lymphatic chain
lymphatic duct
lymphaticostomy
lymphatics
lymphedema

lymphocyte
lymphoid
lymphosarcoma
Lynch curet
Lynch dissector
Lynch electrode
Lynch forceps
Lynch incision
Lynch knife
Lynch laryngoscope
Lynch operation

Lynch scissors
Lynch spatula
Lynch suspension apparatus
Lyon forceps
Lyon-Horgan operation
Lyon tube
lyse
lysed
lysis
lysis of adhesions
Lytle splint

m

ma (milliamperes)
MacAusland chisel
MacAusland dissector
MacAusland-Kelly retractor
MacAusland mallet
MacAusland operation
MacAusland reamer
MacAusland retractor
MacAusland skid
MacDonald clamp
MacDonald dissector
MacDonald periosteal elevator
macerated
Macewen operation
MacFee incision
MacFee neck flap
Machek-Blaskovics operation
Machek-Gifford operation
Machek operation
machine
MacIntosh blade
MacIntosh laryngoscope
MacIntosh operation
MacIntosh prosthesis
Mack tonsillectome
Mackay-Marg tonometer
Mackay retractor
Mackenrodt incision
Mackenrodt operation
MacKenty elevator
MacKenty forceps
MacKenty knife

MacKenty periosteal elevator
MacKenty punch
MacKenty scissors
MacKenty tube
MacKenzie amputation
Mackid operation
Mackler tube
Mackler tube prosthesis
Maclay scissors
macula (*pl.* maculae)
Madden clamp
Madden dissector
Madden hook
Madden ligature carrier
Maddox needle
Maddox rod
Madlener sterilization
Magielski cautery
Magielski chisel
Magielski curet
Magielski elevator
Magielski electrocoagulator
Magielski forceps
Magielski hook
Magielski needle
Magill band
Magill forceps
Magill laryngoscope
Magill tube
Magitot operation
magnet
       Berman

magnet *(continued)*
  bronchoscopic
  Bronson
  electromagnet
  endoscopic
  Equen
  eye
  Grüning
  Haab
  Hirschberg electromagnet
  Holinger
  horseshoe
  Lancaster
  m. extraction
  Mellinger
  permanent
  Ralks
  stomach
  Storz
  Sweet
  temporary
  Thomas
  Wildgren-Reck
magnetic cups
magnetic eye implant
magnetic implant
magnifying loupe
Magnus operation
Magnuson operation
Magnuson saw
Magnuson splint
Magnuson-Stack operation
Magnuson valve
Magovern ball valve prosthesis
Magovern-Cromie ball valve prosthesis
Mahoney dilator
Mahoney speculum

Mahorner-Mead operation
Maier forceps
main-stem bronchus
Maingot hemostat
Mair operation
Maisonneuve amputation
Maisonneuve bandage
Maisonneuve urethrotome
Majewsky operation
major amputation
major connector bar
major operation
major surgery
Makka operation
malacotomy
malaise
malar arch
malar bone
malar elevator
malar incision
malar process
Malbec operation
Malbran operation
Malecot catheter
Malecot drain
malfunction
Malgaigne amputation
Malgaigne apparatus
Malgaigne hook
malignancy
malignant
Maliniac rasp
Maliniac retractor
Malis coagulating unit
Malis coagulator
Malis forceps
Malis scissors
malleable probe

malleable retractor
malleable rod
malleable scoop
malleable screw
malleable spatula
malleolar artery
malleolaris anterior lateralis artery
malleolaris anterior medialis artery
malleolus
malleotomy
mallet
    aluminum
    bakelite
    bone
    Chandler
    Cottle
    Crane
    Gerzog
    Hajek
    Hibbs
    Kirk
    Lucae
    MacAusland
    mastoid
    Meyerding
    orthopedic
    Ralks
    Rush
    Smith-Petersen
    White
malleus
malleus cutter
malleus forceps
malleus nipper
malleus punch
Mallory-Weiss tear
Malm-Himmelstein valvulotome
Maloney bougie

Maloney catheter
Maloney dilator
maloplasty
malpighian bodies
malpighian capsule
Maltz knife
Maltz-Lipsett rasp
Maltz needle
Maltz rasp
Maltz retractor
Maltz saw
malunion
malunited fracture
mamilla (*pl.* mamillae)
mamillary process
mamilliplasty
mamma
mammaplasty
mammary
mammary abscess
mammary artery
mammary duct
mammary glands
mammary prosthesis
mammary support dressing
mammectomy
mammiform
mammogram
mammography
mammoplasia
mammoplasty
mammotomy
Manchester colporrhaphy
Manchester-Donald-Fothergill
    operation
Manchester operation
Manchester uterine suspension
mandible

mandible splint
mandibular
mandibular artery
mandibular articulation
mandibular block
mandibular fossa
mandibular nerve
mandibular prosthesis
mandibularis nerve
mandibulectomy
maneuver
manipulation
manipulation of fracture
manipulation of joint
manipulation of muscle
Mann forceps
mannitol
manometer
    Harvard
    spinal
manometry
Mantz dilator
manual dermatome
manual inspection
manubriogladiolar junction
manubrium
many-tailed bandage
many-tailed dressing
Maquet table
Marcaine hydrochloride
march fracture
Marcks knife
Marcks operation
Marckwald operation
Marcy operation
marginal
marginal chalazion forceps
marginal clamp

marginal ulcer
Margulles coil
Marian operation
Marin bur
Mark IV repair
Markham-Meyerding retractor
marker
    diamond green
    Gonin-Amsler
marking pencil
Marlex bandage
Marlex graft
Marlex mesh
Marlex mesh implant
Marlex prosthesis
Marlex screen
Marlex sheet
Marlex sutures
Marlex tenaculum
marrow
marrow-lymph gland
marrow spoon
Marsan Loop-Loc colostomy bag
    system
Marshall-Marchetti-Krantz opera-
    tion
Marshall-Marchetti operation
Marshall-Marchetti repair
Marshik forceps
marsupial skin flap
marsupialization
marsupialization of abscess
marsupialization of cyst
marsupialization of pilonidal cyst
Martel clamp
Martin and Davy speculum
Martin bandage
Martin clamp

Martin forceps
Martin gouge
Martin hook
Martin needle
Martin operation
Martin pelvimeter
Martin retractor
Martin scissors
Martin snare
Martin speculum
Martin stripper
Martin tube
Martin wire cutter
Martius-Harris operation
Martius operation
Marwedel gastrostomy
Marwedel operation
Maryan forceps
mashed
mask-like facies
Mason-Allen splint
Mason-Auvard speculum
Mason clamp
Mason incision
Mason splint
Mason suction tube
mass
massage
masseter muscle
masseteric artery
masseteric nerve
masseterica artery
massetericus nerve
Massie nail
massive
Masson fascia stripper
Masson-Judd retractor
Masson needle

Masson needle holder
mastadenitis
mastadenoma
mastalgia
mastectomy
mastectomy incision
mastectomy knife
Masterson clamp
masthelcosis
Mastin clamp
mastitis
mastocarcinoma
mastochondroma
mastodynia
mastogram
mastography
mastoid
mastoid antrotomy
mastoid bone
mastoid bur
mastoid canaliculi
mastoid catheter
mastoid chisel
mastoid curet
mastoid dressing
mastoid emissary vein
mastoid fossa
mastoid gouge
mastoid mallet
mastoid operation
mastoid probe
mastoid process
mastoid raspatory
mastoid-retaining retractor
mastoid retractor
mastoid rongeur
mastoid rongeur forceps
mastoid searcher

mastoid suction tube
mastoidectomy
mastoidotomy
mastoidotympanectomy
mastoncus
mastopathia
mastopathia cystica
mastopathy
mastopexy
mastoplastia
mastoplasty
mastoptosis
mastorrhagia
mastorrhaphy
mastoscirrhus
mastosis
mastostomy
mastotomy
Matas band
Matas operation
Matchett-Brown prosthesis
Matchett prosthesis
Mathews speculum
Mathieu forceps
Mathieu raspatory
Mathieu retractor
matrix (*pl.* matrices)
matrix band
Matson elevator
Matson-Mead stripper
Matson operation
Matson periosteal elevator
Matson raspatory
Matson rib stripper
Mattis scissors
mattress sutures
mature cataract
Matzenauer speculum

Mauksch operation
Maumenee erysiphake
Maumenee forceps
Maumenee-Park speculum
Maunoir scissors
Maunsell sutures
Mauriceau-Levret maneuver
Mauriceau maneuver
Mauriceau-Smellie-Veit maneuver
Max Fine forceps
Maxilith pacemaker
maxilla
maxillares veins
maxillaris artery
maxillaris nerve
maxillary
maxillary antrotomy
maxillary artery
maxillary articulation
maxillary dental prosthesis
maxillary nerve
maxillary sinus
maxillary sinusotomy
maxillary veins
maxillofacial
maxillofacial prosthesis
maxillomandibular traction
maximal
maximum
Maxi-Myst vaporizer
Maxitrol
Maydl colostomy
Maydl hernia
Maydl operation
Mayer pessary
Mayer position
Mayer speculum
Mayer splint

Mayfield clip
Mayfield curet
Mayfield forceps
Mayfield-Kees headrest
Mayfield osteotome
Mayfield spatula
Maylard incision
Mayo-Adams retractor
Mayo-Blake forceps
Mayo-Boldt inverter
Mayo cannula
Mayo carrier
Mayo clamp
Mayo-Collins retractor
Mayo forceps
Mayo-Fueth operation
Mayo gastrojejunostomy
Mayo-Guyon clamp
Mayo-Harrington forceps
Mayo-Harrington scissors
Mayo-Hegar needle holder
Mayo herniorrhaphy
Mayo hook
Mayo hysterectomy
Mayo-Kelly inverter
Mayo knife
Mayo-Lovelace clamp
Mayo-Lovelace retractor
Mayo-Lovelace spur crusher
Mayo-Myers stripper
Mayo needle
Mayo needle holder
Mayo-New scissors
Mayo-Noble scissors
Mayo-Ochsner forceps
Mayo operation
Mayo-Péan forceps
Mayo-Péan hemostat

Mayo-Potts scissors
Mayo probe
Mayo retractor
Mayo-Robson forceps
Mayo-Robson incision
Mayo-Robson operation
Mayo-Robson position
Mayo-Robson scoop
Mayo-Russian forceps
Mayo scissors
Mayo scoop
Mayo-Simpson retractor
Mayo-Sims scissors
Mayo-Stille scissors
Mayo stripper
Mayo sutures
Mayo vein stripper
Mayo-Ward hysterectomy
Mays operation
Mazlin spring intrauterine device
    (IUD)
Mazur operation
mc (millicuries)
McAllister needle holder
McAllister scissors
McArthur incision
McArthur method
McArthur operation
McAtee apparatus
McAtee screw
McBride-Akin operation
McBride bunionectomy
McBride cup
McBride-Moore prosthesis
McBride operation
McBride plate
McBurney incision
McBurney operation

McBurney point
McBurney retractor
McBurney sign
McCall operation
McCall-Schumann operation
McCarroll operation
McCarthy-Alcock forceps
McCarthy-Campbell cystoscope
McCarthy cystoscope
McCarthy electrode
McCarthy electrotome
McCarthy evacuator
McCarthy forceps
McCarthy panendoscope
McCarthy-Peterson cystoscope
McCarthy resectoscope
McCarthy telescope
McCash-Randall operation
McCaskey catheter
McCaskey curet
McCleery-Miller clamp
McClure scissors
McCoy forceps
McCrea cystoscope
McCrea sound
McCullough forceps
McCullough retractor
McCurdy needle
McDermott clip
McDonald cerclage
McDonald clamp
McDonald operation
McDowell mouth gag
McDowell operation
McElroy curet
McEvedy operation
McGannon forceps
McGannon retractor

McGavic operation
McGee-Caparosa wire crimper
McGee forceps
McGee piston
McGee wire crimper
McGhan breast prosthesis
McGhan eye implant
McGill forceps
McGill operation
McGill retractor
McGivney ligator
McGoey-Evans cup
McGraw elastic ligature
McGraw sutures
McGuire clamp
McGuire forceps
McGuire operation
McGuire rib spreader
McGuire scissors
McHenry forceps
McHugh knife
McHugh speculum
McIndoe colpocleisis
McIndoe elevator
McIndoe forceps
McIndoe operation
McIndoe scissors
McIntire splint
McIntosh forceps
McIver catheter
McIvor mouth gag
McKay forceps
McKee-Farrar cup
McKee-Farrar prosthesis
McKee-Farrar rasp
McKee prosthesis
McKeever knife
McKeever operation

McKeever prosthesis
McKenty elevator
McKenzie bur
McKenzie clamp
McKenzie clip
McKenzie drill
McKenzie forceps
McKenzie leukotome
McKissock incision
McKissock operation
McKissock sutures
McLane forceps
McLane-Tucker forceps
McLane-Tucker-Luikart forceps
McLaughlin extractor
McLaughlin incision
McLaughlin nail
McLaughlin operation
McLaughlin plate
McLaughlin screw
McLaughlin speculum
McLean clamp
McLean scissors
McLean sutures
McLean tonometer
McMurray knife
McMurray maneuver
McMurray sign
McNaught prosthesis
McNealy-Glassman-Babcock
    forceps
McNealy-Glassman clamp
McNealy-Glassman-Mixter clamp
McNealy-Glassman-Mixter forceps
McNeill-Goldmann scleral ring
McPheeters table
McPherson-Castroviejo scissors
McPherson forceps

McPherson needle holder
McPherson scissors
McPherson spatula
McPherson speculum
McPherson-Vannas scissors
McPherson-Wheeler blade
McPherson-Wheeler knife
McPherson-Ziegler knife
McQuigg clamp
McReynolds driver
McReynolds extractor
McReynolds hook
McReynolds keratome
McReynolds knife
McReynolds operation
McReynolds scissors
McReynolds spatula
McVay herniorrhaphy
McVay incision
McVay operation
McWhinnie dissector
McWhinnie electrode
McWhirter technique
McWhorter hemostat
Mead rongeur
Measuroll sutures
meat forceps
meat-grasping forceps
meatal
meatal clamp
meatal dilator
meatal incision
meatal sound
meatoantrotomy
meatoplasty
meatoscope
meatotome
    Bunge

meatotome *(continued)*
    electric
    Ellik
    Otis
    Riba electric ureteral
    ureteral
meatotomy
meatotomy electrode
meatotomy knife
meatus
meatus acustici externi nerve
meatus clamp
mechanical block
mechanical finger
mechanical ileus
mechanical obstruction
mechanical respirator
Meckel diverticulectomy
Meckel diverticulum
Meckel operation
meconium
Med-Neb respirator
Medallion lens expressor
media (*sing.* medium)
medial
medial border
medial collateral ligament
medial condyle
medial incision
medial ligament
medial malleolus
medial meniscectomy
medial meniscus
medial osteotomy
medial parapatellar incision
medially
median artery
median incision

median laryngotomy
median line
median nerve
median parapatellar incision
mediana antebrachii vein
mediana artery
mediana basilica vein
mediana cephalica vein
mediana cubiti vein
medianus nerve
mediastinal
mediastinal cannula
mediastinal veins
mediastinales veins
mediastinitis
mediastinoscope
mediastinoscopy
mediastinotomy
mediastinum
mediate amputation
medicated bougie
Medi-graft prosthesis
Meding tonsil enucleator
mediocarpal articulation
mediotarsal amputation
Mediplast
Meditape
medium (*pl.* media)
medium chromic sutures
medium forceps
medium screwdriver
Medrafil suture wire
Medtronic pacemaker
medulla (*pl.* medullae)
medullary
medullary canal
medullary canal reamer
medullary pin

medullary tube
medusa
Meek-Wall dermatome
Meeker forceps
meerschaum probe
megacolon
megalogastria
meibomian forceps
meibomian glands
Meigs curet
Meigs operation
Meigs sutures
melanoma
melanotic
melanotic whitlow
melena
Meller operation
Meller retractor
Meller spatula
Mellinger magnet
Mellinger speculum
meloplasty
Meltzer anesthesia
Meltzer nasopharyngoscope
Meltzer punch
membrana tympani
membrane
    alveolodental
    arachnoid
    basement
    basilar
    Bowman's
    Bruch's
    Descemet's
    drum
    false
    fenestrated
    fetal

membrane *(continued)*
    Henle's
    hyaline
    hyoglossal
    m. perforation
    m.-puncturing forceps
    mucous
    nuclear
    olfactory
    placental
    Reissner's
    Scarpa's
    serous
    synovial
    tympanic
    vitreous
membranous
membranous cataract
Menge operation
Menge pessary
Mengert index
Menghini needle
meningea anterior artery
meningea media artery
meningea posterior artery
meningeae mediae veins
meningeae veins
meningeal artery
meningeal veins
meningeorrhaphy
meninges
meningioma
meniscectomy
meniscectomy scissors
meniscofemoral ligaments
meniscotome
    Bowen-Grover
    Smillie

meniscus
meniscus knife
menometrorrhagia
menorrhagia
menstrual extraction
mental artery
mental nerve
mentalis artery
mentalis muscle
mentalis nerve
mentoplasty
Mentor bladder pacemaker
meperidine
mepivacaine hydrochloride
meprobamate
mEq (milliequivalents)
Merchant procedure
Mercier catheter
Mercier operation
Mercier sound
Mercurio position
mercury-filled esophageal bougie
Merindino procedure
Mermingas operation
merocrine gland
Merrifield knife
Mersilene gauze
Mersilene graft
Mersilene sutures
Merthiolate
mesenchymal
mesenchyme
mesenterectomy
mesenteric
mesenteric adenitis
mesenteric artery
mesenteric hernia
mesenteric vein

mesenterica inferior artery
mesenterica inferior vein
mesenterica superior artery
mesenterica superior vein
mesenteriopexy
mesenteriorrhaphy
mesenteriplication
mesentery
mesentorrhaphy
mesh
    Marlex
    Mylar
    Ortho-Mesh
    stainless steel
    tantalum
    Teflon
    Usher Marlex
    Vitallium
    wire
mesial
mesoappendicitis
mesoappendix
mesocecum
mesocolic
mesocolic hernia
mesocolon
mesocoloplication
mesogastrium
mesonephric duct
mesopexy
mesorectum
mesosalpinx
mesosigmoid
mesosigmoidopexy
metacarpal arteries
metacarpal bones
metacarpal saw
metacarpal splint

metacarpal veins
metacarpals
metacarpeae dorsales arteries
metacarpeae dorsales veins
metacarpeae palmares arteries
metacarpeae palmares veins
metacarpectomy
metacarpocarpal articulations
metacarpophalangeal articulations
metal applicator
metal band
metal band sutures
metal cannula
metal catheter
metal clamp
metal clip
metal locator (See also *magnet*)
    Berman
    Berman-Moorhead
    Wildgen-Reck
metal nail
metal pin
metal plate
metal prosthesis
metal rod
metal ruler
metal screw
metal sound
metal splint
metal syringe
metallic sphere introducer
metastasis (*pl.* metastases)
metastatic
metastatic carcinoma
metatarsal
metatarsal arteries
metatarsal bones
metatarsal splint

metatarsal veins
metatarsals
metatarseae dorsales arteries
metatarseae dorsales veins
metararseae plantares arteries
metatarseae plantares veins
metatarsectomy
metatarsophalangeal articulations
method
methohexital sodium
methoxyflurane
methyl methacrylate
methylene blue
meticulous
Metras catheter
metroplasty
metrorrhagia
Metycaine hydrochloride
Metzenbaum chisel
Metzenbaum forceps
Metzenbaum knife
Metzenbaum-Lipsett scissors
Metzenbaum scissors
Metzenbaum-Tyding forceps
Meyer-Halsted incision
Meyer hockey-stick incision
Meyer needle
Meyer retractor
Meyerding chisel
Meyerding curet
Meyerding-Deaver retractor
Meyerding gouge
Meyerding mallet
Meyerding osteotome
Meyerding retractor
Meyerding skid
Meyhoeffer curet
Meyhoeffer knife

MFB (metallic foreign body)
MGH (Massachusetts General Hospital)
MGH forceps
MGH osteotome
MGH periosteal elevator
mHg (millimeters of mercury)
Michel clamp
Michel clip
Michel forceps
Michel trephine
Michelson bronchoscope
Michigan forceps
micro-air drill
microcrimped prosthesis
microcurie
microdermatome
micro-forceps
microgastria
micro-mike
micro-needle
micro-needle holder
microphthalmus
micro-pin
micro-pin forceps
micropoint cautery
micropoint needle
microprobe surgical tape
micro-scissors
microscope
    aural
    Barraquer-Zeiss
    beta ray
    binocular
    capillary
    centrifuge
    color contrast
    comparison

microscope *(continued)*
    compound
    corneal
    darkfield
    Derlacki-Shambaugh
    electron
    epic
    epimicroscope
    fluorescence
    Greenough
    hypodermic
    infrared
    integrating
    interference
    ion
    laser
    light
    Olympus
    Omni operating
    opaque
    operating
    Oto-Microscope
    phase
    phase contrast
    photon
    polarizing
    projector x-ray
    rectified
    rectified polarizing
    reflecting
    Rheinberg
    scanning electron
    schlieren
    Shambaugh-Derlacki
    simple
    slit-lamp
    stereoscopic
    stroboscopic

microscope *(continued)*
    surgical
    television
    trinocular
    ultramicroscope
    ultrasonic
    ultraviolet
    x-ray
    Yasargil
    Zeiss
microscopic hook
microscopic scissors
microscopy
microsurgery
microsurgery retractor
microsurgical scissors
microsurgical spatula
microwave
microwave diathermy
micturition
mid forceps
mid-forceps delivery
midaxillary line
midcarpal joint
Middeldorpf splint
middle ear
middle ear aspirator
middle turbinate
Middleton curet
midfemoral block
midline incision
midportion
midsternum splitting incision
Mikulicz clamp
Mikulicz drain
Mikulicz enterectomy
Mikulicz forceps
Mikulicz gastrectomy

Mikulicz gastrotomy
Mikulicz incision
Mikulicz operation
Mikulicz tarsectomy
Mikulicz-Vladimiroff operation
Milch operation
Miles clamp
Miles operation
Miles proctosigmoidectomy
Milex forceps
Milex retractor
milium *(pl.* milia)
milk ducts
Millard operation
Miller-Abbott tube
Miller curet
Miller forceps
Miller laryngoscope
Miller operation
Miller retractor
Miller scissors
Miller-Senn retractor
Miller speculum
milliamperes (ma)
millicuries (mc)
milliequivalents (mEq)
Milliknit graft
Millin-Bacon retractor
Millin-Bacon spreader
Millin clamp
Millin forceps
Millin-Read operation
Millin retractor
Millin suction tube
Millin tube
milliner's needle
Mills forceps
Milwaukee brace

Mimer table
Miner osteotome
Minerva cast
Mingazzini-Förster operation
miniature electrotome
miniature forceps
miniature sound
minilaparotomy
Minilith pacemaker
minimal
minimum
Minneapolis prosthesis
minor amputation
minor connector bar
minor operation
minor surgery
minor surgery scissors
Minsky operation
Miochol
Mira cautery
Mira photocoagulator
Mira reamer
Mira unit
Mirault-Brown-Blair operation
Mirault operation
mirror cannula
mirror laryngoscope
missed abortion
mist
mist therapy
Mitchell-Diamond forceps
Mitchell knife
Mitchell operation
Mitchell stone basket
mitral commissurotomy
mitral dilator
mitral forceps
mitral insufficiency

mitral knife
mitral regurgitation
mitral stenosis knife
mitral valve
mitral valve dilator
mitral valve hinging operation
mitral valve-holding forceps
mitral valve prosthesis
mitral valve retractor
mitral valve spreader
mitral valvotomy
mitral valvulotomy
mixed amputation
mixed anesthesia
mixed glands
mixed hemorrhoids
mixed joint
mixed tumor
Mixter clamp
Mixter dilator
Mixter forceps
Mixter-McQuigg forceps
Mixter needle
Mixter probe
Mixter punch
Mixter scissors
Mixter tube
mm (millimeter)
MMM (microporous Minnesota
    Mining) (3M)
MMM dressing (3M dressing)
MMM drape (3M drape)
MMM Vi-Drape (3M Vi-Drape)
mobile
mobile cecum
mobility
mobilization
mobilized

mobilizer
    Derlacki
    ear
Mobin-Uddin filter
Mobin-Uddin umbrella
Mobitz heart block
modification
modified
modified flap operation
modified technique
modular knee prosthesis
Moe impactor
Moe plate
Moebius knife
Moehle forceps
Moersch bronchoscope
Moersch electrode
Moersch esophagoscope
Moersch forceps
Mohr clamp
Mohr splint
Mohrenheim fossa
moist dressing
moist gangrene
moist packs
moist tape
moistened tape
molar pregnancy
molars
mold
molded splint
mole
moleskin
Moll's glands
Mollison retractor
Mollo boots
Molt curet
Molt guillotine

Molt mouth gag
Molt periosteal elevator
Moltz-Storz tonsillectome
Moncrieff cannula
Moncrieff irrigator
monitor
monitoring
monitoring cannula
Monks-Esser flap
Monks operation
monocular bandage
monocular dressing
monocular patch
monofilament sutures
monofilament wire
monofilament wire sutures
monomer suction biopsy tube
monopolar cautery
Monroe-Kerr cesarean section
Monroe-Kerr incision
monster rongeur
Montague abrader
Montague proctoscope
Montague sigmoidoscope
Montefiore tube
Monteggia fracture
Montevideo units
Montgomery's glands
Montgomery speculum
Montgomery tapes
Moore-Blount driver
Moore-Blount extractor
Moore-Blount plate
Moore-Blount screwdriver
Moore button
Moore chisel
Moore-Corradi operation
Moore drill

Moore driver
Moore elevator
Moore extractor
Moore forceps
Moore fracture
Moore gouge
Moore hip prosthesis
Moore nail
Moore operation
Moore osteotome
Moore pin
Moore plate
Moore rasp
Moore reamer
Moore retractor
Moore scoop
Moore spoon
Moore thoracoscope
Moore tube
Moorehead clamp
Moorehead dissector
Moorehead elevator
Moorehead knife
Moorehead periosteotome
Moorehead retractor
Morax operation
morcellement
morcellement nephrectomy
Morch tube
Morel-Fatio blepharoplasty
Moreno clamp
Morestin operation
Morgagni foramen
morgagnian cataract
Morison incision
Morison method
Morison pouch
Moritz-Schmidt forceps

morphine
morphine sulfate
morphologic
morphology
Morris cannula
Morris catheter
Morris drain
Morris retractor
Morris splint
Morrison-Hurd dissector
Morrison-Hurd retractor
Morse-Andrews suction tube
Morse-Ferguson suction tube
Morse retractor
Morse scissors
Morse suction tube
Morson forceps
mortise
Morton stone dislodger
Morton's toe
Moschcowitz operation
Mosetig-Moorhof bone wax
Mosher curet
Mosher drain
Mosher esophagoscope
Mosher forceps
Mosher punch
Mosher retractor
Mosher speculum
Mosher suction tube
Mosher-Toti operation
Mosher tube
mosquito clamp
mosquito forceps
Moss tube
Motais operation
motility
Moult curet

Mount forceps
Mount-Mayfield forceps
Mount-Olivecrona forceps
Moure-Coryllos rib shears
Moure esophagoscope
mouse-tooth forceps
mouth gag
    Boyle Davis
    Brophy
    Collis
    Davis
    Davis-Crowe
    Denhardt
    Denhardt-Dingman
    Dingman
    Dingman-Denhardt
    Dott
    Doyen-Jansen
    Green
    Green-Sewall
    Hibbs
    Jennings
    Jennings-Skillern
    Kilner-Dott
    Lane
    Lewis
    McDowell
    McIvor
    Molt
    Ralks-Davis
    Roser
    side
    Sluder-Jansen
    Wesson
mouth-to-mouth resuscitation
movable kidney
moving strip x-ray technique
moxibustion

Moynihan clamp
Moynihan forceps
Moynihan gastrojejunostomy
Moynihan-Navratil forceps
Moynihan operation
Moynihan position
Moynihan probe
Moynihan scoop
Muck forceps
mucobuccal
mucocele
mucocutaneous
mucocutaneous hemorrhoid
mucogingival junction
mucoperichondrium
mucoperiosteal elevator
mucoperiosteum
mucopurulent
mucosa
mucosa elevator
mucosa knife
mucosa speculum
mucosal
mucosal hernia
mucotome
mucous (adjective)
mucous forceps
mucous glands
mucous membrane
mucous membrane graft
mucus (noun)
Mueller-Balfour retractor
Mueller bur
Mueller cautery
Mueller clamp
Mueller curet
Mueller forceps
Mueller-Frazier suction tube

Mueller-Frazier tube
Mueller hip prosthesis
Mueller-Laforce adenotome
Mueller needle
Mueller operation
Mueller-Pool suction tube
Mueller-Pool tube
Mueller-Pynchon suction tube
Mueller-Pynchon tube
Mueller retractor
Mueller saw
Mueller scissors
Mueller speculum
Mueller suction tube
Mueller tongue blade
Mueller tonometer
Mueller trephine
Mueller-Yankauer suction tube
Mueller-Yankauer tube
Muer anoscope
Muir clamp
Muldoon dilator
Muldoon tube
Mules eye implant
Mules implant
Mules operation
Mules scoop
Müller cesarean section
Müller maneuver
Müller sclerectomy
Müller vaginal hysterectomy
müllerian duct
Mulligan prosthesis
multangulum majus
multifidi muscles
multifidus muscles
multifilament sutures
multifilament wire

multifocal
multiholed tube
multi-lead electrode
multilocular
multinodular
multiparity
multiple
multiple-action rongeur
multiple amputation
multiple biopsy
multiple fasciotomies
multiple fractures
multiple-lumen tube
multiple-point electrode
multiple resectoscope
multiple tenotomies
Multipoise headrest
multipurpose forceps
multipurpose instruments
multistrand sutures
Mumford Gigli-saw guide
Mumford-Gurd operation
Mumford operation
Mundie forceps
Munnell operation
Munro retractor
Munro scissors
Murdock speculum
Murdock-Wiener speculum
murmur
Murphy brace
Murphy button
Murphy chisel
Murphy dilator
Murphy forceps
Murphy gouge
Murphy hook
Murphy knife

Murphy-Lane skid
Murphy needle
Murphy punch
Murphy reamer
Murphy retractor
Murphy scissors
Murphy tube
muscle (muscles)*
    abductor
    adductor
    anconeus
    antitragus
    arrector m's of hair
    articular
    aryepiglottic
    arytenoid
    auricular
    biceps
    brachial
    brachioradial
    bronchoesophageal
    buccinator
    bulbocavernous
    canine
    ceratocricoid
    chin
    chondroglossus
    ciliary
    coccygeal
    constrictor
    coracobrachial
    corrugator
    cremaster
    cricoarytenoid
    cricothyroid

*m. = muscle
 m's = muscles

muscle (muscles) *(continued)*
    deltoid
    depressor
    detrusor urinae
    epicranial
    erector
    extensor
    fibular
    flexor
    gastrocnemius
    gemellus
    genioglossus
    geniohyoid
    glossopalatine
    gluteus maximus
    gluteus medius
    gluteus minimus
    gracilis
    hyoglossal
    iliac
    iliococcygeal
    iliocostal
    iliopsoas
    incisive
    infraspinous
    intercostal
    interosseous
    interspinal
    intertransverse
    ischiocavernous
    latissimus dorsi
    levator
    levator ani
    long
    longissimus
    longitudinal
    lumbrical
    masseter

muscle (muscles)* *(continued)*
- multifidus
- m. advancement
- m. clamp
- m. forceps
- m. guarding
- m. hook
- m. incision
- m. of helix
- m. of incisure of helix
- m. of tragus
- m. of uvula
- m.-recession forceps
- m. relaxants
- m. retractor
- m.-splitting hook
- m.-splitting incision
- m. tone
- mylohyoid
- nasal
- oblique
- obturator
- occipitofrontal
- omohyoid
- opposing
- orbicular
- orbital
- palatoglossus
- palatopharyngeal
- palmar
- papillary
- pectinate
- pectineal
- pectoral
- peroneal

*m. = muscle
 m's = muscles

muscle (muscles) *(continued)*
- piriform
- plantar
- platysma
- pleuroesophageal
- popliteal
- procerus
- pronator
- psoas
- pterygoid
- pubococcygeal
- puboprostatic
- puborectal
- pubovaginal
- pubovesical
- pyramidal
- quadrate
- quadriceps
- rectococcygeus
- rectourethral
- rectouterine
- rectovesical
- rectus
- rhomboid
- risorius
- rotator
- sacrococcygeal
- salpingopharyngeal
- sartorius
- scalene
- semimembranous
- semispinal
- semitendinous
- serratus
- soleus
- sphincter
- spinal
- splenius

muscle (muscles)* *(continued)*
- stapedius
- sternal
- sternocleidomastoid
- sternocostal
- sternohyoid
- sternothyroid
- styloglossus
- stylohyoid
- stylopharyngeus
- subclavius
- subcostal
- subscapular
- supinator
- supraspinous
- suspensory
- tarsal
- temporal
- temporoparietal
- tensor
- teres major
- teres minor
- thyroarytenoid
- thyroepiglottic
- thyrohyoid
- tibial
- tracheal
- transverse
- transversospinal
- trapezius
- triangular
- triceps
- vastus
- vertical
- vocal

muscle (muscles) *(continued)*
- zygomatic

muscular

musculature

musculocutaneous

musculocutaneous amputation

musculocutaneous flap

musculocutaneous nerve

musculophrenic artery

musculophrenic veins

musculophrenica artery

musculophrenicae veins

musculoplasty

musculotendinous cuff

musculus (*pl.* musculi)*
- m. abductor digiti minimi manus
- m. abductor digiti minimi pedis
- m. abductor hallucis
- m. abductor pollicis brevis
- m. abductor pollicis longus
- m. adductor brevis
- m. adductor hallucis
- m. adductor longus
- m. adductor magnus
- m. adductor pollicis
- m. anconeus
- m. antitragicus
- mm. arrectores pilorum
- m. articularis cubiti
- m. articularis genus
- m. aryepiglotticus
- m. arytenoideus obliquus
- m. arytenoideus transversus

*m. = muscle
m's = muscles

*m. = musculus [*L.*]
mm. = musculi [*L.*, pl.]

musculus (*pl.* musculi)*
   (continued)
      m. auricularis anterior
      m. auricularis posterior
      m. auricularis superior
      m. biceps brachii
      m. biceps femoris
      m. brachialis
      m. brachioradialis
      m. bronchoesophageus
      m. buccinator
      m. bulbocavernosus
      m. bulbospongiosus
      m. ceratocricoideus
      m. chondroglossus
      m. ciliaris
      m. coccygeus
      m. constrictor pharyngis
        inferior
      m. constrictor pharyngis
        medius
      m. constrictor pharyngis
        superior
      m. coracobrachialis
      m. corrugator supercilii
      m. cremaster
      m. cricoarytenoideus
        lateralis
      m. cricoarytenoideus
        posterior
      m. cricothyroideus
      m. deltoideus
      m. depressor anguli oris
      m. depressor labii inferioris
      m. depressor septi nasi

*m. = musculus [*L.*]
 mm. = musculi [*L.*, pl.]

musculus (*pl.* musculi)*
   (continued)
      m. depressor supercilii
      m. digastricus
      m. dilator pupillae
      m. epicranius
      m. erector spinae
      m. extensor carpi radialis
        brevis
      m. extensor carpi radialis
        longus
      m. extensor carpi ulnaris
      m. extensor digiti minimi
      m. extensor digitorum
      m. extensor digitorum brevis
      m. extensor digitorum
        longus
      m. extensor hallucis brevis
      m. extensor hallucis longus
      m. extensor indicis
      m. extensor pollicis brevis
      m. extensor pollicis longus
      m. flexor carpi radialis
      m. flexor carpi ulnaris
      m. flexor digiti minimi
        brevis manus
      m. flexor digiti minimi
        brevis pedis
      m. flexor digitorum brevis
        pedis
      m. flexor digitorum longus
        pedis
      m. flexor digitorum pro-
        fundus
      m. flexor digitorum super-
        ficialis
      m. flexor hallucis brevis
      m. flexor hallucis longus

musculus (*pl.* musculi)*
  (continued)
    m. flexor pollicis brevis
    m. flexor pollicis longus
    m. gastrocnemius
    m. gemellus inferior
    m. gemellus superior
    m. genioglossus
    m. geniohyoideus
    m. gluteus maximus
    m. gluteus medius
    m. gluteus minimus
    m. gracilis
    m. helicis major
    m. helicis minor
    m. hyoglossus
    m. iliacus
    m. iliococcygeus
    m. iliocostalis
    m. iliocostalis cervicis
    m. iliocostalis lumborum
    m. iliocostalis thoracis
    m. iliopsoas
    m. incisivi labii inferioris
    m. incisivi labii superioris
    m. incisurae helicis
    m. infraspinatus
    mm. intercostales
    mm. intercostales externi
    mm. intercostales interni
    mm. interossei dorsales
      manus
    mm. interossei dorsales
      pedis
    mm. interossei palmares

*m. = musculus [*L.*]
  mm. = musculi [*L.*, pl.]

musculus (*pl.* musculi)*
  (continued)
    mm. interossei plantares
    mm. interspinales
    mm. intertransversarii
    m. ischiocavernosus
    m. latissimus dorsi
    m. levator anguli oris
    m. levator ani
    m. levator glandulae
      thyroideae
    m. levator labii superioris
    m. levator labii superioris
      alaeque nasi
    m. levator palpebrae
      superioris
    m. levator prostate
    m. levator scapulae
    m. levator veli palatini
    mm. levatores costarum
    m. longissimus capitis
    m. longissimus cervicis
    m. longissimus thoracis
    m. longitudinalis superior
      linguae
    m. longus capitis
    m. longus colli
    mm. lumbricales manus
    mm. lumbricales pedis
    m. masseter
    m. mentalis
    mm. multifidi
    m. mylohyoideus
    m. nasalis
    m. obliquus auriculae
    m. obliquus capitis inferior
    m. obliquus capitis superior

musculus (*pl.* musculi)*
    (*continued*)
        m. obliquus externus
          abdominis
        m. obliquus inferior bulbi
        m. obliquus internus
          abdominis
        m. obliquus superior bulbi
        m. obturatorius externus
        m. obturatorius internus
        m. occipitofrontalis
        m. omohyoideus
        m. opponens digiti minimi
          manus
        m. opponens pollicis
        m. orbicularis oculi
        m. orbicularis oris
        m. orbitalis
        m. palatoglossus
        m. palatopharyngeus
        m. palmaris brevis
        m. palmaris longus
        mm. papillares
        mm. pectinati
        m. pectineus
        m. pectoralis major
        m. pectoralis minor
        m. peroneus brevis
        m. peroneus longus
        m. peroneus tertius
        m. piriformis
        m. plantaris
        m. pleuroesophageus
        m. popliteus
        m. procerus

*m. = musculus [*L.*]
 mm. = musculi [*L.*, pl.]

musculus (*pl.* musculi)*
    (*continued*)
        m. pronator quadratus
        m. pronator teres
        m. psoas major
        m. psoas minor
        m. pterygoideus lateralis
        m. pterygoideus medialis
        m. pubococcygeus
        m. puboprostaticus
        m. puborectalis
        m. pubovaginalis
        m. pyramidalis
        m. pyramidalis auriculae
        m. quadratus femoris
        m. quadratus lumborum
        m. quadratus plantae
        m. quadriceps femoris
        m. rectococcygeus
        m. rectourethralis
        m. rectouterinus
        m. rectovesicalis
        m. rectus abdominis
        m. rectus capitis anterior
        m. rectus capitis lateralis
        m. rectus capitis posterior
          major
        m. rectus capitis posterior
          minor
        m. rectus femoris
        m. rectus inferior bulbi
        m. rectus lateralis bulbi
        m. rectus medialis bulbi
        m. rectus superior bulbi
        m. rhomboideus major
        m. rhomboideus minor
        m. risorius
        mm. rotatores

musculus (*pl.* musculi)*
    (continued)

m. sacrococcygeus dorsalis
m. sacrococcygeus ventralis
m. salpingopharyngeus
m. sartorius
m. scalenus anterior
m. scalenus medius
m. scalenus minimus
m. scalenus posterior
m. semimembranosus
m. semispinalis capitis
m. semispinalis cervicis
m. semispinalis thoracis
m. semitendinosus
m. serratus anterior
m. serratus posterior inferior
m. serratus posterior
  superior
m. soleus
m. sphincter
m. sphincter ampullae
  hepatopancreaticae
m. sphincter ani externus
m. sphincter ani internus
m. sphincter ductus
  choledochi
m. sphincter pupillae
m. sphincter pylori
m. sphincter urethrae
m. sphincter vesicae
  urinariae
m. spinalis capitis
m. spinalis cervicis
m. spinalis thoracis

*m. = musculus [*L.*]
 mm. = musculi [*L.*, pl.]

musculus (*pl.* musculi)*
    (continued)

m. splenius capitis
m. splenius cervicis
m. stapedius
m. sternalis
m. sternocleidomastoideus
m. sternohyoideus
m. sternothyroideus
m. styloglossus
m. stylohyoideus
m. stylopharyngeus
m. subclavius
mm. subcostales
m. subscapularis
m. supinator
m. supraspinatus
m. suspensorius
m. tarsalis inferior
m. tarsalis superior
m. temporalis
m. temporoparietalis
m. tensor fasciae latae
m. tensor tympani
m. tensor veli palatini
m. teres major
m. teres minor
m. thyroarytenoideus
m. thyroepiglotticus
m. thyrohyoideus
m. tibialis anterior
m. tibialis posterior
m. trachealis
m. tragicus
m. transversospinalis
m. transversus abdominis
m. transversus auriculae
m. transversus linguae

musculus (*pl.* musculi)*
  (continued)
    m. transversus menti
    m. transversus nuchae
    m. transversus perinei
      profundus
    m. transversus perinei
      superficialis
    m. transversus thoracis
    m. trapezius
    m. triceps brachii
    m. triceps surae
    m. uvulae
    m. vastus intermedius
    m. vastus lateralis
    m. vastus medialis
    m. verticalis linguae
    m. vocalis
    m. zygomaticus major
    m. zygomaticus minor
Museholdt forceps
mushroom catheter
Musken tonometer
mustache dressing
Mustard intra-atrial operation
Mustarde otoplasty
myasthenia
mydriasis
myectomy
myelogram
myelography
myelotomy
Myers forceps
Myers punch
Myers retractor

*m. = musculus [*L.*]
  mm. = musculi [*L.*, pl.]

Myers vein stripper
Myerson electrode
Myerson forceps
Myerson punch
Myerson saw
Myerson trocar
Mylar mesh
Myles adenotome
Myles cannula
Myles clamp
Myles curet
Myles forceps
Myles punch
Myles snare
Myles speculum
Myles tonsillectome
mylohyoid line
mylohyoid muscle
mylohyoid nerve
mylohyoideus muscle
mylohyoideus nerve
myocardial clamp
myocardial electrode
myocardial infarction
myocardiectomy
myocardiotomy
myocardium
myoma (*pl.* myomata)
myomata uteri
myomectomy
myometrium
myonephropexy
myoneural junction
myopia
myoplasty
myorrhaphy
myosuture
myotasis

myotenontoplasty
myotenotomy
myotomy
myotonic cataract
myringectomy
myringodectomy
myringoplasty
myringoplasty knife

myringostapediopexy
myringotome
myringotome knife
myringotomy
myringotomy incision
myrintotomy knife
myringotomy tube
myxoglobulosis appendicitis

n

Nabatoff vein stripper
nabothian cyst
nabothian follicle
Nachlas tube
nadbath anesthetic
nadir
Naffziger operation
Naffziger-Poppen Crain orbital
   decompression
Nagamatsu incision
nail
       adjustable
       Augustine
       Badgley
       Barr
       boat
       cannulated
       cloverleaf
       Curry hip
       diamond
       Dooley
       Engel-May
       four-flanged
       fracture
       Hansen-Street
       hip
       hooked
       intramedullary
       Jewett
       K-nail
       Ken
       Knowles pin

nail *(continued)*
       Küntscher
       Lottes
       Massie
       McLaughlin
       metal
       Moore
       n. bed
       n. extractor
       n. plate
       Neufeld
       noncannulated
       osteotomy
       Pugh
       Richards
       Rush
       Sampson
       Schneider
       self-adjusting
       self-broaching
       Smillie
       Smith-Petersen
       Steinmann
       Temple University
       Thatcher
       Thornton
       three-flanged
       Tiemann
       triflange intramedullary
       V-medullary
       Venable-Stuck
       Vesely-Street

nail *(continued)*
      Vitallium
      Webb
nailing
Nalline
nanogram (ng)
naphthalinic cataract
napkin-ring lesion
Narath omentopexy
Narath operation
narcosis
narcotic agents
narcotic antagonists
naris (*pl.* nares)
narrow elevator
narrow retractor
narrowing
nasal arteries
nasal bone
nasal chisel
nasal curet
nasal-cutting forceps
nasal-dressing forceps
nasal duct
nasal elevator
nasal forceps
nasal fossa
nasal gouge
nasal-grasping forceps
nasal hump-cutting forceps
nasal incision
nasal knife
nasal muscle
nasal-packing forceps
nasal polyp
nasal polyp forceps
nasal polyp hook
nasal polypectomy

nasal probe
nasal punch
nasal rasp
nasal reconstruction
nasal retractor
nasal rongeur
nasal saw
nasal scissors
nasal septoplasty
nasal septum
nasal snare
nasal speculum
nasal splint
nasal suction tip
nasal suction tube
nasal tube
nasal veins
nasales externae veins
nasales posteriores laterales et
      septi arteries
nasalis muscle
nasociliaris nerve
nasociliary nerve
naso-endotracheal anesthesia
nasofrontal vein
nasofrontalis vein
nasogastric
nasogastric feeding tube
nasogastric suction
nasogastric tube
nasolabial
nasolacrimal duct
nasolacrimal tube
nasomaxillary suture
nasopalatine nerve
nasopalatinus nerve
nasopharyngeal applicator
nasopharyngeal pack

nasopharyngeal retractor
nasopharyngeal speculum
nasopharyngeal tube
nasopharyngoscope
     ACMI
     Broyles
     Holmes
     Meltzer
     Yankauer
nasopharynx
nasotracheal catheter
nasotracheal intubation anesthesia
nasotracheal tube
natal cleft
Nathan pacemaker
National cautery
National cystoscope
National instruments
National proctoscope
National speculum
nausea
navel
navicular bone
navicular fossa
Neal cannula
Neal catheter
near-and-far sutures
Nebinger-Praun operation
neck extension position
necro-purulent appendicitis
necropsy
necrosis (*pl.* necroses)
necrotic
needle (See also *suture needle.*)
     abdominal
     Abrams
     abscission
     Adson

needle *(continued)*
     Adson-Murphy
     Agnew
     Alexander
     Amsler
     aneurysm
     angiography
     angular
     antrum
     aortic vent
     aortogram
     aortography
     arterial
     arteriogram
     artery
     aspirating
     atraumatic
     Babcock
     Barker
     Barrett
     Beyer
     biopsy
     bipolar
     Blair-Brown
     blunt
     bone biopsy
     Bonney
     Bovie
     Bowman
     brain biopsy
     Brockenbrough
     Brophy
     Brophy-Deschamps
     Brown
     Bunnell
     Calhoun
     Calhoun-Merz
     Campbell

needle *(continued)*

- cataract
- catheter
- caudal
- cerebral angiography
- cervical
- Charles
- Charlton
- chemopallidectomy
- Child-Phillips
- Clagett
- cleft palate
- Cloquet
- Colver
- cone
- Conrad-Crosby
- Cooper
- Cope
- corneal
- couching
- Cournand
- Cournand-Grino
- Craig
- Curry
- curved
- Cushing
- cutting
- cyclodiathermy
- dacryocystorhinostomy
- Damshek
- Dandy
- Davis
- Dean
- debridement
- Dees
- Deknatel
- Denis Browne
- DePuy-Weiss

needle *(continued)*

- Deschamps
- Deschamps-Navratil
- desiccation
- desiccation-fulguration
- Desmarres
- diathermy
- Dingman
- discission
- Dix
- Docktor
- Dorsey
- Dos Santos
- Doyen
- Drapier
- Durham
- Emmet
- epilation
- Epstein
- exploring
- fascia
- Fein
- Ferguson
- Fischer
- fish-hook
- fistula
- Floyd
- Flynt
- Frackelton
- Francke
- Frankfeldt
- Franklin-Silverman
- Frazier
- Frederick
- French-eye
- Gallie
- Gardner
- gastrointestinal

needle *(continued)*
- Gillmore
- Goldbacher
- Graefe
- Grantham
- Grieshaber
- Hagedorn
- Hajek
- Halle
- Halsey
- harelip
- Harken
- heart
- hemorrhoidal
- Henton
- Hoen
- Holinger
- Hourin
- House
- House-Barbara
- House-Rosen
- Hunt
- Hutchins
- hypodermic
- Illinois
- Ingersoll
- injection
- intestinal
- intestinal plication
- iris
- iris knife
- Jameson
- Jamshidi
- Jelco
- Kader
- Kalt
- Kaplan
- Karras

needle *(continued)*
- Keith
- Kelly
- King
- Klatskin
- Knapp
- knife
- Kobak
- Kohn
- Kronecker
- lacrimal
- Lahey
- Lane
- Lapides
- Lewy-Rubin
- Lichtwicz
- ligature
- Lindeman
- Linton-Blakemore
- liver biopsy
- lobotomy
- lock
- long
- Longdwel
- Lowsley
- Luer
- lumbar aortography
- lumbar puncture
- Lundy
- Lundy-Irving
- Luongo
- Maddox
- Magielski
- Maltz
- Martin
- Masson
- Mayo
- McCurdy

needle *(continued)*
    Menghini
    Meyer
    micro-needle
    micropoint
    milliner's
    Mixter
    Mueller
    Murphy
    n. biopsy
    n. electrode
    n. holder (see separate listing)
    n. probe
    Nelson
    New's
    Newman
    Overholt
    palpating
    Paparella
    paracentesis
    Parhad-Poppen
    Parker
    Penfield
    percutaneous
    Pereyra
    Pitkin
    pleural biopsy
    pneumothorax
    pneumothorax injection
    Poppen
    Potter
    Potts
    prostatic biopsy
    puncture
    radium
    rectal
    rectal injection
    renal

needle *(continued)*
    Retter
    Reverdin
    rib
    ribbon gut
    Riedel
    Riley
    Robb
    Rochester
    Rolf lance
    Rosen
    Roser
    Ross
    Rubin
    Ruskin
    Sachs
    Salah
    Sanders-Brown-Shaw
    Saunders
    Saunders-Paparella
    Schuknecht
    Scoville
    Sedlinger
    septum
    Shambaugh
    Sheldon-Spatz
    Sheldon-Swann
    Shirodkar
    short
    Silverman
    ski
    Sluder
    Smiley-Williams
    spatula
    spinal
    staphylorrhaphy
    sternal
    sternal puncture

needle *(continued)*

    Stocker
    stop
    strabismus
    Strauss
    Sturmdorf
    suction biopsy
    suture (see separate listing)
    suturing
    Sutton
    swaged
    taper-point
    Tapercut
    tattooing
    Teflon-covered
    THI
    Titus
    Todd
    tonsil
    Travenol
    trocar-point
    TruCut
    Tuohy
    Turkel
    University of Illinois
    Updegraff
    uterine
    vacuuming
    Veenema-Gusberg
    venipuncture
    venoclysis
    ventricular
    Verres
    Vim
    Vim-Silverman
    von Graefe
    Voorhees
    Walker

needle *(continued)*

    Wangensteen
    Ward
    Ward-French
    Watson-Williams
    Weeks
    Wertheim-Navratil
    Wood
    Yankauer
    Ziegler
    Zoellner

needle holder

    Adaptic
    adhesive
    Adson
    angular
    angulated
    Barraquer
    boomerang
    Boynton
    Bozeman-Wertheim
    Castroviejo
    Castroviejo-Kalt
    Collier
    Crile
    Crile-Murray
    Crile-Wood
    curved
    Davis
    DeBakey
    Derf
    Diamond
    dry
    Ellis
    Finochietto
    French-eye
    Gardner
    Gillies

needle holder *(continued)*
    Grant
    Green
    Grieshaber
    Halsey
    Heaney
    Hegar
    Johns Hopkins
    Johnson
    Julian
    K-S adhesive
    Kalt
    Lapides
    Masson
    Mayo
    Mayo-Hegar
    McAllister
    McPherson
    micro-needle holder
    Neivert
    Paton
    plastic
    prostatic
    Sarot
    Stille-French
    Stratte
    taper-point
    Troutman-Barraquer
    vascular
    Wangensteen
    Young
    Young-Millin
needling
needling of lens
Neef hammer
Neer shoulder prosthesis
Negus bronchoscope
Negus telescope

Neisser syringe
Neisseria
Neisseria gonorrhea
Neivert dissector
Neivert-Eves snare
Neivert hook
Neivert knife
Neivert needle holder
Neivert retractor
Neivert snare
Nélaton catheter
Nélaton operation
Nélaton probe
Nelson-Bethune rib shears
Nelson forceps
Nelson needle
Nelson rib spreader
Nelson rib stripper
Nelson-Roberts stripper
Nelson scissors
Nelson trocar
Nembutal
Neo-Synephrine
neocystostomy
neodymium laser
neomycin
neoplasia
neoplasm
neoplastic
neoplastic fracture
neoplasty
Neosporin
neostigmine
neo-ureterocystotomy
neovascularization
nephrectomy
nephrocolic ligament
nephrocolopexy

nephrocystanastomosis
nephrogram
nephrography
nephrolithiasis
nephrolithotomy
nephrolithotomy forceps
nephrolysis
nephropexy
nephroplasty
nephroptosis
nephropyelolithotomy
nephropyeloplasty
nephropyeloureterostomy
nephrorrhaphy
nephroscopy
nephrostomy
nephrostomy catheter
nephrostomy clamp
nephrostomy hook
nephrostomy tube
nephrotome plate
nephrotomogram
nephrotomography
nephrotomy
nephroureterectomy
nephroureterocystectomy
nerve (nerves)*
    abducens (cranial nerve VI)
    abducent
    accessory (cranial nerve XI)
    acoustic
    alveolar
    ampullary
    anococcygeal
    auditory

nerve (nerves) *(continued)*
    auricular
    axillary
    buccal
    cardiac
    caroticotympanic
    carotid
    cavernous n's of clitoris
    cavernous n's of penis
    cerebral
    cervical
    ciliary
    clunial
    coccygeal
    cochlear
    cranial
    cranial nerve I (olfactory)
    cranial nerve II (optic)
    cranial nerve III (oculo-
      motor)
    cranial nerve IV (trochlear)
    cranial nerve V (trigeminal)
    cranial nerve VI (abducens)
    cranial nerve VII (facial)
    cranial nerve VIII (vestibulo-
      cochlear)
    cranial nerve IX (glosso-
      pharyngeal)
    cranial nerve X (vagus)
    cranial nerve XI (accessory)
    cranial nerve XII (hypo-
      glossal)
    cubital
    cutaneous
    digital
    dorsal n. of clitoris
    dorsal n. of penis
    ethmoidal

*n. = nerve
 n's = nerves

nerve (nerves)* *(continued)*

facial (cranial nerve VII)
femoral
fibular
frontal
genitofemoral
glossopharyngeal (cranial
  nerve IX)
gluteal
hemorrhoidal
hypogastric
hypoglossal (cranial nerve
  XII)
iliohypogastric
ilioinguinal
infraoccipital
infraorbital
infratrochlear
intercostobrachial
intermediate
interosseous
ischiadic
jugular
labial
laryngeal
lingual
lumbar
mandibular
masseteric
maxillary
median
mental
musculocutaneous
mylohyoid
nasociliary

*n. = nerve
 n's = nerves

nerve (nerves) *(continued)*

nasopalatine
n. block
n. blocking anesthesia
n. fibers
n. graft
n. hook
n. of pterygoid canal
n. of tensor tympani
n. of tensor veli palatini
n. retractor
n. root
n. root resection
n. root-retractor
n. root transection
n. separator
n. stimulator
n. sutures
n. tract
obturator
occipital
oculomotor (cranial nerve
  III)
olfactory (cranial nerve I)
ophthalmic
optic (cranial nerve II)
palatine
perineal
peroneal
petrosal
phrenic
plantar
pneumogastric
pterygoid
pterygopalatine
pudendal
radial
rectal

nerve (nerves)* *(continued)*
- recurrent
- saccular
- sacral
- saphenous
- sciatic
- scrotal
- spinal
- splanchnic
- stapedius
- subclavian
- subcostal
- sublingual
- suboccipital
- subscapular
- supraclavicular
- supraorbital
- suprascapular
- supratrochlear
- sural
- temporal
- thoracic
- thoracodorsal
- tibial
- trigeminal (cranial nerve V)
- trochlear (cranial nerve IV)
- tympanic
- ulnar
- utricular
- vaginal
- vagus (cranial nerve X)
- vertebral
- vestibulocochlear (cranial nerve VIII)
- vidian

nerve (nerves) *(continued)*
- zygomatic

nervus (*pl.* nervi)*
- n. abducens
- n. accessorius
- nn. alveolares superiores
- n. alveolaris inferior
- n. ampullaris anterior
- n. ampullaris lateralis
- n. ampullaris posterior
- nn. anococcygei
- nn. auriculares anteriores
- n. auricularis magnus
- n. auricularis posterior
- n. auriculotemporalis
- n. axillaris
- n. buccalis
- n. canalis pterygoidei
- nn. cardiaci thoracici
- n. cardiacus cervicalis inferior
- n. cardiacus cervicalis medius
- n. cardiacus cervicalis superior
- nn. carotici externi
- n. caroticotympanici
- n. caroticus internus
- nn. cavernosi clitoridis
- nn. cavernosi penis
- nn. cervicales
- nn. ciliares breves
- nn. ciliares longi
- nn. clunium inferiores
- nn. clunium medii

*n. = nerve
 n's = nerves

*n. = nervus [*L.*]
 nn. = nervi [*L.*, pl.]

nervus (*pl.* nervi)* *(continued)*
    nn. clunium superiores
    n. coccygeus
    nn. craniales
    n. cutaneus antebrachii
        lateralis
    n. cutaneus antebrachii
        medialis
    n. cutaneus antebrachii
        posterior
    n. cutaneus brachii lateralis
        inferior
    n. cutaneus brachii lateralis
        superior
    n. cutaneus brachii medialis
    n. cutaneus brachii posterior
    n. cutaneus dorsalis inter-
        medius
    n. cutaneus dorsalis lateralis
    n. cutaneus dorsalis medialis
    n. cutaneus femoris lateralis
    n. cutaneus femoris
        posterior
    n. cutaneus surae lateralis
    n. cutaneus surae medialis
    nn. digitales dorsales hallucis
        lateralis et digiti secundi
        medialis
    nn. digitales dorsales nervi
        radialis
    nn. digitales dorsales nervi
        ulnaris
    nn. digitales dorsales pedis
    nn. digitales palmares com-
        munes nervi mediani

*n. = nervus [*L.*]
 nn. = nervi [*L.*, pl.]

nervus (*pl.* nervi)* *(continued)*
    nn. digitales palmares com-
        munes nervi ulnaris
    nn. digitales palmares pro-
        prii nervi mediani
    nn. digitales palmares pro-
        prii nervi ulnaris
    nn. digitales plantares com-
        munes nervi plantaris
        lateralis
    nn. digitales plantares com-
        munes nervi plantaris
        medialis
    nn. digitales plantares pro-
        prii nervi plantaris lateralis
    nn. digitales plantares pro-
        prii nervi plantaris medialis
    n. dorsalis clitoridis
    n. dorsalis penis
    n. dorsalis scapulae
    n. ethmoidalis anterior
    n. ethmoidalis posterior
    n. facialis
    n. femoralis
    n. fibularis
    n. frontalis
    n. genitofemoralis
    n. glossopharyngeus
    n. gluteus inferior
    n. gluteus superior
    n. hypogastricus dexter
    n. hypogastricus sinister
    n. hypoglossus
    n. iliohypogastricus
    n. ilioinguinalis
    n. infraorbitalis
    n. infratrochlearis
    nn. intercostobrachiales

nervus (*pl.* nervi)* *(continued)*
- n. intermedius
- n. interosseus anterior
- n. interosseus cruris
- n. interosseus posterior
- n. ischiadicus
- n. jugularis
- nn. labiales anteriores
- nn. labiales posteriores
- n. lacrimalis
- n. laryngeus inferior
- n. laryngeus recurrens
- n. laryngeus superior
- n. lingualis
- nn. lumbales
- n. mandibularis
- n. massetericus
- n. maxillaris
- n. meatus acustici externi
- n. medianus
- n. mentalis
- n. musculocutaneus
- n. mylohyoideus
- n. nasociliaris
- n. nasopalatinus
- n. obturatorius
- n. occipitalis major
- n. occipitalis minor
- n. occipitalis tertius
- n. oculomotorius
- nn. olfactorii
- n. ophthalmicus
- n. opticus
- nn. palatini minores
- n. palatinus major

nervus (*pl.* nervi)* *(continued)*
- nn. perineales
- n. peroneus communis
- n. peroneus profundus
- n. peroneus superficialis
- n. petrosus major
- n. petrosus minor
- n. petrosus profundus
- nn. phrenici accessorii
- n. phrenicus
- n. plantaris lateralis
- n. pterygoideus lateralis
- n. pterygoideus medialis
- nn. pterygopalatini
- n. pudendus
- n. radialis
- nn. rectales inferiores
- n. saccularis
- nn. sacrales
- n. saphenus
- nn. scrotales anteriores
- nn. scrotales posteriores
- nn. spinales
- nn. splanchnici lumbales
- nn. splanchnici pelvini
- nn. splanchnici sacrales
- n. splanchnicus imus
- n. splanchnicus major
- n. splanchnicus minor
- n. stapedius
- n. subclavius
- n. subcostalis
- n. sublingualis
- n. suboccipitalis
- n. subscapularis
- nn. supraclaviculares intermedii

*n. = nervus [*L.*]
 nn. = nervi [*L.*, pl.]

nervus (*pl.* nervi)* *(continued)*
    nn. supraclaviculares laterales
    nn. supraclaviculares mediales
    n. supraorbitalis
    n. suprascapularis
    n. supratrochlearis
    n. suralis
    nn. temporales profundi
    n. tensoris tympani
    n. tensoris veli palatini
    nn. thoracici
    n. thoracicus longus
    n. thoracodorsalis tibialis
    n. transversus colli
    n. trigeminus
    n. trochlearis
    n. tympanicus
    n. ulnaris
    n. utricularis
    n. utriculoampullaris
    nn. vaginales
    n. vagus
    n. vertebralis
    n. vestibulocochlearis
    n. zygomaticus
Nesacaine
Nesacaine-CE
Nesbit cystoscope
Nesbit electrode
Nesbit electrotome
Nesbit hemostatic bag
Nesbit operation
Nesbit resectoscope

Nesbit snare
nested trocar
Nettleship-Wilder dilator
Neubeiser splint
Neuber operation
Neuber tube
Neufeld driver
Neufeld nail
Neufeld plate
Neufeld screw
Neurain drill
Neurairtome drill
neural
neurectasia
neurectomy
neurexeresis
neuroanastomosis
neurogenic fracture
neurological
neurological scissors
neurolysis
neuroma
neuromuscular junction
neuroplasty
neurorrhaphy
neurosurgery
neurosurgical bur
neurosurgical headrest
neurosurgical light
neurotome
    enucleation
    Hall
neurotomy
neurotripsy
neurovascular bundle
neutral electrode
neutral position

*n. = nervus [*L.*]
  nn. = nervi [*L.*, pl.]

nevus (*pl.* nevi)
New-Lamobtte osteotome
New Orleans Eye and Ear forceps
New Orleans loupe
New Orleans stripper
New's electrode
New's forceps
New's hook
New's needle
New's scissors
New's tube
Newman forceps
Newman hook
Newman knife
Newman needle
Newman proctoscope
Newman tenaculum
ng (nanogram)
NG (nasogastric)
NG tube
niche
Nichols clamp
Nichols rongeur
Nichols speculum
Nicola clamp
Nicola gouge
Nicola operation
Nicola raspatory
Nida operation
Niebauer prosthesis
Niedner clamp
Niedner forceps
Niedner knife
Niedner valvulotome
night splint
NIH catheter
Nikon camera

nipper
    House-Dieter
    malleus
Nisentil
Nissen forceps
Nissen gastrectomy
Nissen rib spreader
Nissen sutures
nitrazine test
nitrogen
nitrous oxide
Nizetic operation
no-absorption anesthesia
Nobis aortic occluder
Noble forceps
Noble operation
Noble position
Noble scissors
nocturia
node
node dissection
nodose
nodular
nodular goiter
nodule
Noel-Thompson operation
Noland-Budd curet
nonabsorbable surgical sutures
nonabsorbable sutures
noncannulated nail
noncrushing clamp
noncutting suture needle
nonfenestrated forceps
nonfunctioning
noninversion
nonpenetrating keratoplasty
nonperforating
nonradiating

nonrebreathing anesthesia
nonrebreathing valve
nonslipping forceps
nonstress test (NST)
nontoothed forceps
nonunion
nonviable
non-weightbearing brace
noose
normal saline
North-South retractor
Northbent scissors
Norwood forceps
Norwood snare
nose-bridge prosthesis
nostril
nostril elevator
notch
notched rotation osteotomy
notched ruler
Nott-Guttmann speculum
Nott speculum
Nourse syringe
Novak curet
Novocain
Noyes forceps
Noyes punch
Noyes rongeur
Noyes scissors
Noyes-Shambaugh scissors
Noyes speculum
NPO (nothing by mouth)
NST (nonstress test)

nuchal ligament
nuchal line
Nuck's canal
nuclear cataract
nuclear membrane
nucleus
nucleus pulposus
Nu-gauze dressing
Nugent forceps
Nugent-Gradle scissors
Nugent-Green-Dimitry erysiphake
Nugent hook
nulligravida
nullipara
numbness
Nunez clamp
Nunez-Nunez knife
Nunez sternal approximator
Nunez tube
nupercaine hydrochloride
Nurolon sutures
Nussbaum clamp
Nussbaum narcosis
nutmeg liver
nutriciae humeri arteries
nutrient arteries of humerus
Nuttall operation
Nuttall retractor
Nylok bolt
nylon monofilament sutures
nylon sutures
nylon vascular prosthesis
nystagmus

O

oat cell carcinoma
Ober operation
Ober tendon passer
Ober-Yount operation
Oberhill retractor
Oberst operation
O'Beirne sphincter
O'Beirne tube
obliqua atrii sinistri vein
oblique
oblique amputation
oblique bandage
oblique fracture
oblique hernia
oblique incision
oblique muscle
oblique relaxing incision
oblique vein of left atrium
obliquus auriculae muscle
obliquus capitis inferior muscle
obliquus capitis superior muscle
obliquus externus abdominis
    muscle
obliquus inferior bulbi muscle
obliquus internus abdominis
    muscle
obliquus superior bulbi muscle
obliterate
obliteration
O'Brien akinesia
O'Brien block
O'Brien forceps

obstetric delivery
obstetric forceps
obstetric position
obstetrical forceps
obstetrical hysterectomy
obstetrical position
obstetrical spoon
obstetrical stirrups
obstipation
obstruction
obturator
    Alcock
    Alcock-Timberlake
    Cripps
    esophagoscope
    o. arteries
    o. hernia
    o. muscle
    o. nerve
    o. veins
    Timberlake
    ureteral catheter
obturatoria accessoria artery
obturatoria artery
obturatoriae veins
obturatorius externus muscle
obturatorius internus muscle
obturatorius nerve
obtuse angle
obtuse angle knife
Obwegeser incision
Obwegeser osteotomy

Obwegeser retractor
occipital artery
occipital bone
occipital emissary vein
occipital nerve
occipital triangle
occipital vein
occipitalis artery
occipitalis major nerve
occipitalis minor nerve
occipitalis tertius nerve
occipitalis vein
occipitoatlantal articulation
occipitofrontal muscle
occipitofrontalis muscle
occipitomastoid suture
occlude
occluder
    aortic
    Nobis aortic
occluding clamp
occluding forceps
occluding fracture frame
occlusal mold
occlusal rest bar
occlusal surface
occlusion
occlusion clamp
occlusion forceps
occlusive
occlusive disease
occlusive dressing
occlusive ileus
occult
occult blood
occult fracture
Ochsner clamp
Ochsner-Dixon forceps

Ochsner forceps
Ochsner position
Ochsner probe
Ochsner retractor
Ochsner scissors
Ochsner trocar
Ochsner tube
Ockerblad clamp
O'Connor clamp
O'Connor finger cup
O'Connor forceps
O'Connor hook
O'Connor operation
O'Connor-O'Sullivan retractor
O'Connor-Peter operation
O'Connor retractor
O'Conor nephropexy
ocular prosthesis
oculomotor nerve (cranial nerve III)
oculomotorius nerve
Oddi sphincter
Odman-Ledin catheter
O'Donaghue splint
odontectomy
odontexesis
odontogenic tumor
odontoid process
odontoma
odontoplasty
odontoscopy
odontotomy
O'Dwyer tube
Oertli knife
Oertli silk
offset hand retractor
offset hinge prosthesis
offset reamer

Ogilvie herniorrhaphy
Ogilvie operation
Ogston-Luc operation
Ogston operation
O'Hanlon forceps
O'Hara forceps
O'Hara operation
Oldberg dissector
Oldberg forceps
Oldberg retractor
Oldberg rongeur
olecranon
olecranon process
oleothorax
olfactorii nerves
olfactory
olfactory glands
olfactory membrane
olfactory nerve (cranial nerve I)
olive dilator
olive-tip bougie
olive-tip catheter
olive-tipped bougie
Olivecrona clip
Olivecrona dissector
Olivecrona forceps
Olivecrona rongeur
Olivecrona scissors
Olivecrona spatula
Oliver retractor
Ollier incision
Ollier operation
Ollier raspatory
Ollier retractor
Ollier-Thiersch graft
Ollier-Thiersch operation
Olshausen operation
Olympus fiberscope

Olympus microscope
Olympus panendoscope
O'Malley knife
Ombrédanne operation
omental
omental hernia
omental tuber
omentectomy
omentofixation
omentopexy
omentoplasty
omentorrhaphy
omentosplenopexy
omentotomy
omentum
Omni-Atricor pacemaker
Omni-Ectocor pacemaker
Omni operating microscope
Omni-Stanicor pacemaker
omohyoid muscle
omohyoideus muscle
omphalectomy
omphalelcosis
omphalic
omphalitis
omphalocele
omphalotomy
on-edge mattress sutures
O'Neill clamp
O'Neill scissors
one-stage operation
onlay graft
onychauxis
onychectomy
onychia
onychomycosis
onychoplasty
onychorrhexis

onychotomy
oophorectomy
oophorocystectomy
oophorohysterectomy
oophoropexy
oophoroplasty
oophororrhaphy
oophorosalpingectomy
oophorostomy
oophorotomy
oothecectomy
Op-Temp cautery
opacification
opacity
opaque
opaque microscope
open amputation
open anesthesia
open angle glaucoma
open drainage
open drop anesthesia
open-end aspirating tube
open endotracheal inhalation
    anesthesia
open fracture
open inhalation anesthesia
open operation
open reduction
open reduction and fixation
open reduction and internal fixa-
    tion (ORIF)
open reduction of dislocation
open reduction of fracture
open reduction of fracture-
    dislocation
open reduction with internal
    fixation
open thimble splint

opening
opening snap
operable
operating gastroscope
operating microscope
operating otoscope
operating room
operating scissors
operating suite
operating telescope
operative
operative amputation
operative cholangiogram
operative cholangiography
operative enteroscope
operative field
operative findings
operative incision
operative site
operation
operculectomy
operculum (*pl.* opercula)
Ophthaine
ophthalmectomy
ophthalmic artery
ophthalmic cautery
ophthalmic knife
ophthalmic nerve
ophthalmic pick
ophthalmic vein
ophthalmica artery
ophthalmica inferior vein
ophthalmica superior vein
ophthalmicus nerve
ophthalmodynamometer
    Bailliart
    suction
ophthalmodynamometry

ophthalmometer
ophthalmoplegia
ophthalmoscope
    binocular
    direct
    Friedenwald
    ghost
    Gullstrand
    halogen
    indirect
    Loring
    luminous
    reflecting
ophthalmoscopy
ophthalmotomy
Oppenheim brace
opponens digiti minimi manus
    muscle
opponens pollicis muscle
opponens splint
opponensplasty
opposing muscle
optic canal
optic foramen
optic iridectomy
optic nerve (cranial nerve II)
optical esophagoscope
optical iridectomy
optical laryngoscope
opticus nerve
OR (operating room)
ora
ora serrata
oral
oral cavity
oral fistula
oral forceps
oral mucosa

oral panendoscope
oral restorative surgery
oral urogram
oral urography
orbicular incision
orbicular muscle
orbicularis block
orbicularis oculi muscle
orbicularis oris muscle
orbit
orbital
orbital akinesia
orbital bone
orbital cavity
orbital contents
orbital enucleation compressor
orbital floor prosthesis
orbital fracture reduction
orbital implant
orbital muscle
orbital retractor
orbitalis muscle
orbitotomy
orchectomy
orchidectomy
orchidoepididymectomy
orchidopexy
orchidoplasty
orchidorrhaphy
orchidotomy
orchiectomy
orchiopexy
orchioplasty
orchiorrhaphy
orchiotomy
Ord operation
organ
organomegaly

ORIF (open reduction and internal fixation)
orifice
Orlon vascular prosthesis
oronasal
oropharynx
orotracheal
orotracheal tube
Orr incision
Orsi-Grocco method
Ortho-Mesh
orthodontic band
orthopedic drill
orthopedic mallet
orthopedic wrench
Orthoplast dressing
orthopnea
orthopnea position
orthoroentgenogram
orthoroentgenography
orthostatic
Ortolani sign
Ortved stone dislodger
os (*pl.* ossa)*
    o. calcis
    o. calcis clamp
    o. capitatum
    oo. carpi
    o. costale
    o. coccygis
    o. coxae
    o. cuboideum
    o. cuneiforme intermedium
    o. cuneiforme laterale
    o. cuneiforme mediale

*o. = os [*L.*]
  oo. = ossa [*L.*, pl.]

os (*pl.* ossa)* *(continued)*
    oo. digitorum
    o. ethmoidale
    o. frontale
    o. hamatum
    o. hyoideum
    o. ilium
    o. ischii
    o. lacrimale
    o. lunatum
    o. magnum
    oo. metacarpalia
    oo. metatarsalia
    o. nasale
    o. naviculare
    o. occipitale
    o. palatinum
    o. parietale
    o. pisiforme
    o. pubis
    o. sacrum
    o. scaphoideum
    oo. sesamoidea
    o. sphenoidale
    oo. tarsi
    o. temporale
    o. trapezium
    o. trapezoideum
    o. triquetrum
    o. zygomaticum
Osborne operation
oscillating saw
oscillation
oscillatory saw
oscillometrics
oscillometry
Osgood operation
O'Shaughnessy clamp

O'Shaughnessy forceps
osmostat
osseous
ossicle
ossicle-holding forceps
ossicular chain
ossicular replacement prosthesis
ossiculectomy
ossiculotomy
ossification
ostearthrotomy
ostectomy
ostectomy plate
osteoarthritis
osteoarthrotomy
osteochondritis dissecans
osteoclasis
osteoclast
    Collin
    Phelps-Gocht
    Rizzoli
osteolysis
osteomyelitis
osteopathic manipulation
osteoperiosteal graft
osteoplastic amputation
osteoplastic flap
osteoplastic flap clamp
osteoplasty
osteoporosis
osteorrhaphy
osteosuture
osteosynthesis
osteotome
    alar
    Albee
    Alexander
    Army

osteotome *(continued)*
    articular
    articulation
    bayonet
    Blount
    bone
    Bowen
    Buck
    Campbell
    Carroll
    Carroll-Legg
    Carroll-Smith-Petersen
    Cavin
    Cherry
    Clayton
    Cloward
    Cobb
    Compere
    Converse
    Cottle
    Crane
    Dingman
    Epstein
    Frazier
    Hibbs
    Hoke
    Hough
    Howorth
    Kezerian
    Lahey
    Lambotte
    Lambotte-Henderson
    Legg
    Leinbach
    Mayfield
    Meyerding
    MGH
    Miner

osteotome *(continued)*
    Moore
    New-Lambotte
    perforating
    Roos
    Rowland
    scoliosis
    Sheehan
    Silver
    single-guarded
    Smith-Petersen
    spinal fusion
    Stille
    thin
    U.S. Army
osteotomy
osteotomy nail
osteotomy pin
osteotomy plate
ostium *(pl.* ostia)
O'Sullivan-O'Connor retractor
O'Sullivan-O'Connor speculum
O'Sullivan retractor
otectomy
Otis anoscope
Otis bougie
Otis-Brown cystoscope
Otis meatotome
Otis sound
Otis urethrotome
otitis
otitis externa
otitis media
Oto-Microscope
otonecrectomy
otopexy
otoplasty
otosclerectomy

otoscleronectomy
otosclerosis
otosclerotic processes
otoscope
    Bruening
    Brunton
    halogen
    operating
    pneumatic
    Politzer
    Siegle
    Toynbee
    Welch Allyn
otoscopy
Ottenheimer dilator
outer layer
outflow
outfolding
outfracture
outlay operation
outlet
output
outrigger splint
oval amputation
oval esophagoscope
oval incision
oval speculum
oval window
oval-window hook
ovarian
ovarian abscess
ovarian artery
ovarian cyst
ovarian cystectomy
ovarian fossa
ovarian hernia
ovarian ligament
ovarian trocar

ovarian vein
ovarica artery
ovarica dextra vein
ovarica sinistra vein
ovariectomy
ovariocentesis
ovariosalpingectomy
ovary
over-and-over sutures
overdistention
overhang
overhead fracture frame
overhead light
Overholt elevator
Overholt-Finochietto rib spreader
Overholt forceps
Overholt-Jackson bronchoscope
Overholt needle
Overholt operation
Overholt periosteal elevator
Overholt raspatory
Overholt retractor
Overholt rib spreader
overlapping closure
overlapping sutures
overripe cataract
oversewing

oversewn
Overstreet forceps
oviduct
ovoid
ovoid packing
ovoid radium application
ovoids
ovum forceps
Owen position
Owens catheter
Owens hemostatic bag
Owens operation
Owens silk sutures
Owens sutures
Oxaine
oxethazaine
Oxford operation
oxycel cotton
oxycel pack
oxygen
oxygen therapy
oxygenation
oxygenator
oxytocin
oxyuriasis
Oyloidin sutures

p

P loop
Pace knife
pacemaker
    Amtech-Killeen
    Arco lithium
    artificial
    asynchronous
    Biotronik
    bipolar
    bipolar Medtronic
    cardiac
    Chardack
    Chardack-Greatbatch
    Coratomic
    Cordis
    Cordis Atricor
    Cordis Ectocor
    Cordis fixed-rate
    Cordis Ventricor
    CPI Maxilith
    CPI Minilith
    demand
    dual pass
    Ectocor
    electric cardiac
    Electrodyne
    endocardial bipolar
    external
    external asynchronous
    external demand
    external-internal
    fixed-rate

pacemaker *(continued)*
    General Electric
    implantable
    implanted
    Intermedics Thinlith II
    Lambda
    lithium
    Maxilith
    Medtronic
    Minilith
    Nathan
    Omni-Atricor
    Omni-Ectocor
    Omni-Stanicor
    p. catheter
    p. electrode
    permanent transvenous
    radio-frequency
    single-pass
    Stanicor
    Starr-Edwards
    synchronous
    Telectronic
    temporary transvenous
    transpericardial
    transvenous
    transvenous catheter
    Ventricor
    ventricular-suppressed
    ventricular-triggered
    wandering
    Zoll

Paci operation
pacing catheter
pacing electrode wire
pacing wire electrode
pack
packer
packing
pad electrode
padded clamp
padded splint
padding
Padgett dermatome
Padgett graft
Padgett-Hood electrodermatome
Page forceps
Page knife
Pagenstecher linen thread sutures
Pagenstecher operation
Pagenstecher scoop
Paget disease
pain
painful
paint
Pajot hook
Pajot maneuver
palatal bar
palate elevator
palate hook
palate lengthening
palate pusher hook
palate retractor
palatina ascendens artery
palatina descendens artery
palatina externa vein
palatina major artery
palatinae minores arteries
palatine
palatine artery

palatine bone
palatine nerve
palatine process
palatine tonsils
palatine vein
palatini minores nerves
palatinus major nerve
palatoethmoid suture
palatoglossus muscle
palatopharyngeal muscle
palatopharyngeus muscle
palatoplasty
palatorrhaphy
Palfyn sutures
palliation
palliative
palliative procedure
pallidectomy
pallidotomy
pallidum
palm
palmar fascia
palmar muscle
palmaris brevis muscle
palmaris longus muscle
Palmer dilator
Palmer-Widen operation
palpating needle
palpation probe
palpebra (*pl.* palpebrae)
palpebral
palpebral arteries
palpebral veins
palpebrales inferiores veins
palpebrales laterales arteries
palpebrales mediales arteries
palpebrales superiores veins
palpebrales veins

palsy
pampiniform plexus
Panas operation
Panas ptosis correction technique
Pancoast operation
Pancoast sutures
pancolectomy
pancreas
pancreatectomy
pancreatic
pancreatic duct
pancreatic pseudocyst
pancreatic ranula
pancreatic veins
pancreaticae veins
pancreaticocystoduodenostomy
pancreaticocystoenterostomy
pancreaticocystogastrostomy
pancreaticocystojejunostomy
pancreaticoduodenal arteries
pancreaticoduodenal veins
pancreaticoduodenales inferiores
    arteries
pancreaticoduodenales veins
pancreaticoduodenectomy
pancreaticoduodenostomy
pancreaticoenterostomy
pancreaticogastrostomy
pancreaticoileostomy
pancreaticojejunostomy
pancreaticosplenic
pancreaticosplenic ligament
pancreatitis
pancreatoduodenectomy
pancreatogram
pancreatography
pancreatolithectomy
pancreatolithotomy

pancreatotomy
pancreolithotomy
panendoscope
    Foroblique
    French-McCarthy
    Olympus
    oral
    p. electrode
    Stern-McCarthy
panendoscopy
Pang forceps
panhysterectomy
panhystero-oophorectomy
panhysterosalpingectomy
panhysterosalpingo-oophorectomy
panniculectomy
panniculotomy
panniculus (*pl.* panniculi)
pannus
Panorex x-ray
panproctocolectomy
pantaloon hernia
pantaloon operation
Pantopaque
pants-over-vest repair
panus
Panzer scissors
Pap smear
Papanicolaou smear
Paparella catheter
Paparella curet
Paparella elevator
Paparella fenestrometer
Paparella knife
Paparella needle
Paparella pick
Paparella retractor
Paparella scissors

Paparella tube
papaverine
paper tape
papilla (*pl.* papillae)
papilla of Vater
papillares muscles
papillary
papillary duct
papillary muscles
papillate
papillectomy
papilloma (*pl.* papillomas, papillo-
    mata)
papilloma forceps
papillomata (*sing.* papilloma)
papillomatous goiter
papillosphincterotomy
Paquelin cautery
para (1, 2, 3, etc.)
paracentesis (*pl.* paracenteses)
paracentesis abdominis
paracentesis cordis
paracentesis knife
paracentesis needle
paracentesis pericardii
paracentesis pulmonis
paracentesis thoracis
paracentesis vesicae
paracervical block
paracostal incision
paraduodenal
paraduodenal hernia
paraesophageal
paraesophageal hernia
paraffin
paraffin dressing
paraffin implant
parainguinal incision

paraldehyde
parallel
parallel incision
parallel-jaw spring clip
paralysis
paralytic
paralytic ileus
paramedian incision
paramesonephric duct
parametrial curettage
parametrial fixation
parametritis
parametrium
parametrium clamp
parametrium forceps
paramuscular incision
paraneural anesthesia
parapatellar incision
paraperitoneal
paraperitoneal hernia
pararectal incision
pararectus incision
parasaccular
parasaccular hernia
parasacral anesthesia
parasagittal incision
parascapular incision
parasitology
parasternal
parathyroid
parathyroid gland
parathyroidectomy
paratrooper fracture
paraumbilical veins
paraumbilicales veins
paraurethral duct
paravaginal hysterectomy
paravaginal incision

paravertebral anesthesia
Paré sutures
parenchyma
parenchymal
parenchymatous
parenchymatous goiter
parenteral
parenteral alimentation
parenteral hyperalimentation
paresis
paresthesia
Parhad-Poppen needle
Parham band
Parham-Martin band
Parham-Martin clamp
parietal
paries (*pl.* parietes)
parietal bone
parietal emissary vein
parietal hernia
parietal peritoneum
parietal pleura
parietes (*sing.* paries)
parietomastoid suture
Park-Guyton speculum
Park-Maumenee speculum
Park speculum
Parker clamp
Parker-Heath cautery
Parker incision
Parker-Kerr "basting stitch"
Parker-Kerr forceps
Parker-Kerr sutures
Parker knife
Parker-Mott retractor
Parker needle
Parker retractor
Parkhill operation

Parkinson position
paronychia
parotid
parotid capsule
parotid duct
parotid gland
parotid veins
parotideae veins
parotidectomy
parotitis
parous
parovarian
paroxysmal nocturnal dyspnea
    (PND)
parry fracture
pars (*pl.* partes)
pars plana
pars pylorica
pars superior duodeni
partes (*sing.* pars)
partial amputation
partial anesthesia
partial breech delivery
partial excision
partial occlusion forceps
partial ossicular replacement
    prosthesis (PORP)
partial rebreathing anesthesia
partial thickness skin graft
partially occluding clamp
Partipilo clamp
Partsch operation
parumbilical
parumbilical hernia
parumbilical incision
passage
passage of sound
passive

paste
patch (see also *graft* and
    prosthesis)
    Dacron
    Edwards
    felt
    intracardiac
    Ivalon
    p. angioplasty
    p. closure of defect
    p. dressing
    Teflon
patella
patella cap prosthesis
patella dislocation
patellapexy
patellar hook
patellar ligament
patellar tendon
patellectomy
patellofemoral prosthesis
patency
patent
patent ductus
patent ductus clamp
patent ductus forceps
patent ductus retractor
Paterson cannula
Paterson forceps
pathologic fracture
pathological amputation
Paton forceps
Paton knife
Paton needle holder
Paton spatula
Paton trephine
Patrick test
Patterson forceps

Patterson trocar
patties
Patton cannula
Patton dilator
Patton speculum
patulent
patulous
paucity
Paufique knife
Paufique operation
Paufique trephine
Paul-Mixter tube
Paul retractor
Pauwels operation
Payne-Ochsner forceps
Payne-Péan forceps
Payne-Rankin forceps
Payr clamp
PBI (protein-bound iodine)
PE (polyethylene) tube
PE (pressure-equalization) tube
Peabody splint
Péan amputation
Péan clamp
Péan forceps
Péan hysterectomy
Péan incision
Péan operation
Péan position
peanut forceps
peanut-grasping forceps
pear-shaped bur
Pearsall silk sutures
peau d'orange
pectenotomy
pectinate
pectinate ligament
pectinate line

pectinate muscles
pectinati muscles
pectineal
pectineal fascia
pectineal hernia
pectineal ligament
pectineal line
pectineal muscle
pectineus muscle
pectoral
pectoral muscles
pectoralis major muscle
pectoralis minor muscle
pedal pulse
Pedersen speculum
pediatric bronchoscope
pediatric forceps
pediatric scissors
pedicle
pedicle clamp
pedicle flap
pedicle graft
pedis pulse
peduncle
pedunculated
PEEP (positive end expiratory pressure)
pelvectomy
pelves (*sing.* pelvis)
pelvic
pelvic bone
pelvic clamp
pelvic colon
pelvic examination
pelvic floor
pelvic inflammatory disease (PID)
pelvic organ exenteration
pelvic organs

pelvic splint
pelvic traction
pelvic version
pelvifixation
pelvilithotomy
pelvimeter
    Barbara
    Breisky
    Collin
    Collyer
    DeLee
    DeLee-Breisky
    Martin
    Thoms
    William
pelvimetry
pelviolithotomy
pelvioplasty
pelviostomy
pelviotomy
pelvirectal
pelvirectal achalasia
pelvis (*pl.* pelves)
pelvisection
pelviureteroplasty
Pemberton clamp
Pemberton forceps
Pemberton operation
Pemberton retractor
pencil
    electrosurgery
    marking
    skin
pendulous
penectomy
penetrating drill
penetrating keratoplasty
Penfield clip

Penfield dissector
Penfield elevator
Penfield forceps
Penfield needle
Penfield retractor
penicillin
penile clamp
penile implant
penile prosthesis
penis
penis clamp
penlight cautery
Pennington clamp
Pennington elevator
Pennington forceps
Pennington speculum
penoplasty
Penrose drain
Penrose tube
Penthrane
pentobarbital
Pentothal
peptic
peptic glands
peptic ulcer
per primam healing
per primam intentionem
per secundum healing
per secundum intentionem
Percaine
percolator irrigator
percutaneous
percutaneous arteriogram
percutaneous arteriography
percutaneous needle
percutaneous transluminal
   coronary angioplasty
Percy cautery

Percy forceps
Percy retractor
Percy-Wolfson retractor
Pereyra bladder suspension
Pereyra cannula
Pereyra needle
Pereyra operation
perforantes arteries
perforantes veins
perforated ulcer
perforating
perforating appendicitis
perforating arteries
perforating bur
perforating drill
perforating forceps
perforating fracture
perforating osteotome
perforating ulcer
perforating veins
perforation
perforative
perforator
     antrum
     Bishop
     Blot
     cranial
     Cushing
     DeLee-Perce
     D'Errico
     Hillis
     Joseph
     Lempert
     membrane
     p. drill
     Royce
     Smellie
     Stein

perforator *(continued)*
    Thornwald
    tympanum
    Wellaminski
perfusion
perfusion cannula
perianal
perianal abscess
perianal incision
periappendicitis
periareolar incision
periarterial sympathectomy
periarticular fracture
pericardectomy
pericardiac veins
pericardiaceae veins
pericardiacophrenic artery
pericardiacophrenic veins
pericardiacophrenica artery
pericardiacophrenicae veins
pericardial
pericardial baffle
pericardial raspatory
pericardicentesis
pericardiectomy
pericardiocentesis
pericardiolysis
pericardioplasty
pericardiorrhaphy
pericardiostomy
pericardiotomy
pericardium
perichondrial elevator
pericostal suture
peridectomy
peridural anesthesia
perigastric
perilimbal

perilimbal incision
perilymph
perimetry
perinatal
perineal
perineal artery
perineal bandage
perineal dissection
perineal lithotomy
perineal needle biopsy
perineal nerve
perineal retractor
perineal support sutures
perineales nerves
perinealis artery
perineoplasty
perineorrhaphy
perineotomy
perinephric
perineum
perineural anesthesia
perinuclear cataract
periocular
periodontal anesthesia
periodontal ligament
periodontal probe
periosteal
periosteal elevator
    Adson
    Allis
    Aufranc
    Bethune
    blunt
    Bowen
    Bristow
    Brophy
    Cameron
    Cameron-Haight

periosteal elevator *(continued)*
- Campbell
- Carroll
- Carroll-Legg
- Cheyne
- Cloward
- Cobb
- Coryllos
- Coryllos-Doyen
- costal
- curved
- Cushing-Hopkins
- Davidson
- Davis
- D'Errico
- Dingman
- double-ended
- Doyen
- Dunning
- Farabeuf
- Fomon
- Freer
- Haight
- Hibbs
- Hoen
- Iowa
- Joseph
- Key
- Kinsella
- Kirmisson
- Kocher
- Lane
- Langenbeck
- long
- Love-Adson
- MacDonald
- MacKenty
- Matson

periosteal elevator *(continued)*
- MGH
- Molt
- mucoperiosteal
- Overholt
- Poppen
- Raney
- Richardson
- Sayre
- Sedillot
- Sewall mucoperiosteal
- Spurling
- Steele
- Turner

periosteal graft

periosteal raspatory

periosteal stripping

periosteoplastic amputation

periosteorrhaphy

periosteotome
- Alexander
- Alexander-Farabeuf
- Ballenger
- Brophy
- Brown
- costal
- Dean
- Fomon
- Freer
- Jansen
- Joseph
- Moorehead
- Potts

periosteotomy

periosteum

periosteum elevator

periosteum stripper

periostotomy

peripad
peripalpebral
peripheral
peripheral blood vessels
peripheral cataract
peripheral iridectomy
peripheral iridectomy forceps
peripheral iridotomy
peripheral pulses
peripheral vascular forceps
periphery
perirectal
perirectal abscess
perirenal tissues
periscapular incision
peristalsis
peristaltic
peristaltic rushes
peritectomy
peritomy
peritoneal
peritoneal button
peritoneal cavity
peritoneal clamp
peritoneal incision
peritoneal shunt
peritonealization
peritonealize
peritoneocentesis
peritoneoplasty
peritoneoscope
peritoneoscopy
peritoneotomy
peritoneum
peritonitis
peritonization
peritonize
peritonsillar

peritonsillar abscess
perityphlitis
perityphlitis actinomycotica
periumbilical
periurethral tissues
Perkins tractor
Perma-hand silk sutures
permanent implant
permanent magnet
permanent transvenous pacemaker
permeation anesthesia
peronea artery
peroneae veins
peroneal
peroneal artery
peroneal muscle
peroneal nerve
peroneal veins
peroneal vessels
peroneus brevis muscle
peroneus communis nerve
peroneus longus muscle
peroneus profundus nerve
peroneus superficialis nerve
peroneus tertius muscle
peroral
peroxide
perpendicular
perpendicular plate
Perritt forceps
Perthes incision
pertrochanteric fracture
pes planus operation
pessary
    Chambers
    cup
    diaphragm
    doughnut

pessary *(continued)*
  Emmert-Gellhorn
  Gariel
  Gehrung
  Gellhorn
  Gynefold
  Hodge
  intrauterine
  lever
  lucite
  Mayer
  Menge
  prolapsus
  retrodisplacement
  retroversion
  ring
  Smith
  Smith-Hodge
  stem
  Thomas
  Wylie
  Zwanck
petechia *(pl.* petechiae)
Peter operation
Petersen bag
Petersen lithotomy
Petersen operation (urol.)
Peterson operation (gyn.)
Petit hernia
Petit's ligament
Petit sutures
petrolatum gauze
petrolatum gauze dressing
petrosal nerve
petrosquamous suture
petrosus major nerve
petrosus minor nerve

petrosus profundus nerve
petrous bone
petrous pyramid
petrous pyramid air cells
Petz clamp
Peyton brain spatula
Pezzer catheter
Pezzer drain
Pfannenstiel incision
Pfau forceps
Pfau punch
Pfeifer operation
Pfister-Schwartz stone basket
Pfister stone basket
pH
phacocystectomy
phacoemulsification
phacoerysis
phacolysis
phalangeal articulations
phalangectomy
phalanges (*sing.* phalanx)
phalangization
phalangophalangeal amputation
phalanx (*pl.* phalanges)
phalanx distalis
phalanx media
phalanx proximalis
Phalen sign
phalloplasty
phallus
Phaneuf clamp
Phaneuf forceps
phantom limb pain
Pharmaseal catheter
Pharmaseal drain
pharyngea ascendens artery
pharyngeae veins

pharyngeal artery
pharyngeal flap operation
pharyngeal insufflation anesthesia
pharyngeal mirror
pharyngeal tube
pharyngeal veins
pharyngectomy
pharyngoesophageal diverticulec-
    tomy
pharyngogram
pharyngorrhaphy
pharyngolaryngectomy
pharyngoplasty
pharyngorraphy
pharyngoscopy
pharyngotomy
pharynx
phase-contrast microscope
phase microscope
Pheasant operation
Pheifer-Young retractor
Phelps-Gocht osteoclast
Phelps operation
Phelps splint
Phemister elevator
Phemister incision
Phemister onlay bone graft
Phemister operation
Phemister punch
Phemister raspatory
Phemister reamer
phenol
phenopeel
pheochromocytoma
Phillips bougie
Phillips catheter
Phillips clamp
Phillips screw

Phillips screwdriver
phimosis
phimosis forceps
pHisoDerm
pHisoHex
phlebectomy
phlebitis
phlebogram
phlebography
phlebolith
phlebolithiasis
phleboplasty
phleborrhaphy
phlebosclerosis
phlebothrombosis
phlebotomy
phlegm
phlegmon
phlegmonous
phonation
phonocardiogram
phonocardiography
Phoropter
photochemotherapy
photocoagulation
photocoagulator
photoculdoscope
photomotogram
photon microscope
photophobia
photo-strobe
phototherapy
phrenemphraxis
phrenic
phrenic arteries
phrenic nerve
phrenic retractor
phrenic veins

phrenicae inferiores arteries
phrenicae inferiores veins
phrenicae superiores arteries
phrenicectomized
phrenicectomy
phrenicectomy forceps
phrenici accessorii muscle
phreniclasis
phrenicocolic ligament
phrenicoexeresis
phrenicolienal ligament
phreniconeurectomy
phrenicosplenic ligament
phrenicotomy
phrenicotripsy
phrenicus nerve
phrenoplegia
Physick operation
physiotherapy
phytobezoar
pia mater
PICA (posterior inferior cerebellar
    artery)
pick
    Burch
    House
    ophthalmic
    Paparella
    Rhein
    right-angle
    small
    stapes
    Wells
pick-up screw
Picot retractor
Picot speculum
PID (pelvic inflammatory disease)
piecemeal

piecemeal removal of kidney
Pierce cannula
Pierce dissector
Pierce elevator
Pierce forceps
Pierce-Hoskins forceps
Pierce-O'Connor operation
Pierce retractor
Pierce rongeur
Pierce syringe
Pierce trocar
Pierce tube
Piffard curet
pigment
pigmented nevus
pigtail catheter
pigtail probe
Pilcher catheter
Pilcher hemostatic bag
pile clamp
pile forceps
piles
pill-rolling motion
pillar
pillar forceps
pillar-grasping forceps
pillar retractor
Pilling bronchoscope
Pilling tube
pillion fracture
pillow splint
pilocarpine
pilojection
pilonidal cyst
pilonidal dimple
pilonidal sinus
Pilopaque
pilot drill

piloting trocar
pin
    Austin Moore
    Böhler
    Bohlman
    Breck
    calibrated guide
    cloverleaf
    Compere
    Craig
    Davis
    DePuy
    Deyerle
    duodenal
    Fahey
    fixation
    Furniss-Clute
    guide
    Hagie
    Hansen-Street
    Hatcher
    Haynes
    hip
    intramedullary
    Jones
    Knowles
    Kuntscher
    Lottes
    medullary
    metal
    micro-pin
    Moore
    osteotomy
    pin-bending forceps
    p. clamp
    p. chuck handle
    p. fixation
    p. punch

pin *(continued)*
    p. retractor
    p. sutures
    Pischel
    Pischel micro-pin
    Roger Anderson
    Rush
    safety
    Schneider
    self-broaching
    skeletal
    Smith-Petersen
    Steinmann
    Street
    threaded
    trochanter
    Turner
    Venable-Stuck
    von Saal
    Walker
    Zimmer
pinch graft
pinchcock clamp
pineal body
pineal gland
pinealectomy
pinealoma
pinealotomy
ping-pong fracture
pinna
pinning operation
Piper forceps
piperocaine hydrochloride
pipette
piriform muscle
piriformis muscle
Pirogoff amputation
Pirogoff operation

Pischel electrode
Pischel elevator
Pischel forceps
Pischel micro-pin
Pischel pin
pisiform bone
piston
piston prosthesis
Pitha forceps
Pitkin needle
Pitocin
pituitary
pituitary ablation
pituitary body
pituitary capsulectomy
pituitary capsulectomy knife
pituitary curet
pituitary elevator
pituitary forceps
pituitary fossa
pituitary gland
pituitary rongeur
pituitectomy
pivot joint
placenta
placenta clamp
placenta curet
placenta forceps
placenta previa
placenta previa forceps
placental forceps
placental fragments
placental membrane
placentogram
placentography
Placido disk
plafond
plain catgut sutures

plain films
plain forceps
plain gauze
plain gauze ABDs
plain gut sutures
plain interrupted sutures
plain screwdriver
plain ties
plain tissue forceps
plane
planing
plantar
plantar artery
plantar flexion
plantar muscle
plantar nerve
plantar wart
plantaris lateralis artery
plantaris lateralis nerve
plantaris medialis artery
plantaris muscle
plantation
plaque
plasma exchange
plasma transfusion
plaster bandage
plaster cast
plaster cast knife
plaster dressing
plaster knife
plaster-of-Paris dressing
plaster-of-Paris scissors
plaster saw
plaster shears
plaster spline
plaster splint
plastic ball eye implant
plastic cannula

plastic catheter
plastic closure
plastic conformer
plastic construction
plastic curet
plastic drape
plastic dressing
plastic implant
plastic needle holder
plastic operation
plastic reconstruction
plastic repair
plastic scissors
plastic Silastic
plastic sphere eye implant
plastic sphere implant
plastic splint
plastic suction tip
plastic surgery
plastic sutures
plastic syringe
plastic tube
Plastipore ossicular replacement
   prosthesis
plasty
plate
     anchor
     Badgley
     bent blade
     blade
     Blount
     bone
     Brophy
     coaptation
     dental
     DePuy
     Deyerle
     die

plate *(continued)*
     double-angle blade
     dural
     Eggers
     Elliott
     femoral condyle
     finger
     Foley
     fracture
     Hansen-Street
     Hoen
     Hubbard
     intertrochanteric
     Ishihara
     Jaeger
     Jewett
     Ken
     Kessel
     knee
     L-plate
     Laing
     Lane
     Lawson-Thornton
     lid
     lugged
     McBride
     McLaughlin
     metal
     Moe
     Moore
     Moore-Blount
     nail
     nephrotome
     Neufeld
     ostectomy
     osteotomy
     p. punch
     polyethylene

plate *(continued)*
    serpentine
    Sherman
    Silastic
    silicone
    six-hole stainless steel
    skull
    slotted
    Smith-Petersen
    SMO
    spinal fusion
    spring
    steel
    suction
    tarsal
    Teflon
    Temple University
    Thornton
    trochanteric
    V-blade
    Venable
    Vitallium
    vulcanite
    Wilson
    Wright
    Y-bone
    Zuelzer
platinum blade electrode
platysma
platysma muscle
pleating
pledget
plethysmogram
plethysmography
Pleur-evac suction tube
Pleur-evac tube
pleura
pleura dissector

pleuracotomy
pleural biopsy needle
pleural biopsy punch
pleural cavity
pleural suction tube
pleurectomy
pleurectomy forceps
pleurocentesis
pleurodesis
pleuroesophageal muscle
pleuroesophageus muscle
pleurolysis
pleuropexy
pleurotomy
plexectomy
Plexiglas eye implant
Plexiglas implant
plexus *(pl.* plexus or plexuses)
plexus anesthesia
plexus of Santorini
Pley forceps
plica *(pl.* plicae)
plica duodenalis
plica duodenojejunalis
plica duodenomesocolica
plica epigastrica
plica gastropancreatica
plica ileocecalis
plica paraduodenalis
plica umbilicalis
plicae *(sing.* plica)
plicating sutures
plication sutures
plicotomy
pliers
        Allen
        Bailey
        Berbecker

pliers *(continued)*
    crown-crimping
    dental
    dressing
    Fisherman
    root
    vice-grip
plombage
plug
    Air-Lon
    Alcock
    catheter
    decannulation
    Dittrich
    gastrostomy
    Johnston
    Reich-Nechtow
    Sims
Plummer bougie
Plummer dilator
Plummer-Vinson dilator
Plummer-Vinson radium
    applicator
PND (paroxysmal nocturnal
    dyspnea)
pneumatic
pneumatic dilator
pneumatic otoscope
pneumatic tonometer
pneumatic tourniquet
pneumocentesis
pneumocisternogram
pneumocisternography
pneumoconiosis
pneumoencephalogram
pneumoencephalography
pneumogastric nerve
pneumogram

pneumography
pneumogynogram
pneumogynography
pneumomediastinogram
pneumomediastinography
pneumonectomy
pneumonocentesis
pneumonolysis
pneumonotomy
pneumoperitoneum
pneumothorax
pneumothorax apparatus
pneumothorax injection needle
pneumothorax needle
pneumoventriculogram
pneumoventriculography
pocket probe
pockmark
podalic version
point
point electrode
point forceps
point tenderness
pointed scissors
pointed-tip electrode
polar cataract
polarizing microscope
Polaroid camera
pole
polio laryngoscope
Polisar-Lyons tube
polishing brush
Politzer knife
Politzer operation
Politzer otoscope
Politzer speculum
politzerization
Polley-Bickel trephine

pollicization
Pollock amputation
Polya anastomosis
Polya gastrectomy
Polya gastroenterostomy
Polya gastrojejunostomy
Polya operation
Polyak operation
polycentric prosthesis
polycystic kidney
Polydek sutures
polyester sutures
polyethylene cannula
polyethylene catheter
polyethylene cement
polyethylene collar button
polyethylene drain
polyethylene eye implant
polyethylene implant
polyethylene plate
polyethylene prosthesis
polyethylene snare
polyethylene sutures
polyethylene tube
polyethylene vein stripper
polyfilament sutures
polymyxin
polyp
polyp forceps
polypectomy
polypoid
polyposis
polyposis gastrica
polyposis intestinalis
polyposis ventriculi
polypotome
polypropylene sutures
polypus

polypus forceps
polystan catheter
polystan shunt
polystyrene foam
polyunguia
polyurethane implant
polyurethane packing
polyuria
polyvinyl alcohol
polyvinyl curet
polyvinyl drain
polyvinyl implant
polyvinyl sponge
polyvinyl tubing
Pomeroy operation
Poncet operation
pond fracture
Pond splint
pons (*pl.* pontes)
pons cerebelli
pons hepatis
pontes (*sing.* pons)
pontine
Pontocaine
pool sucker
Pool suction tube
Pool tube
pooling
poorly differentiated carcinoma
poplitea artery
poplitea vein
popliteal
popliteal artery
popliteal incision
popliteal muscle
popliteal vein
popliteus muscle
Poppen-Blalock clamp

Poppen-Blalock-Salibi clamp
Poppen clamp
Poppen coagulator
Poppen elevator
Poppen forceps
Poppen needle
Poppen periosteal elevator
Poppen rongeur
Poppen scissors
porcine graft
poroplastic splint
porotomy
PORP (partial ossicular replacement prosthesis)
Porro cesarean hysterectomy
Porro cesarean section
Porro operation
Porro-Veit operation
porta
porta hepatis
porta lienis
portacaval
portacaval anastomosis
portacaval shunt
portal
portal obstruction
portal vein
portea vein
Porter forceps
Portex speaking tube
portosystemic anastomosis
Porto-vac suction tube
Porzett splint
Posey belt
position
    Adams
    Albert
    anatomical

position *(continued)*
  arm extension
  Bonner
  Boyce
  Bozeman
  Brickner
  Buie
  Caldwell
  Casselberry
  chest
  coiled
  decortical
  decubitus
  Depage
  dorsal
  dorsal decubitus
  dorsal elevated
  dorsal inertia
  dorsal lithotomy
  dorsal recumbent
  dorsal rigid
  dorsodecubitus
  dorsolithotomy
  dorsorecumbent
  dorsosacral
  dorsosupine
  Edebohls
  Elliot
  English
  face-down
  fetal
  Fowler
  frog-legged
  Fuchs
  genucubital
  genufacial
  genupectoral
  head dependent
  head-low

position *(continued)*
- hinge
- horizontal
- hornpipe
- inverted jackknife
- jackknife
- Jones
- Jonge
- kidney
- knee-chest
- knee-elbow
- kneeling-squatting
- Kraske
- Lange
- lateral
- lateral decubitus
- lateral prone
- lateral recumbent
- Law
- leapfrog
- left lateral
- lithotomy
- lithotomy Trendelenburg
- Mayer
- Mayo-Robson
- Mercurio
- Moynihan
- neck extension
- neutral
- Noble
- obstetric
- obstetrical
- Ochsner
- orthopnea
- Owen
- Parkinson
- Péan
- Proetz

position *(continued)*
- prone
- prone jackknife
- recumbent
- rest
- reverse Trendelenburg
- right lateral
- Robson
- Rose
- Samuel
- Schuller
- Scultetus
- semi-Fowler
- semiprone
- semireclining
- shock
- Simon
- Sims
- sitting
- steep Trendelenburg
- Stenver
- stern
- supine
- tonsil
- Trendelenburg
- upright
- Valentine
- Walcher
- Waters
- Waters-Waldron
- Williams
- Wolfenden

positrocephalogram
positrocephalography
Post-Harrington erysiphake
postaural approach
postauricular
postauricular approach

postauricular incision
postcaval
postcaval shunt
posterior bone block
posterior cervical lip
posterior chamber
posterior colporrhaphy
posterior forceps
posterior horn
posterior incision
posterior iridodialysis
posterior jejunostomy
posterior palate hook
posterior pillar
posterior rectus sheath
posterior rhizotomy
posterior splint
posterior stab incision
posterior urethroscope
posterior vein of left ventricle
posterior ventriculi sinistri cordis
    vein
posterior vitrectomy
posterolateral
posterolateral incision
postmenopausal
postmortem
postnasal balloon
postnasal dressing
postnasal tube
postoperative
postpartum sterilization
postplaced sutures
postural drainage
postural version
postvoiding cystogram
postvoiding cystography
postvoiding residual (PVR)

Potain apparatus
Potain aspirator
Potain trocar
potential cautery
Poth operation
Pott fracture
Pott splint
Potter needle
Potter version
Potts anastomosis
Potts clamp
Potts dilator
Potts dissector
Potts elevator
Potts forceps
Potts knife
Potts needle
Potts-Neidner clamp
Potts periosteotome
Potts rib shears
Potts-Riker dilator
Potts-Riker valvulotome
Potts-Satinsky clamp
Potts scissors
Potts-Smith forceps
Potts-Smith-Gibson operation
Potts-Smith operation
Potts-Smith scissors
Potts-Smith tenaculum
Potts tenaculum
Potts valvulotome
pouch
pouch of Douglas
pouch of Hartmann
pouch of Morison
pouch of Munro
poudrage
Poulard operation

Poupart's ligament
Poutasse clamp
Poutasse forceps
Power operation
Pozzi operation
Pozzi tenaculum
Prague maneuver
pramoxine hydrochloride
Pratt anoscope
Pratt curet
Pratt dilator
Pratt director
Pratt forceps
Pratt hook
Pratt probe
Pratt scissors
Pratt-Smith forceps
Pratt sound
Pratt speculum
pre-existing
prefrontal lobotomy
preinvasive carcinoma
preliminary iridectomy
premedicate
premedication
premolars
preparation
preplaced sutures
prepped and draped
prepubic
prepubic fascia
prepuce
prepuce forceps
preputial
preputial gland
preputiotomy
prepyloric
prepyloric sphincter

prepyloric vein
prepylorica vein
presacral anesthesia
presacral neurectomy
Presbyterian Hospital instruments
presection sutures
presentation
Preshaw clamp
pressure anesthesia
pressure bandage
pressure dressing
pressure elevator
pressure equalization tube
pressure forceps
pressure fracture
presumptive
Price-Thomas clamp
Price-Thomas forceps
Price-Thomas rib stripper
Priessnitz bandage
prilocaine hydrochloride
primary amputation
primary anastomosis
primary carcinoma
primary closure
primary colostomy
primary procedure
primary sutures
primipara
Prince cautery
Prince clamp
Prince forceps
Prince knife
Prince-Potts scissors
Prince rongeur
Prince scissors
princeps pollicis artery
principal artery of thumb

Pringle clamp
Pringle incision
prism
prism diopters
Pritchard cannula
Pritchard speculum
Pritchard syringe
Pritikin punch
probang
probe

    Amoils cryoprobe
    Amussat
    Anel lacrimal
    angled
    Arbuckle
    Bakes
    Barr
    Bermenam-Werner
    blood-flow
    blunt
    Bowman
    Brackett
    Brock
    Brodie
    bronchoscopic
    Buck
    Buie
    bullet
    Bunnell
    cataract
    Cherry
    Coakley
    common duct
    cryogenic
    cryoprobe
    Desjardin
    dilaprobe
    dilating

probe *(continued)*
    dissecting
    drum
    ear
    Earle
    electric
    Emmet
    Esmarch
    eustachian
    eyed
    Fenger
    fiberoptic
    fistula
    flexible
    Fogarty
    fragmentation
    Fränkel
    frontal sinus
    gall duct
    gallstone
    Gilmore
    Girard
    Girdner
    Hotz
    intrauterine
    Jackson
    Jansen-Newhart
    Kistner
    Knapp iris repositor
    Kron
    lacrimal
    Larry
    Lilienthal
    Lillie
    Lucae
    malleable
    mastoid
    Mayo

probe *(continued)*
  meerschaum
  Mixter
  Moynihan
  nasal
  needle
  Nélaton
  Ochsner
  palpation
  periodontal
  pigtail
  pocket
  Pratt
  p. director
  p. scissors
  rectal
  Rockey
  Rosen
  salpingeal
  scissors
  Sims
  sinus
  Skillern
  Spencer
  sphenoid
  spiral
  tactile
  telephone
  Theobald
  thermistor
  tin-bullet
  uterine
  vacuum intrauterine
  vertebrated
  Vibrodilator
  Wasko
  Welch Allyn
  Williams

probe *(continued)*
  wire
  Yankauer
  Ziegler
probing
procaine hydrochloride
procerus muscle
process
  acromial
  acromion
  alveolar
  basilar
  caudate
  ciliary
  clinoid
  condyloid
  coracoid
  coronoid
  ensiform
  ethmoid
  frontal
  frontonasal
  malar
  mamillary
  mastoid
  odontoid
  palatine
  pterygoid
  spinous of vertebra
  styloid
  uncinate
  xiphoid
  zygomatic
procidentia
proctalgia
proctalgia fugax
proctectasia
proctectomy

procteurynter
procteurysis
proctitis
proctoclysis
proctococcypexy
proctocolectomy
proctocolitis
proctocolonoscopy
proctocolpoplasty
proctocystoplasty
proctocystotomy
Proctodone
proctoelytroplasty
proctologic
proctology
proctolysis
proctoperineoplasty
proctorrhaphy
proctopexy
proctoplasty
proctoptosis
Proctor elevator
Proctor retractor
proctorrhaphy
proctoscope
    ACMI
    Boehm
    Fansler
    Gabriel
    Goldbacher
    Hirschman
    Hirschman-Martin
    Kelly
    Lieberman
    Montague
    National
    Newman
    Pruitt

proctoscope *(continued)*
    Strauss
    Turell
    Tuttle
    Vernon-David
    Welch Allyn
    Yeomans
proctoscopic speculum
proctoscopy
proctosigmoidectomy
proctosigmoiditis
proctosigmoidopexy
proctosigmoidoscope
proctosigmoidoscopy
proctostenosis
proctostomy
prototome
proctotomy
proctovalvotomy
production
products of conception
Proetz position
profilometer
profunda brachii artery
profunda clitoridis artery
profunda femoris artery
profunda femoris vein
profunda linguae artery
profunda linguae vein
profunda penis artery
profundae clitoridis veins
profundae penis veins
progesterone
prognathism
progressive
projectile
projector x-ray microscope
prolapse

prolapse of uterus
prolapsed hemorrhoid
prolapsus
prolapsus ani
prolapsus pessary
prolapsus recti
prolene sutures
proliferation
prominence
promontory
pronation
pronator muscle
pronator quadratus muscle
pronator teres muscle
prone
prone jackknife position
prone position
Proneze pad
Proneze pillow
prong
pronged retractor
prop graft
proparacaine hydrochloride
properitoneal
properitoneal hernia
prophylaxis
propoxycaine hydrochloride
propranolol
proptosed
proptosis
propylene dressing
prostaglandin suppository
prostate
prostate gland
prostatectomy
prostatectomy bag
prostatic biopsy needle
prostatic capsule

prostatic catheter
prostatic dissector
prostatic driver
prostatic ducts
prostatic enucleator
prostatic forceps
prostatic hook
prostatic lobe-holding forceps
prostatic needle holder
prostatic punch
prostatic retractor
prostatic scissors
prostatic tractor
prostatic trocar
prostatic urethra
prostatism
prostatitis
prostatocystotomy
prostatolithotomy
prostatotomy
prostatovesiculectomy
prosthesis (*pl.* prostheses) (see
    also *graft* and *patch*)
    Acrax
    Akiyama
    Alvarez
    Anametric
    Angelchik anti-reflux
    anti-incontinence
    aortic valve
    arterial
    Aufranc hip
    Aufranc-Turner hip
    Austin Moore
    ball-type
    ball valve
    Bateman
    Beall mitral valve

prosthesis *(continued)*
>	Bechtel
>	bifurcated seamless
>	bifurcation
>	Bjork-Shiley mitral valve
>	Braunwald-Cutter
>	breast
>	Bucholz
>	bypass
>	CAD (computerized assisted design)
>	Cape Town
>	carpal
>	Carrion penile
>	Cartwright heart
>	Cartwright valve
>	Cartwright vascular
>	Causse-Shea
>	Celestin
>	Charnley
>	Charnley-Mueller
>	cleft palate
>	collagen tape
>	compartmental total knee
>	Cooley-Bloodwell-Cutter
>	Cooley-Cutter
>	crimped Dacron
>	crimped woven
>	Cutter SCDK
>	Cutter-Smeloff cardiac valve
>	Dacron
>	DeBakey
>	DeBakey valve
>	DeBakey vascular
>	dental
>	DePalma hip
>	DePuy hip
>	discoid aortic

prosthesis *(continued)*
>	discoid valve
>	ear pinna
>	ear piston
>	Edwards
>	Edwards Teflon intracardiac
>	Eicher hip
>	endoesophageal
>	F. R. Thompson hip
>	fascia lata
>	femoral
>	femoral head
>	finger joint
>	4-A Magovern
>	Freeman-Swanson
>	gel-filled
>	Geomedic
>	geometric
>	Giliberty
>	gliding
>	Gor-Tex
>	Gott
>	Guepar
>	Hammersmith
>	Harken
>	Harris
>	Harrison
>	heart
>	Helanca
>	Herbert
>	Heyer-Schulte breast
>	hinged leaflet vascular
>	hingeless heart valve
>	hip
>	hollow sphere
>	House
>	Hufnagel valve
>	hybrid

prosthesis *(continued)*
    incus replacement
    inflatable mammary
    interlocked mesh
    intraluminal tube
    Jewett
    Joplin toe
    Judet
    Kaufman penile
    Kay-Shiley valve
    Kay-Suzuki valve
    Kinematic
    knitted vascular
    L-type nose-bridge
    Leinbach
    Lippman hip
    London
    Lorenzo SMO
    low profile valve
    MacIntosh
    Mackler tube
    Magovern ball valve
    mammary
    mandibular
    Marlex
    Matchett
    Matchett-Brown
    maxillary dental
    maxillofacial
    McBride-Moore
    McGhan breast
    McKee
    McKee-Farrar
    McKeever
    McNaught
    Medi-graft
    metal
    microcrimped

prosthesis *(continued)*
    Minneapolis
    mitral valve
    modular knee
    Moore hip
    Mueller hip
    Mulligan
    Neer shoulder
    Niebauer
    nose bridge
    nylon vascular
    ocular
    offset hinge
    orbital floor
    orlon vascular
    ossicular replacement
    partial ossicular replacement
    patellar cap
    patellofemoral
    penile
    piston
    Plastipore
    polycentric
    polyethylene
    PORP (partial ossicular
        replacement prosthesis)
    Richards
    Rosi bridge
    Sampson
    Sauerbruch
    Sauvage
    Sbarbaro
    SCDT heart valve
    Schuknecht piston
    seamless
    seamless tube
    Sheehy-House
    Shier knee

prosthesis *(continued)*
- Silastic
- Silastic mammary
- Silastic penile
- Silastic testicular
- silicone
- Sivash
- Small-Carrion penile
- Smeloff-Cutter valve
- Smith-Petersen
- SMO
- solid silicone orbital
- Speed
- stainless steel
- stainless steel wire
- stapes
- Starr-Edwards valve
- steel-wire
- stem
- Stenzel rod
- straight-stem
- surgical
- sutureless valve
- Swanson
- tantalum
- tantalum stapes
- Teflon
- Thompson
- tibial
- tibial plateau
- tibiofemoral
- titanium
- total hip
- total knee
- Townley
- trial
- tri-leaflet aortic
- Turner

prosthesis *(continued)*
- two-prong stem finger
- UCI
- umbrella-type
- Usher Marlex mesh
- valve
- Vanghetti
- vascular
- vessel
- Vitallium
- Vitallium Moore
- Wada valve
- Walldius knee
- Weavenit
- Wesolowski
- wire piston
- woven-tube vascular
- wire stapes
- Zimaloy
- Zimmer

prosthetic
prosthetic device
prosthetic replacement arthro-
    plasty
protamine
protective bandage
protective dressing
protecto splint
protein-bound iodine (PBI)
proteinuria
prothrombin time
protrusion
Providence clamp
Providence forceps
Providence Hospital clamp
Providence Hospital forceps
proximal
proximal incision

Pruitt anoscope
Pruitt proctoscope
pruritus
pruritus ani
Pryor-Péan retractor
PSCE (presurgical clotting evalua-
    tion)
pseudarthrosis
pseudocapsule
pseudocyst
pseudoligamentous
pseudomembrane
pseudomembranous
psoas major
psoas minor
psoas muscle
psoas retractor
psychogenic
PTCA (percutaneous transluminal
    coronary angioplasty)
pterygium
pterygium keratome
pterygium knife
pterygium operation
pterygium transplant
pterygoid muscle
pterygoid nerve
pterygoid process
pterygoideus lateralis muscle
pterygoideus lateralis nerve
pterygoideus medialis muscle
pterygoideus medialis nerve
pterygopalatine nerves
pterygopalatini nerves
ptosis
ptosis clamp
ptosis correction
ptosis forceps

ptosis knife
ptosis operation
ptosis sling
ptotic
ptyalectasis
ptyalolithiasis
ptyalolithotomy
pubes (*sing.* pubis)
pubic
pubic bone
pubic ramus
pubic tubercle
pubioplasty
pubiotomy
pubis (*pl.* pubes)
pubococcygeal muscle
pubococcygeoplasty
pubococcygeus muscle
puboprostatic muscle
puboprostaticus muscle
puborectal muscle
puborectalis muscle
pubovaginal muscle
pubovaginalis muscle
pubovesical muscle
pubovesicalis muscle
pudenda interna artery
pudenda interna vein
pudendae externae arteries
pudendae externae veins
pudendal anesthesia
pudendal arteries
pudendal block
pudendal hernia
pudendal nerve
pudendal vein
pudendal vessel
pudendus nerve

Pudenz shunt
Pudenz tube
Pudenz valve
pudic
pudic vessel
Puestow operation
Pugh nail
pull-out wire
pull-through abdominoperineal
    resection
pull-through procedure
pull-through proctectomy
pulled tendon
pulley sutures
pulmonalis dextra artery
pulmonalis inferior dextra vein
pulmonalis inferior sinistra vein
pulmonalis sinistra artery
pulmonalis superior dextra vein
pulmonalis superior sinistra vein
pulmonary aortic anastomosis
pulmonary artery
pulmonary artery banding
pulmonary artery catheter
pulmonary artery clamp
pulmonary artery forceps
pulmonary clamp
pulmonary embolism clamp
pulmonary function studies
pulmonary innominate anasto-
    mosis
pulmonary ligament
pulmonary resection
pulmonary retractor
pulmonary subclavian anastomosis
pulmonary toilet
pulmonary trunk
pulmonary valve knife

pulmonary valvulotome
pulmonary valvulotomy
pulmonary vein
pulmonary vessel clamp
pulmonary vessel forceps
pulmonic clamp
pulp
pulp amputation
pulp canal
pulpectomy
pulpotomy
pulsatile
pulsating aneurysm
pulsation
pulse
pulse generator
pulsion
pulsion hernia
pump
        Carmody
        drainage
        Emerson
        gastrostomy
        Gomco
        Hakim-Cordis
        hand
        Harvard
        IVAC
        p. oxygenator
        Stedman suction
        suction
        suction-pressure
        vacuum hand
punch
        Abrams biopsy
        adenoid
        Adler
        Ainsworth

punch *(continued)*
    Mixter
    Mosher
    Murphy
    Myers
    Myerson
    Myles
    nasal
    Noyes
    oval
    Peau
    Phemister
    pin
    plate
    pleural biopsy
    Pritikin
    prostatic
    p. biopsy
    p. curet
    p. forceps
    p. resection
    p. sclerectomy
    p. technique
    Raney
    Reaves
    Rhoton
    Rubin-Holth
    Sachs
    Schlesinger
    Schmeden
    Schubert biopsy
    scleral
    sclerectomy
    Seiffert
    Seletz
    semicircular
    skull cone
    Spencer

punch *(continued)*
    sphenoid
    Spies
    Spurling-Kerrison
    square
    sternal
    Stevenson
    Storz
    Struyken
    Sweet
    Takahashi
    Thompson
    Thoms-Gaylor biopsy
    Tischler
    tonsil
    Turkel
    uterine biopsy
    Van Struycken
    Veenema-Gusberg
    vessel
    Wagner
    Walton
    Walton-Schubert
    Watson-Schubert
    Watson-Williams
    Whitcomb-Kerrison
    Wilde
    Wittner biopsy
    Yankauer
    Yeomans
punctate
punctate cataract
punctate electrode
punctate electrotome
punctum
punctum dilator
punctum snip
puncture

puncture incision
puncture needle
puncture wound
pupil
pupillary block
pupillotomy
Purcell retractor
Purlon sutures
pursestring cervical closure
pursestring sutures
purulence
purulent
pus
pus tube
push-back palatoplasty
pusher
    Geomedic femoral
    suture
Pusto dilatation
pustule
Putti approach
Putti gouge
Putti operation
Putti-Platt director
Putti-Platt operation
Putti rasp
Putti raspatory
Putti splint
Puusepp operation
PVR (postvoiding residual)
pyelectasia
pyelectasis
pyelogram
pyelography
pyeloileocutaneous anastomosis
pyeloileostomy
pyelolithotomy
pyelonephritis

pyeloplasty
pyelorrhaphy
pyeloscopy
pyelostomy
pyelotomy
pyelotomy incision
pyeloureterogram
pyeloureterography
pyeloureteroplasty
pylon
pylorectomy
pyloric
pyloric antrum
pyloric glands
pyloric occlusion operation
pyloric stenosis dilator
pyloric vein
pyloristenosis
pylorodilator
pylorodiosis
pyloroduodenitis
pyloroduodenotomy
pylorogastrectomy
pyloromyotomy
pyloroplasty
pyloroptosis
pyloroscopy
pylorospasm
pylorostenosis
pylorostomy
pylorotomy
pylorus
pylorus clamp
pylorus separator
Pynchon applicator
Pynchon cannula
Pynchon-Lillie tongue depressor
Pynchon speculum

Pynchon suction tube
Pynchon tongue depressor
Pynchon tube
pyocele
pyocelia
pyogenic
pyogenic abscess
pyoktanin sutures
pyorrhea
pyosalpinx
pyramid
pyramid of thyroid
pyramidal

pyramidal cataract
pyramidal eye implant
pyramidal fracture
pyramidal lobe of thyroid
pyramidal muscle
pyramidal trocar
pyramidal tube
pyramidialis auriculae muscle
pyramidialis muscle
Pyrex tube
Pyridium
pyriform sinus
pyuria

q

Q-tips
quadrangular
quadrant
quadrate muscle
quadratus femoris muscle
quadratus lumborum muscle
quadratus plantae muscle
quadriceps femoris muscle
quadriceps muscle
quadricepsplasty
quadrilateral
quadriplegia
quadriplegic
quadruple amputation
Quaglino operation
quarantine

Queckenstedt maneuver
Queckenstedt test
Queen Anne dressing
Quelicin
Quenu-Mayo operation
quenuthoracoplasty
Quervain forceps
Quervain fracture
Quervain-Sauerbruch retractor
Quevedo forceps
quilled sutures
quilt sutures
quilted sutures
Quinton tube
Quisling hammer
quotient

r

rachicentesis
rachitomy
racket incision
raclage
radial
radial artery
radial artery of index finger
radial incision
radial iridotomy
radial nerve
radial nerve splint
radial veins
radiales veins
radialis artery
radialis indicis artery
radialis nerve
radiate arteries of kidney
radiation
radiation therapy
radical
radical antrum operation
radical excision
radical excision of lesion
radical gastrectomy
radical glossectomy
radical groin dissection
radical hemorrhoidectomy
radical herniorrhaphy
radical hysterectomy
radical lymphadenectomy
radical mastectomy
radical mastoidectomy

radical neck dissection
radical operation
radical sinusotomy
radicle
radicotomy
radicular
radiculectomy
radiculopathy
radio-frequency pacemaker
radioactive
radioactive applicator
radioactive cobalt
radioactive iodine
radioactive uptake
radiocarpal articulation
radiocarpal ligament
radiogram
radiography
radioisotope
radioisotope applicator
radiology
radiopaque bougie
radiopaque intestinal tube
radiopaque substance
radioresistant
radiosensitive
radiotherapy
radioulnar articulation
radium
radium application
radium applicator
radium implant

radium insertion
radium needle
radius
railway catheter
rainbow fracture frame
rake
    amputation
    Blake
    r. retractor
    Volkmann
rales
Ralks applicator
Ralks clamp
Ralks-Davis mouth gag
Ralks drill
Ralks elevator
Ralks forceps
Ralks knife
Ralks magnet
Ralks mallet
Ramdohr sutures
rami (*sing.* ramus)
ramification
Ramirez shunt
ramisection
Ramsbotham hook
Ramsbotham knife
Ramsbotham sickle
Ramsey County pyoktanin sutures
Ramstedt dilator
Ramstedt operation
Ramstedt pyloromyotomy
Ramstedt pyloroplasty
ramus (*pl.* rami)
Randall curet
Randall forceps
Randall operation
Randolph cannula

Raney clip
Raney curet
Raney-Crutchfield tongs
Raney dissector
Raney drill
Raney forceps
Raney Gigli-saw guide
Raney periosteal elevator
Raney punch
Raney retractor
Raney rongeur
range of motion
ranine artery
ranine vein
Rankin clamp
Rankin-Crile forceps
Rankin forceps
Rankin operation
Rankin retractor
Rankin tractor
Ransohoff operation
ranula
Ranzewski clamp
Rapaport dilator
raphe
Rashkind procedure
rasp (see also *raspatory*)
    antrum
    Aufricht
    Aufricht-Lipsett
    Austin Moore
    Beck
    Berne
    bone
    Brawley
    Brown
    Charnley-Mueller
    Cohen

rasp *(continued)*
    Converse
    corneal
    Cottle
    Dean
    Eicher
    Epstein
    F. R. Thompson
    facet
    femoral shaft
    Fisher
    Fomon
    frontal
    Good
    Israel
    Joseph
    Lamont
    Lewis
    Lundsgaard
    Lundsgaard-Burch
    Maliniac
    Maltz
    Maltz-Lipsett
    McKee-Farrar
    Moore
    nasal
    Putti
    Ritter
    Saunders-Paparella
    Schmidt
    sinus
    Spratt
    stem
    Thompson
    trochanter
    Watson-Williams
    Wiener
    Wiener-Pierce

rasp *(continued)*
    window
    Woodward
raspatory (see also *rasp*)
    Alexander
    Babcock
    Bacon
    Ballenger
    Bastow
    Beck
    Berry
    Brunner
    Coryllos
    Davis
    Doyen
    Farabeuf
    Friedrich
    Hedblom
    Hoen
    Hopkins
    Jansen
    Joseph
    Kirmisson
    Kocher
    Ladd
    Lambert-Berry
    laminectomy
    Lane
    Langenbeck
    Langenbeck-O'Brien
    Lebsche
    Lewis
    mastoid
    Mathieu
    Matson
    Nicola
    Ollier
    Overholt

raspatory *(continued)*
    pericardial
    periosteal
    Phemister
    Putti
    r. elevator
    rib
    Sauerbruch
    Sayre
    Schneider
    Sedillot
    Semb
    Trélat
    Willauer
    xyster
    Yasargil
    Zoellner
Rastelli operation
rat-tooth forceps
ratchet
Ratliff-Blake forceps
Ratliff-Mayo forceps
Raverdino operation
Ravich cystoscope
Ravich dilator
Ravich lithotriptoscope
raw surface
Ray curet
Ray forceps
Ray-Parsons-Sunday elevator
Ray speculum
Ray spoon
Rayner-Choyce eye implant
Raytec gauze
Raytec sponge
razor scalpel
reach-and-pin forceps
reaction

reactive
readjustment
ream
reamer
    acetabular
    adjustable cup
    Aufranc
    Austin Moore
    ball
    bone
    cannulated
    chamfer
    Charnley
    deepening
    DePuy
    engine
    expanding
    femoral head
    femoral neck
    finishing ball
    finishing cup
    grooving
    Indiana
    Jergeson
    Jewett
    Küntscher
    Lorenzo
    Lottes
    MacAusland
    medullary canal
    Mira
    Moore
    Murphy
    offset
    Phemister
    Reiswig
    Rush
    shaft

reamer *(continued)*
    shelf
    Smith-Petersen
    spherical
    spiral
    Sturmdorf
    trochanter
reamputation
reanastomosis
reapproximate
reattachment
reattachment of retina
reattachment of tendon
Reaves punch
rebound tenderness
rebreathing anesthesia
recalcitrant
Recamier curet
Recamier operation
recanalize
recessed-head screw
recessing of tendon
recession forceps
recession of ocular muscle
recipient
Recklinghausen tonometer
reclosure
reconstruction
reconstruction operation
reconstructive arthroplasty
reconstructive technique
recontour
recording
recovery
recovery room (RR)
rectal
rectal anesthesia
rectal artery

rectal biopsy forceps
rectal bougie
rectal catheter
rectal curet
rectal cutter
rectal dilator
rectal director
rectal hernia
rectal hook
rectal injection cannula
rectal injection needle
rectal needle
rectal nerves
rectal polyps
rectal probe
rectal pull-through operation
rectal retractor
rectal scissors
rectal snare
rectal speculum
rectal stricture
rectal trocar
rectal tube
rectal vein
rectales inferiores nerves
rectales inferiores veins
rectales mediae veins
rectalis inferior artery
rectalis media artery
rectalis superior artery
rectalis superior vein
rectangular
rectangular amputation
rectectomy
rectified microscope
rectified polarizing microscope
rectocele
rectocele repair

rectococcygeus muscle
rectopexy
rectoplasty
rectorectostomy
rectoromanoscopy
rectorrhaphy
rectoscopy
rectosigmoid
rectosigmoidectomy
rectosigmoidoscope
rectosigmoidoscopy
rectosigmoidostomy
rectostomy
rectotomy
rectourethral muscle
rectourethralis muscle
rectouterine ligament
rectouterine muscle
rectouterinus muscle
rectovaginal
rectovaginal fistula
rectovesical
rectovesical muscle
rectovesicalis muscle
rectum
rectus
rectus abdominis muscle
rectus capitis anterior muscle
rectus capitis lateralis muscle
rectus capitis posterior major
    muscle
rectus capitis posterior minor
    muscle
rectus femoris muscle
rectus incision
rectus inferior bulbi muscle
rectus lateralis bulbi muscle
rectus medialis bulbi muscle

rectus muscle
rectus muscle hook
rectus muscle splitting incision
rectus superior bulbi muscle
recumbent position
recurrens radialis artery
recurrens tibialis anterior artery
recurrens tibialis posterior artery
recurrens ulnaris artery
recurrent
recurrent artery
recurrent nerve
red reflex
red Robinson catheter
red rubber catheter
red-tip aspirator
red-top tube
Redi hemodialysis machine
Redivac drain
reducible
reducible hernia
reducing fracture frame
reducing valve
reduction
reduction mammaplasty
reduction of fracture
reduction of hernia
reduction of intussusception
reduction of torsion
reduction of volvulus
reduction technique
reductive mammaplasty
redundancy
redundant
reefing
re-entry operation
Reese dermatome
Reese forceps

Reese knife
Reese operation
Reese stimulator
re-establishment
reference electrode
referral
referred
reflected
reflecting microscope
reflecting ophthalmoscope
reflection
reflex
reflexes
reflux
refraction
refractive error
refracture of bone
refrigeration anesthesia
refusion of blood
regional anesthesia
regional block anesthesia
regional ileitis
regional node
Regnoli operation
regular sinus rhythm
regurgitation
Rehfuss tube
Rehn-Delorme operation
Reich-Nechtow clamp
Reich-Nechtow curet
Reich-Nechtow dilator
Reich-Nechtow forceps
Reich-Nechtow plug
Reichenheim-King operation
reimplantation
Reiner-Beck snare
Reiner curet
Reiner knife

Reiner-Knight forceps
Reiner rongeur
reinforcement
reinforcing
Reinhoff-Finochietto rib spreader
Reinhoff rib spreader
reinnervation
reinsertion
reintubation
Reisinger forceps
Reissner's membrane
Reiswig reamer
relaxation
relaxation sutures
relaxing incision
release
release of tendo Achillis
release of trigger finger
relief incision
Reliquet lithotrite
Relton-Hall frame
remnant
remobilization
removal
removal of calculus
removal of drain
removal of dressing
removal of emboli
removal of embryo
removal of fetal structures
removal of foreign body
removal of hydatidiform mole
removal of pack
removal of packing
removal of placental fragments
removal of retained placenta
removal of retained placenta and
    membranes

removal of sequestrum
renal
renal arteries
renal capsule
renal capsulectomy
renal clamp
renal colic
renal needle
renal pedicle clamp
renal veins
renales veins
renalis artery
renis arteries
Renografin
rent
reopening
repacking
repair
repair of defect
repair of septal defect
reperitonealize
replacement
replacement graft
replacement prosthesis
replacement transfusion
Replogle tube
reposition
reprepped
resecting fracture
resection
resection clamp
resection-recession of eye muscles
resectoscope
    Bard
    Baumrucker
    Bumpus
    cold-punch
    French-Iglesias

resectoscope *(continued)*
    Gray
    Green
    Iglesias
    McCarthy
    miniature
    multiple
    Nesbit
    r. sheath
    rotating
    Scott
    Stern-McCarthy
    Storz-Iglesias
    Thompson
    Timberlake
resectoscopy
residual
Resifilm
respiration
respiration assisted anesthesia
respiration bronchoscope
respiration pyelogram
respiration pyelography
respiration unassisted anesthesia
respirator
respiratory
respiratory embarrassment
response
rest position
restoration
restricted
restriction
restrictor
resulting defect
resuscitation
resuscitator
resuture
retained placenta

retained placenta and membranes
retaining device
retaining retractor
retention
retention catheter
retention cyst
retention sutures
retina
retinaculotomy
retinaculum (*pl.* retinacula)
retinal cryopexy
retinal detachment
retinal detachment repair
retinal puncture cautery
retinoscope
    Copeland
    electric
    Welch Allyn
retinoscopy
retract
retraction
retractor
    abdominal
    abdominal-vascular
    Adams
    Adson
    Adson-Beckman
    Agrikola
    alar
    Alden
    Allen
    Allison
    Allport
    Allport-Babcock
    Alm
    Alter
    aluminum cortex
    Amoils

retractor *(continued)*
    amputation
    anal
    Anderson-Adson
    Andrews
    Ann Arbor
    anterior
    Anthony
    antrum
    aorta
    aortic valve
    apicolysis
    appendectomy
    Army
    Army-Navy
    Arruga
    atrial
    Aufranc
    Aufricht
    Austin
    automatic skin
    Babcock
    baby
    Bacon
    Badgley
    Bahnson
    Balfour
    Ballen-Alexander
    Bankhart
    Baron
    Barr
    Barrett-Adson
    Beaver
    Becker
    Beckman
    Beckman-Adson
    Beckman-Eaton
    Beckman-Weitlaner

retractor *(continued)*

Beneventi
Bennett
Berens
Berna
Bernay
Bethune
Bicek
bifid
biliary
bivalve
Black
bladder
Blair
Blair-Brown
Blakesley
Blount
blunt
blunt rake
Bosworth
bowel
Boyes-Goodfellow hook
Braastad
brain
Brantley-Turner
Brawley
Brewster
Brompton Hospital
Bronson-Turz
Brown
Brunner
Brunschwig
Bucy
Buie-Smith
bulb
Burford
Burford-Finochietto
button-hook

retractor *(continued)*

Byford
Cairns
Campbell
capsule
Cardillo
Carter
Castallo
Castroviejo
Cave
cecostomy
cerebellum
cerebral
cervical
chalazion
Chandler
Charnley
cheek
Cherry
Cloward
Cloward-Hoen
cobra
Cole
Colver
Cone
contour
Converse
Cook
Cooley
corner
cortex
Coryllos
costal arch
Cottle
Cottle-Neivert
Crafoord
Craig-Sheehan
cranial

retractor *(continued)*
- Crile
- Crotti
- Cushing
- dacryocystorhinostomy
- Davidoff
- Davidson
- Davis
- Deaver
- DeBakey-Balfour
- DeBakey-Cooley
- Decker
- decompression
- deep
- Delaney
- Delee
- DeMartel
- DePuy
- D'Errico
- D'Errico-Adson
- Desmarres
- Dingman
- Dingman-Senn
- Dorsey
- Dott
- double-ended
- Downing
- Doyen
- dull
- dull-pronged
- Dumont
- duodenal
- dural
- East-West
- Eastman
- Edinburgh
- Elschnig
- Emmet

retractor *(continued)*
- endaural
- epiglottis
- erector spinae
- examination
- externo-frontal
- eye
- eyelid
- Falk
- Farabeuf
- Farr
- Favoloro
- Feldman
- femoral neck
- Ferguson
- Ferguson-Moon
- Ferris Smith
- Ferris Smith-Sewall
- finger
- Fink
- Finochietto
- Fisher
- Fisher-Nugent
- flexible
- flexible shaft
- Flexsteel
- Fomon
- Foss
- four-prong
- Franklin
- Franz
- Frater
- Frazier
- Freer
- Freiberg
- French
- French-Stern-McCarthy
- Friedman

retractor *(continued)*
- Fritsch
- Fulton
- gallbladder
- gastric resection
- Gelpi
- Gibson-Balfour
- Gifford
- Gilvernet
- Glaser
- Glenner
- Goelet
- goiter
- Goldstein
- Good
- Goodhill
- Goodyear
- Gosset
- Gradle
- Grant
- Green
- Grieshaber
- Groenholm
- Gross
- Gross-Pomeranz-Watkins
- Gruenwald
- Guttmann
- Haight
- Hajek
- half-moon
- Hamby
- Hamby-Hibbs
- hand
- Harken
- Harrington
- Harrington-Pemberton
- Harrison
- Hartstein

retractor *(continued)*
- Haslinger
- Haverfield
- Haverfield-Scoville
- Hayes
- Heaney
- Heaney-Simon
- Hedblom
- Heifitz
- Helfrick
- hemilaminectomy
- Henderson
- Henner
- Hibbs
- Hill-Ferguson
- Hillis
- Himmelstein
- hip
- Hoen
- Hohmann
- Holman
- hook
- horizontal
- House
- House-Urban
- Howorth
- Hudson
- Hunt
- Hupp
- Hurd
- hysterectomy
- infant abdominal
- intestinal occlusion
- intracardiac
- iris
- Israel
- Jackson
- Jacobson

retractor *(continued)*
 Jaeger
 Jannetta
 Jansen
 Jansen-Gifford
 Jansen-Wagner
 Jefferson
 Johns Hopkins
 Johnson
 Jones
 Jorgenson
 Judd-Masson
 Kelly
 Kelly-Sims
 Kerrison
 kidney
 Killian-King
 King
 King-Hurd
 Kirby
 Kirkland
 Klemme
 Knapp
 knee
 knife
 Kocher
 Kocher-Crotti
 Kraske
 Kristeller
 Kronfeld
 lacrimal
 lacrimal sac
 Lahey
 laminectomy
 Lane
 Lange
 Langenbeck
 Laplace

retractor *(continued)*
 laryngeal
 laryngofissure
 Latrobe
 Legueu
 Lemmon
 Lempert
 Lempert-Colver
 Lewis
 lid
 lighted
 Lilienthal-Sauerbruch
 Lillie
 Linton
 lip
 Little
 liver
 Lorie
 Lothrop
 Love
 Lowsley
 Luer
 Lukens
 lung
 Luongo
 MacAusland
 MacAusland-Kelly
 Mackay
 Maliniac
 malleable
 Maltz
 Markham-Meyerding
 Martin
 Masson-Judd
 mastectomy
 mastoid
 mastoid-retaining
 Mathieu

retractor *(continued)*

- Mayo
- Mayo-Adams
- Mayo-Collins
- Mayo-Lovelace
- Mayo-Simpson
- McBurney
- McCullough
- McGannon
- McGill
- Meller
- Meyer
- Meyerding
- Meyerding-Deaver
- microsurgery
- Milex
- Miller
- Miller-Senn
- Millin
- Millin-Bacon
- mitral valve
- Mollison
- Moore
- Moorehead
- Morris
- Morrison-Hurd
- Morse
- Mosher
- Mueller
- Mueller-Balfour
- Munro
- Murphy
- muscle
- Myers
- narrow
- nasal
- nasopharyngeal
- Neivert

retractor *(continued)*

- nerve
- nerve root
- North-South
- Nuttall
- OB
- Oberhill
- Obwegeser
- Ochsner
- O'Connor
- O'Connor-O'Sullivan
- offset
- Oldberg
- Oliver
- Ollier
- orbital
- O'Sullivan
- O'Sullivan-O'Connor
- Overholt
- palate
- Paparella
- Parker
- Parker-Mott
- patent ductus
- Paul
- Pemberton
- Penfield
- Percy
- Percy-Wolfson
- perineal
- Pheifer-Young
- phrenic
- Picot
- Pierce
- pillar
- pin
- Proctor
- pronged

retractor *(continued)*

- prostatic
- Pryor-Péan
- psoas
- pulmonary
- Purcell
- Quervain-Sauerbruch
- rake
- Raney
- Rankin
- rectal
- retaining
- retropubic
- rib
- ribbon
- Richardson
- Richardson-Eastman
- Rigby
- right-angle
- Rizzo
- Rizzuti
- Robinson
- Rochester
- Rochester-Ferguson
- Rollet
- Roos
- Ross
- Roux
- S-shaped
- Sachs
- Sauerbruch
- Sauerbruch-Zukschwerdt
- Sawyer
- scalp
- scapula
- Schuknecht
- Schwartz
- Scoville

retractor *(continued)*

- Seletz-Gelpi
- self-retaining
- self-retaining spring
- Semb
- Senn
- Senn-Dingman
- Senturia
- serrated
- serrefine
- Sewall
- Shambaugh
- sharp-pronged
- Shearer
- Sheehan
- Sheldon
- Shurly
- Sims
- Sims-Kelly
- Sistrunk
- six-prong rake
- skid
- skin-flap
- Sloan
- Sluder
- Smillie
- Smith
- Smith-Buie
- Smith-Petersen
- Snitman
- soft-palate
- spike
- spinal
- spinal cord
- splanchnic
- spring
- spring wire
- St. Luke

retractor *(continued)*
  sternal
  sternum
  Stevenson
  Stookey
  Strully
  submucous
  suprapubic
  Sweeney
  Sweet
  Taylor
  Temple-Fay
  Theis
  three-prong
  thymus
  thyroid
  tibia
  tissue
  tonsil
  tonsil pillar
  toothed
  Tower
  tracheal
  trigeminal
  Tuffier
  Tuffier-Raney
  two-prong rake
  two-pronged
  U.S. Army
  Ullrich
  universal
  uvula
  vacuum
  vaginal
  vagotomy
  vascular
  Veenema
  vein

retractor *(continued)*
  ventriculogram
  vertical
  vesical
  visceral
  Volkman
  Walker
  Walter-Deaver
  Webb
  Webb-Balfour
  Weber
  Webster
  Weder
  Weder-Solenberger
  weighted posterior
  Weinberg
  Weitlaner
  Wesson
  White-Proud
  Wilmer
  Wilson
  wire
  Wolfson
  Wullstein
  Yasargil
  Young
retrenchment
retroauricular incision
retrobulbar
retrobulbar anesthesia
retrobulbar block
retrobulbar injection
retrocecal
retrocecal hernia
retrocolic
retrodisplaced pessary
retrodisplacement
retrodisplacement of uterus

retroflexed
retroflexion
retrogasserian neurotomy
retrograde
retrograde bougie
retrograde electrode
retrograde flow
retrograde hernia
retrograde pyelogram
retrograde pyelography
retrograde urogram
retrograde urography
Retrografin dye
retromammary
retromandibular vein
retromandibularis vein
retroperitoneal
retroperitoneal hernia
retroperitoneal injection of air
retroperitoneal space
retropubic prostatectomy
retropubic retractor
retropubic space
retropulsion
retrospective telescope
retroversion
retroversion of uterus
retroversion pessary
retroverted
Retter needle
return-flow cannula
return-flow hemostatic catheter
Reuter bobbins
Reuter button
Reuter stainless steel bobbins
Reuter tube
revascularize
revascularization

Reverdin graft
Reverdin needle
Reverdin operation
reverse
reverse-angle skid curet
reverse bandage
reverse-bevel laryngoscope
reverse-curve clamp
reverse cutting sutures
reverse Kingsley splint
reverse-shape eye implant
reverse Trendelenburg position
reversed bandage
reversible knife
revision
revision of graft
revision of scar
Reynolds clamp
Reynolds scissors
Reynolds tongs
Reynolds tube
Rezek forceps
rhegmatogenous retinal detachment
Rhein pick
Rheinberg microscope
Rheinstaedter curet
rheumatoid arthritis
Rhinelander clamp
rhinocheiloplasty
rhinokyphectomy
rhinomanometer
rhinomanometry
rhinommectomy
rhinoplastic correction
rhinoplasty
rhinoplasty saw
rhinorrhaphy

rhinorrhea
rhinoscopy
rhinoseptoplasty
rhinostomy
rhinotomy
rhizodontropy
rhizotomy
RhoGAM
rhomboid ligament
rhomboid muscle
rhomboideus major muscle
rhomboideus minor muscle
rhonchus (*pl.* rhonchi)
Rhoton punch
rhytidectomy
rhytidoplasty
rib
rib cage
rib contractor
    Bailey
    Bailey-Gibbon
    Graham
    Sellor
    Waterman
rib cutter
rib drill
rib edge stripper
rib elevator
rib guillotine
rib needle
rib raspatory
rib retractor
rib rongeur
rib shears (see also *shears*)
    Bacon
    Bethune
    Bethune-Coryllos
    Brunner

rib shears *(continued)*
    Coryllos-Bethune
    Coryllos-Moure
    Coryllos-Shoemaker
    Doyen
    Duval-Coryllos
    Giertz-Shoemaker
    Gluck
    Harrington-Mayo
    infant
    Moure-Coryllos
    Nelson-Bethune
    Potts
    Roberts
    Roberts-Nelson
    Sauerbruch
    Sauerbruch-Coryllos
    Semb
    Shoemaker
    Stille
    Stille-Giertz
    Tudor-Edwards
    Walton
rib spreader (see also *spreader*)
    Burford
    Burford-Finochietto
    child's
    Davis
    DeBakey
    Finochietto
    Gerbode
    Haight
    Harken
    infant
    Lemmon
    Lilienthal
    Lilienthal-Sauerbruch
    McGuire

rib spreader *(continued)*
    Nelson
    Nissen
    Overholt
    Overholt-Finochietto
    Reinhoff
    Reinhoff-Finochietto
    Sweet
    Sweet-Burford
    Thies
    Tuffier
    Weinberg
    Wilson
rib stripper (See *stripper.*)
Riba electric ureteral meatotome
Ribble bandage
ribbon gut
ribbon gut needle
ribbon retractor
Ricard amputation
Richard forceps
Richards clamp
Richards curet
Richards nail
Richards prosthesis
Richards screw
Richardson-Eastman retractor
Richardson operation
Richardson periosteal elevator
Richardson retractor
Richardson sutures
Richet bandage
Richet operation
Richter forceps
Richter hernia
Richter sutures
Rickham reservoir
ridge

riding-pants deformity
Ridlon knife
Ridlon operation
Ridpath curet
Riecker bronchoscope
Riedel disease
Riedel lobe
Riedel needle
Riedel struma
Rienhoff clamp
Rienhoff dissector
Rienhoff forceps
Ries-Wertheim hysterectomy
Riex hernia
Rigal sutures
Rigaud operation
Rigby retractor
Rigg cannula
right-angle clamp
right-angle curet
right-angle mattress sutures
right-angle pick
right-angle retractor
right-angle scissors
right-angle telescope
right-angled bone cutter
right-angled erysiphake
right coronary artery
right lateral position
right lower quadrant (RLQ)
right rectus incision
right upper lobe (RUL)
right upper quadrant (RUQ)
rigidity
Riley needle
rim incision
rima (*pl.* rimae)

ring
 Abbe
 Bonaccolto scleral
 centering
 Coats
 Falope
 fixation
 Fleischer
 Flieringa scleral
 Gräfenberg
 Kayser-Fleischer
 Lowe
 McNeill-Goldmann scleral
 r. clamp
 r. curet
 r. cutter
 ring-end forceps
 r. finger
 r. forceps
 r. graft
 r. pessary
 r. rotation forceps
 Schatzki
 Thiersch
 wire
Ringenberg electrode
Ringer's lactate solution
Ringer's solution
ripe cataract
Ripstein operation
Risdon incision
Risdon wire
Rish chisel
Rish knife
risorius muscle
Ritchie tenaculum
Ritgen maneuver
Ritisch sutures

Ritter coagulator
Ritter dilator
Ritter drain
Ritter forceps
Ritter rasp
Ritter sound
Rives splenectomy
Rizzo retractor
Rizzoli operation
Rizzoli osteoclast
Rizzuti lens expressor
Rizzuti-McGuire scissors
Rizzuti retractor
RLQ (right lower quadrant)
Robb cannula
Robb forceps
Robb knife
Robb needle
Robb syringe
Robert Jones dressing
Robert operation
Robert snare
Roberts applicator
Roberts chisel
Roberts esophagoscope
Roberts forceps
Roberts laryngoscope
Roberts-Nelson rib shears
Roberts-Nelson rib stripper
Roberts-Nelson tourniquet
Roberts rib shears
Roberts speculum
Robertson forceps
Robertson knife
Robinson catheter
Robinson retractor
Robinson stone basket
Robinson stone dislodger

Robson position
Rochester awl
Rochester-Carmalt forceps
Rochester clamp
Rochester elevator
Rochester-Ewald forceps
Rochester-Ferguson retractor
Rochester-Ferguson scissors
Rochester forceps
Rochester-Harrington forceps
Rochester knife
Rochester-Mixter forceps
Rochester needle
Rochester-Ochsner forceps
Rochester-Péan clamp
Rochester-Péan forceps
Rochester-Rankin forceps
Rochester retractor
Rochester-Russian forceps
Rochester syringe
Rochester tube
rocker bottom foot
Rockey cannula
Rockey clamp
Rockey endoscope
Rockey forceps
Rockey probe
Rockey scoop
Rocky-Davis incision
rocking leg splint
rod
    colostomy
    compression
    Corti
    distraction
    enamel
    fracture
    glass

rod *(continued)*
    Harrington
    House
    intramedullary
    Küntscher
    Maddox
    malleable
    metal
    r. electrode
    Rush
    Schneider
    Stenzel
    Y-glass
Rodman incision
Rodriguez-Alvarez catheter
Roe clamp
Roe solution
Roeder clamp
Roeder forceps
roentgen
roentgenogram
roentgenography
Roger Anderson apparatus
Roger Anderson operation
Roger Anderson pin
Roger Anderson splint
Rogers amputation
Rogers dissector
Rokitansky hernia
Rolf forceps
Rolf lance
Rolf lance needle
Rolf punctum dilator
rolled Colles splint
roller
roller bandage
roller dressing
roller forceps

roller knife
Rollet incision
Rollet irrigator
Rollet retractor
rollflap operation
rolling of conjunctiva
Rommel cautery
Rommel-Hildreth cautery
rongeur
    Adson
    Andrews-Hartmann
    angular
    antrum
    aortic valve
    Bacon
    Bailey
    Bane
    bayonet
    Beyer
    bone
    bone-cutting
    bone-nibbling
    bony
    Bruening-Citelli
    Cairns
    Campbell
    chicken-bill
    Cicherelli
    Citelli
    Cloward
    Converse
    cranial
    Cushing
    Dean
    Depuy
    DeVilbiss
    double-action
    duckbill

rongeur *(continued)*
    Dufourmentel
    ear
    endaural
    Ferris Smith
    Ferris Smith-Gruenwald
    Ferris Smith-Kerrison
    Ferris Smith-Takahashi
    Fulton
    Garrison
    Glover
    gooseneck
    Gruenwald
    Hajek
    Hartmann
    Hartmann-Herzfeld
    Henny
    Hoen
    Horsley
    Hudson
    Husks
    infundibulectomy
    intervertebral disk
    IV disk
    Ivy
    Jansen
    Juers-Lempert
    Kerr
    Kerrison
    Killian
    laminectomy
    Lebsche
    Leksell
    Lempert
    Lillie
    Liston
    Littauer
    Lombard

rongeur *(continued)*
- Lombard-Beyer
- Lombard-Boies
- Love-Gruenwald
- Love-Kerrison
- Luer
- Luer-Hartmann
- mastoid
- Mead
- monster
- multiple-action
- nasal
- Nichols
- Noyes
- Oldberg
- Olivecrona
- Pierce
- pituitary
- Poppen
- Prince
- Raney
- Reiner
- rib
- r. forceps
- Rowland
- Ruskin
- Sauerbruch
- Sauerbruch-Lebsche
- Schlesinger
- Schwartz-Kerrison
- Selverstone
- Semb
- Semb-Sauerbruch
- Shearer
- side-curved
- Smith-Petersen
- Spurling
- Spurling-Kerrison

rongeur *(continued)*
- St. Luke
- Stille
- Stille-Leksell
- Stille-Luer
- Stookey
- straight
- Struempel
- Strully-Kerrison
- taper jaw
- Tobey
- up-cutting
- Walton
- Watson-Williams
- Weil
- Weingartner
- Whiting

Roos osteotome
Roos retractor
Roosevelt clamp
root amputation
root canal
root-canal broach
root-canal spreader
root pliers
root sheath
Roper cannula
ropy mass
ropy tumor
rosary bougie
Rose cleft lip repair
Rose operation
Rose position
Rose-Thompson cleft lip repair
Rosen curet
Rosen dissector
Rosen elevator
Rosen incision

Rosen knife
Rosen needle
Rosen probe
Rosen separator
Rosen suction tube
Rosen tube
Rosenburg operation
Rosenmueller curet
Rosenmueller fossa
Rosenthal speculum
Roser mouth gag
Roser needle
rosette
Rosi bridge prosthesis
Ross catheter
Ross needle
Ross retractor
Rosser hook
Rostan shunt
rotary dissector
rotating anoscope
rotating forceps
rotating laryngoscope
rotating resectoscope
rotating transilluminator
rotation
rotation forceps
rotation osteotomy
rotation skin flap
rotator muscles
rotatores muscles
rotatory
rotatory hammer
Rouge operation
round-blade scissors
round bur
round counterbore
round ligament of femur

round ligament of liver
round ligament of uterus
round ligaments
round punch forceps
round-tip catheter
Routier operation
routine urinalysis (RUA)
Routte operation
Roux-en-Y anastomosis
Roux-en-Y gastrectomy
Roux-en-Y incision
Roux-en-Y operation
Roux-Goldthwait operation
Roux operation
Roux retractor
Roux sign
Roux spatula
Roux-Y anastomosis
Roux-Y gastrectomy
Rovsing operation
Rovsing sign
Rowinski operation
Rowland forceps
Rowland keratome
Rowland osteotome
Rowland rongeur
Royalite body jacket
Royce knife
Royce perforator
RR (recovery room)
RUA (routine urinalysis)
rubber airway
rubber bolster
rubber-bulb syringe
rubber catheter
rubber dam
rubber-dam clamp
rubber-dam clamp forceps

rubber-dam drain
rubber drain
rubber padding
rubber pegs
rubber-shod clamp
rubber-shod hook
rubber sutures
Rubbrecht operation
rubella
Rubin-Brandborg tube
Rubin cannula
Rubin clamp
Rubin-Holth punch
Rubin needle
Rubin operation
Rubin test
Rubin tube
Rubovits clamp
ruby laser
rudimentary
ruga (*pl.* rugae)
rugae gastricae
Rugby forceps
Rugger-Jersey spine
Ruiz-Mora operation
RUL (right upper lobe)
ruler
    Berndt hip
    hip
    Joseph
    metal
    notched
    scleral
Rumel-Belmont tourniquet
Rumel clamp
Rumel forceps
Rumel splint
Rumel tourniquet

run-off
running chromic sutures
running continuous sutures
running lock sutures
running subcuticular sutures
Ruotte operation
rupture
ruptured
ruptured aneurysm
ruptured disk
ruptured disk curet
RUQ (right upper quadrant)
Rusch catheter
Rusch-Foley catheter
Rusch laryngoscope
Rusch tube
Ruschelit bougie
Ruschelit catheter
Rush clamp
Rush driver
Rush extractor
Rush mallet
Rush nail
Rush pin
Rush reamer
Rush rod
rushes
Rushkin balloon
Ruskin forceps
Ruskin-Liston forceps
Ruskin needle
Ruskin rongeur
Ruskin trocar
Russe incision
Russe operation
Russell-Buck tractor
Russell dilator
Russell forceps

Russell traction
Russell tractor
Russian forceps
Russian-Péan forceps

Ryerson operation
Ryerson tenotome
Ryle tube

S

"S" cannula
S-shaped incision
S-shaped retractor
Saalfield extractor
saber-back scissors
saber-cut approach
saber-cut incision
sac
saccular
saccular aneurysm
saccular nerve
saccularis nerve
sacculation
saccule
sacculus (*pl.* sacculi)
Sachs bur
Sachs cannula
Sachs elevator
Sachs forceps
Sachs hook
Sachs needle
Sachs punch
Sachs retractor
Sachs separator
Sachs spatula
Sachs suction tube
Sachs tube
sacral anesthesia
sacral arteries
sacral block
sacral canal
sacral nerves

sacral veins
sacral vertebrae
sacrales laterales arteries
sacrales laterales veins
sacrales nerves
sacralis mediana artery
sacralis mediana vein
sacrectomy
sacrococcygeal articulation
sacrococcygeal cyst
sacrococcygeal muscle
sacrococcygeal sinus
sacrococcygeus dorsalis muscle
sacrococcygeus ventralis muscle
sacrogenital ligament
sacroiliac
sacroiliac articulation
sacrospinous ligament
sacrouterine ligament
sacrum
saddle-block anesthesia
saddle-block spinal anesthesia
saddle deformity
saddle nose
saddlebàg hernia
Saemisch operation
Saenger operation
Saenger sutures
Safar bronchoscope
safety belt
safety pin
safety pin closer

Sage snare
sagittal suture
Saint (See *St.*)
Sakler erysiphake
Salah needle
Salem sump
Salem sump tube
Salibi clamp
saline
saline compress
saline infusion
saline irrigation
saline-moistened sponge
salivary
salivary ducts
salivary glands
salmon backcut incision
Salmon catheter
salpingeal curet
salpingeal probe
salpingectomy
salpingography
salpingo-oophorectomy
salpingo-oophoroplasty
salpingo-oophororrhaphy
salpingo-oophorostomy
salpingo-oophorotomy
salpingopexy
salpingopharyngeal muscle
salpingopharyngeus muscle
salpingoplasty
salpingorrhaphy
salpingoscopy
salpingostomy
salpingotomy
Salter operation
salvarsan tube
Salvatore-Maloney tracheotome

Sam Roberts esophagoscope
Sam Roberts forceps
Sam Roberts headrest
Sam Roberts laryngoscope
sampling
Sampson nail
Sampson prosthesis
Samuel position
sandbag
Sanders-Brown-Shaw needle
Sanders forceps
Sanders incision
Sanders laryngoscope
sandpaper dermabrader
sandpapering
sandwich flap
sanguineous
Sani-dril sutures
Santorini duct
Santorini plexus
Santulli clamp
Santy forceps
saphena accessoria vein
saphena magna vein
saphena parva vein
saphenectomy
saphenofemoral
saphenofemoral juncture
saphenous
saphenous nerve
saphenous vein
saphenous vein ligation and stripping
Saratoga sump
sarcoid
sarcoma (*pl.* sarcomas, sarcomata)
Sarmiento cast
Sarnoff clamp

Sarns cannula
Sarns saw
Sarot clamp
Sarot forceps
Sarot needle holder
Sarot thoracoscope
sartorius muscle
satellite
Satinsky clamp
Satinsky forceps
Satinsky scissors
Sato knife
Satterlee saw
saturate
saturation
saucerization
saucerize
Sauer-Bacon operation
Sauer debrider
Sauer forceps
Sauer-Sluder tonsillectome
Sauer speculum
Sauer tonsillectome
Sauerbruch-Coryllos rib shears
Sauerbruch forceps
Sauerbruch-Lebsche rongeur
Sauerbruch prosthesis
Sauerbruch raspatory
Sauerbruch retractor
Sauerbruch rib shears
Sauerbruch rongeur
Sauerbruch-Zukschwerdt retractor
Saunders needle
Saunders-Paparella hook
Saunders-Paparella needle
Saunders-Paparella rasp
Sauvage graft
Sauvage prosthesis

Savin operation
saw
    Adams
    Albee
    amputating
    amputation
    angular
    Arruga
    bayonet
    Beaver
    Bishop
    bone
    Brown
    Butcher
    chain
    Charriere
    circular
    circular twin
    Clerf
    Converse
    Cottle
    counter-rotating
    crosscut
    crown
    crurotomy
    electric
    Engel
    Farabeuf
    Gigli
    Gottschalk
    hand
    Hey
    hole
    hub
    Jesse-Stryker
    Joseph
    Joseph-Maltz
    Lamont

saw *(continued)*
  Langenbeck
  laryngeal
  laryngectomy
  laryngofissure
  Lell
  Luck
  Magnuson
  Maltz
  metacarpal
  Mueller
  Myerson
  nasal
  oscillating
  oscillatory
  plaster
  rhinoplasty
  Sarns
  Satterlee
  s. conductor
  s. guide
  Shrady
  single circular
  skull
  Slaughter
  Stille Gigli
  Stryker
  subcutaneous
  transverse
  universal
  Wigmore
  wire
  Woakes
Sawtell applicator
Sawtell-Davis forceps
Sawtell-Davis hemostat
Sawtell forceps
Sawyer retractor

Saxtorph maneuver
Sayoc operation
Sayre apparatus
Sayre bandage
Sayre cast application
Sayre elevator
Sayre periosteal elevator
Sayre raspatory
Sayre splint
Sbarbaro operation
Sbarbaro prosthesis
SBE (subacute bacterial endo-
    carditis)
scalene
scalene elevator
scalene muscle
scalene node
scalene node biopsy
scalenectomy
scalenotomy
scalenus
scalenus anterior muscle
scalenus medius muscle
scalenus minimus muscle
scalenus posterior muscle
scaling
scalp clip
scalp forceps
scalp hemostat
scalp incision
scalp retractor
scalp tourniquet
scalpel (see *knife*)
scalpel blade
scan
scanner
scanning
scanning electron microscope

Scanzoni maneuver
scaphoid
scaphoid gouge
scaphoid screw guide
scaphoid spatula
scapula
scapula retractor
scapular artery
scapulectomy
scapuloclavicular articulation
scapulopexy
scar
scar tissue
scarf bandage
scarifier
scarification
scarifying curet
Scarpa operation
Scarpa's fascia
Scarpa's membrane
Scarpa's sheath
Scarpa's triangle
SCDT heart valve prosthesis
Schaeffer curet
Schall tube
Schamberg extractor
Schanz brace
Schanz operation
Schatz maneuver
Schatzki ring
Schauffler operation
Schauta-Amreich operation
Schauta operation
Schauta-Wertheim operation
Schede curet
Schede operation
Schede sequestrectomy
Schede thoracoplasty

Scheie cautery
Scheie knife
Scheie operation
Scheinmann forceps
Schiller iodine
Schiller test
Schimek operation
Schindler esophagoscope
Schindler gastroscope
Schiøtz tonometer
scirrhous carcinoma
schistosomiasis
Schlange sign
Schlatter operation
Schlein arthroplasty
Schlemm's canal
Schlesinger forceps
Schlesinger Gigli-saw guide
Schlesinger punch
Schlesinger rongeur
schlieren microscope
Schmalz operation
Schmeden punch
Schmeden scissors
Schmidt clamp
Schmidt rasp
Schneider nail
Schneider pin
Schneider raspatory
Schneider rod
Schnidt forceps
Schnidt hemostat
Schobinger incision
Schoemaker anastomosis
Schoemaker-Billroth II gastrectomy
Schoemaker clamp
Schoemaker gastrectomy

Schoemaker gastroenterostomy
Schoemaker scissors
Schoenberg forceps
Scholl knife
Scholl solution
Schonander x-ray changer
Schönbein operation
Schroeder-Braun forceps
Schroeder curet
Schroeder forceps
Schroeder operation
Schroeder scissors
Schroeder tenaculum
Schrotter catheter
Schubert biopsy punch
Schubert forceps
Schuchardt incision
Schuchardt operation
Schuchardt-Pfeifer operation
Schuknecht chisel
Schuknecht elevator
Schuknecht excavator
Schuknecht gouge
Schuknecht hook
Schuknecht knife
Schuknecht needle
Schuknecht operation
Schuknecht piston prosthesis
Schuknecht retractor
Schuknecht scissors
Schuknecht spatula
Schuknecht speculum
Schuknecht trephine
Schuller position
Schulte valve
Schultze knife
Schutz clamp
Schutz clip

Schutz forceps
Schwartz clip
Schwartz curet
Schwartz forceps
Schwartz hook
Schwartz-Kerrison rongeur
Schwartz knife
Schwartz retractor
Schwartze operation
Schwartze-Stacke operation
Schweigger forceps
Schweizer forceps
sciatic
sciatic artery
sciatic hernia
sciatic nerve
sciatica
scimitar-blade knife
scintigram
scintiphoto
scintiphotography
scintiscan
scirrhous
scissor dissection
scissors
    abdominal
    Adson
    Aebli
    alligator
    American umbilical
    angled
    angular
    aortic
    arterial
    arteriotomy
    artery
    backward-cutting
    ball-tipped

scissors *(continued)*
>   ballpoint
>   bandage
>   Bard-Parker
>   Barraquer
>   Barraquer-DeWecker
>   Baruch
>   Becker
>   Bellucci
>   Berbridge
>   Berens
>   blunt
>   Boettcher
>   Bowman
>   Boyd
>   brain
>   Braun
>   Brooks
>   Brophy
>   Brown
>   Buerger-McCarthy
>   Buie
>   bulldog
>   Burnham
>   Busch
>   canalicular
>   cannula
>   capsule
>   capsulotomy
>   cardiac
>   cartilage
>   Castroviejo
>   cataract
>   Caylor
>   chemopallidectomy
>   Cherry
>   Chevalier Jackson
>   Church

scissors *(continued)*
>   circumcision
>   Classon
>   Converse
>   Cooley
>   cornea
>   corneal
>   corneal transplant
>   corneoscleral
>   Cottle
>   Crafoord
>   Craig
>   craniotomy
>   curved
>   curved-on-flat
>   Dandy
>   Dean
>   Deaver
>   DeBakey
>   DeBakey-Metzenbaum
>   decapitation
>   deep-surgery
>   delicate
>   DeMartel
>   DeWecker
>   DeWecker-Pritikin
>   diamond-edge
>   dissecting
>   dorsal
>   Doyen
>   Dubois
>   Duffield
>   Dumont
>   dura
>   dural
>   Emmet
>   endarterectomy
>   enucleation

scissors *(continued)*
- episiotomy
- Esmarch
- esophageal
- Essrig
- eye
- Ferguson
- Ferguson-Metzenbaum
- fine
- fine dissecting
- fine suture
- Finochietto
- flap
- Fomon
- Fox
- Frahur
- Frazier
- Fulton
- gallbladder
- gauze
- Gill
- Gillies
- goiter
- Good
- Graham
- Guggenheim
- Guilford-Schuknecht
- guillotine
- Guist
- gum
- Guyton
- Harrington
- Harrison
- Heath
- hernia
- Heyman
- Heyman-Paparella
- Hoen

scissors *(continued)*
- Holinger
- hook
- Hooper
- House
- House-Bellucci
- House-Metzenbaum
- Huey
- intestinal
- iridocapsulotomy
- iris
- Irvine
- Jackson
- Jacobson
- Jones
- Jorgenson
- Joseph
- Joseph-Maltz
- Kahn
- Katzin
- Kazanjian
- Keith
- Kelly
- keratoplasty
- Kilner
- Kirby
- Knapp
- Knight
- Knowles
- Kreuscher
- Lagrange
- Lahey
- laminectomy
- laryngeal
- laryngofissure
- Lawton
- Lejeune
- Lexer

scissors *(continued)*

- Lillie
- Lincoln
- Lister
- Liston
- Littauer
- Littler
- Litwak
- Litwin
- lobectomy
- long
- lung
- Lynch
- MacKenty
- Maclay
- Malis
- Martin
- Mattis
- Maunoir
- Mayo
- Mayo-Harrington
- Mayo-New
- Mayo-Noble
- Mayo-Potts
- Mayo-Sims
- Mayo-Stille
- McAllister
- McClure
- McGuire
- McIndoe
- McLean
- McPherson
- McPherson-Castroviejo
- McPherson-Vannas
- McReynolds
- meniscectomy
- Metzenbaum
- Metzenbaum-Lipsett

scissors *(continued)*

- micro-scissors
- microscopic
- microsurgical
- Miller
- minor surgery
- Mixter
- Morse
- Mueller
- Munro
- Murphy
- nasal
- Nelson
- neurological
- New's
- Noble
- Northbent
- Noyes
- Noyes-Shambaugh
- Nugent-Gradle
- Ochsner
- Olivecrona
- O'Neill
- operating scissors
- Panzer
- Paparella
- pediatric
- plaster-of-Paris
- plastic
- pointed
- Poppen
- Potts
- Potts-Smith
- Pratt
- Prince
- Prince-Potts
- probe
- prostatic

scissors *(continued)*
- rectal
- Reynolds
- right-angle
- Rizzuti-McGuire
- Rochester-Ferguson
- round-blade
- saber-back
- Satinsky
- Schmeden
- Schoemaker
- Schroeder
- Schuknecht
- s. probe
- Seiler
- semilunar cartilage
- septum
- serrated
- Shortbent
- Sims
- Sistrunk
- Smart
- Smellie
- Southbent
- Spencer
- Stevens
- Stevenson
- stitch
- strabismus
- straight
- Strully
- suture
- Sweet
- sympathectomy
- Taylor
- tenotomy
- thoracic
- Thorek

scissors *(continued)*
- Thorek-Feldman
- Thorpe
- Thorpe-Castroviejo
- Thorpe-Westcott
- throat
- Toennis
- tonsil
- tracheal
- tracheostomy
- trigeminus
- Troutman
- turbinate
- umbilical
- uterine
- Vannas
- vascular
- vena cava
- Verhoeff
- Vezien
- von Graefe
- Waldman
- Walker
- Walker-Apple
- Walker-Atkinson
- Walton
- Weber
- Westcott
- Wester
- White
- Willauer
- Wilmer
- Wincor
- wire
- wire-cutting
- Wullstein
- Wutzler
- Yankauer

scissors *(continued)*
      Yasargil
      Zoellner
sclera
sclera marker
      Amsler
      Gonin-Amsler
scleral buckle eye implant
scleral buckling
scleral cauterization
scleral eye implant
scleral fistula operation
scleral hook
scleral marker
scleral punch
scleral ring
scleral ruler
scleral shortening operation
scleral trephine
sclerectoiridectomy
sclerotome
      Curdy
      Guyton-Lundsgaard
      Lancaster
      Lundsgaard
      Lundsgaard-Burch
sclerectomy by punch
sclerectomy by scissors
sclerectomy by trephining
sclerectomy punch
scleriritomy
sclerocorneal junction
scleronyxis
scleroplasty
sclerosed
sclerosing
sclerosis
sclerostomy

sclerotherapy
scleroticectomy
scleroticonyxis
scleroticopuncture
sclerotomy
sclerotomy knife
Scobee-Allis forceps
Scobee hook
scoliosis
scoliosis brace
scoliosis osteotome
scoop
      Abbott
      abdominal
      Arlt
      Beck
      Berens
      common duct
      cystic duct
      Daviel
      Desjardin
      Elschnig
      enucleation
      fenestrated lens
      Ferguson
      Ferris
      gall duct
      gallstone
      gastrostomy
      Green
      Hess
      Knapp
      Lang
      lens
      Lewis
      Luer
      Luer-Korte
      malleable

scoop *(continued)*
>   Mayo
>   Mayo-Robson
>   Moore
>   Moynihan
>   Mules
>   Pagenstecher
>   Rockey
>   Wells
>   Wilder
>   Yasargil

scope

scopolamine

scotometer

scotometry

Scott cannula

Scott operation

Scott resectoscope

Scott speculum

Scott splint

Scott suction tube

Scoville curet

Scoville forceps

Scoville-Greenwood forceps

Scoville hook

Scoville-Lewis clip

Scoville needle

Scoville retractor

Scoville spatula

Scoville trephine

scraping

scratch incision

screen

screw
>   afterloading
>   Allen
>   arthrodesis
>   Basile

screw *(continued)*
>   Bechtel
>   bone
>   Bosworth
>   Collison
>   compression
>   coracoclavicular
>   cortical
>   cruciate head
>   cruciform
>   Cubbins
>   Doyen
>   Eggers
>   eyelet lag
>   fixing
>   hip
>   Jewett
>   Kristiansen
>   lag
>   Leinbach
>   Lorenzo
>   malleable
>   McAtee
>   McLaughlin
>   metal
>   Neufeld
>   Phillips
>   pick-up
>   recessed head
>   Richards
>   scaphoid
>   s. compressor
>   s. elevator
>   screw-holding forceps
>   screw-holding screwdriver
>   Sherman
>   stainless steel
>   Stryker

screw *(continued)*
    Thatcher
    Thornton
    tonsil
    Townley
    transfixion
    tumor
    Venable
    Vitallium
    Zimmer
screwdriver
    automatic
    Becker
    bone
    Children's Hospital
    Collison
    cruciform
    Cubbins
    DePuy
    Dorsey
    Johnson
    Lane
    medium
    Moore-Blount
    Phillips
    plain
    screw-holding
    Sherman
    Stryker
    White
    Williams
    Zimmer
Scribner shunt
scrotal
scrotal compartment
scrotal dressing
scrotal hernia
scrotal incision

scrotal nerves
scrotal veins
scrotales anteriores nerves
scrotales anteriores veins
scrotales posteriores nerves
scrotales posteriores veins
scrotectomy
scrotocele
scrotoplasty
scrotum
Scudder clamp
Scudder forceps
Scudder skid
Scultetus bandage
Scultetus binder
Scultetus dressing
Scultetus position
scutum
scybalous
scybalum (*pl.* scybala)
seamless prosthesis
searcher
    Allport
    Allport-Babcock
    mastoid
Searcy erysiphake
Searcy forceps
Searcy hook
Searcy tonsillectome
Searcy trephine
sebaceous
sebaceous glands
secobarbital
Seconal
second-degree burn (2nd degree burn)
secondary
secondary amputation

secondary carcinoma
secondary closure of wound
secondary fracture
secondary infection
secondary membrane forceps
secondary sutures
secretion
secretory
section
sector iridectomy
sedative
Seddon operation
Sedillot elevator
Sedillot operation
Sedillot periosteal elevator
Sedillot raspatory
sedimentary cataract
sedimentation rate
Sedlinger needle
Sedlinger operation
segment
segmental
segmental fracture
segmental lung resection
segmental orifices
segmental pulmonary resection
segmental resection
Segond forceps
Segond spatula
segregator
      Cathelin
      Harris
      Luys
Sehrt clamp
Sehrt compressor
Seiffert forceps
Seiffert punch
Seiler knife

Seiler scissors
Seletz cannula
Seletz catheter
Seletz forceps
Seletz-Gelpi retractor
Seletz punch
self-adjusting nail
self-broaching nail
self-broaching pin
self-retaining catheter
self-retaining laryngoscope
self-retaining retractor
self-retaining spring retractor
self-retaining speculum
Selker reservoir
Sellor clamp
Sellor knife
Sellor rib contractor
Sellor valvulotome
Selman clamp
Selman clip
Selman forceps
selvage edge
Selverstone clamp
Selverstone hook
Selverstone rongeur
SEM (systolic ejection murmur)
Semb forceps
Semb operation
Semb raspatory
Semb retractor
Semb rib shears
Semb rongeur
Semb-Sauerbruch rongeur
Semb shears
semicircular canals
semicircular ducts
semicircular incision

semicircular punch
semi-closed anesthesia
semi-closed endobronchial
    anesthesia
semi-closed endotracheal
    anesthesia
semicompressive dressing
semiflexed incision
semi-Fowler position
semilunar bone
semilunar cartilage
semilunar cartilage knife
semilunar cartilage scissors
semilunar incision
semilunar line
semimembranosus muscle
semimembranous muscle
seminal ducts
seminal sutures
seminiferous tubules
seminoma
semi-open anesthesia
semi-open endotracheal inhalation
    anesthesia
semi-pressure dressing
semiprone position
semireclining position
semishell eye implant
semispinal muscle
semispinalis capitis muscle
semispinalis cervicis muscle
semispinalis thoracis muscle
semitendinosus muscle
semitendinous muscle
Semken forceps
Sengstaken balloon
Sengstaken-Blakemore tube
Sengstaken tube

senile cataract
senile entropion
Senn-Dingman retractor
Senn forceps
Senn operation
Senn retractor
Senning baffle
Senning clamp
Senning operation
sensitivity
sensorineural
sentinel gland
sentinel pile
Senturia forceps
Senturia retractor
Senturia speculum
separating wire
separator
    bayonet
    Benson
    curved zonule
    cylindrical zonule
    Davis
    Dorsey
    double-ball
    dura
    dural
    flat zonule
    Frazier
    Grant
    Harris
    Hoen
    Horsley
    House
    Hunter
    Kirby
    Luys
    nerve

separator *(continued)*
    pylorus
    Rosen
    Sachs
    tonsil
    zonule
sepsis
septa (*sing.* septum)
septal compression forceps
septal defect
septal elevator
septal ridge forceps
septectomy
septi pellucidi veins
septic
septic abortion
septoplasty
septorhinoplasty
septostomy
septotomy
septum (*pl.* septa)
septum chisel
septum clamp
septum compression forceps
septum-cutting forceps
septum elevator
septum femorale
septum forceps
septum knife
septum needle
septum scissors
septum speculum
septum splint
septum straightener
septum-straightening forceps
septum trephine
sequela (*pl.* sequelae)
sequestrectomy

sequestrum (*pl.* sequestra)
sequestrum forceps
Serature clip
seromucous glands
seromuscular
seromuscular sutures
seropurulent
serosa
serosanguineous
seroserosal
seroserosal silk
seroserous sutures
serositis
serous
serous glands
serous membrane
serous otitis media
serpentine incision
serpentine plate
serrated curet
serrated forceps
serrated knife
serrated retractor
serrated scissors
serratus anterior muscle
serratus muscle
serratus posterior inferior muscle
serratus posterior superior muscle
serrefine (see *forceps*)
serrefine clamp
serrefine forceps
serrefine implant
serrefine retractor
serum
serum transfusion
sesamoid
sesamoid bones
sessile

sessile polyp
seton drain
seton operation
seton sutures
seton tube
Seutin bandage
sever
Sever-L'Episcopo operation
Sever operation
severance
severing
Sewall-Boyden operation
Sewall cannula
Sewall chisel
Sewall elevator
Sewall forceps
Sewall mucoperiosteal elevator
Sewall retractor
Sewall trocar
sex glands
Sexton knife
sexual glands
SGOT (serum glutamic oxalo-
    acetic transaminase)
Shaaf forceps
shadow-free laryngoscope
shaft
shaft reamer
Shaldon tube
Shallcross forceps
Shallcross hemostat
Shambaugh adenotome
Shambaugh-Derlacki chisel
Shambaugh-Derlacki elevator
Shambaugh-Derlacki microscope
Shambaugh elevator
Shambaugh hook
Shambaugh incision

Shambaugh irrigator
Shambaugh knife
Shambaugh-Lempert knife
Shambaugh needle
Shambaugh retractor
Shantz osteotomy
Shapleigh curet
sharp curet
sharp dissection
sharp elevator
sharp hook
sharp incision
sharp-pointed forceps
sharp-pronged retractor
sharp spoon
sharp-toothed tenaculum
Sharrard operation
shave biopsy
shaving
Shaw clot stripper
Shea-Anthony balloon
Shea bur
Shea curet
Shea drill
Shea hook
Shea incision
Shea irrigator
Shea knife
Shea stapedectomy
Shea tube
Shearer forceps
Shearer retractor
Shearer rongeur
shears (see also *rib shears*)
    Bethune
    Clayton
    Cooley-Pontius
    Diertz

shears *(continued)*
- Dubois
- Esmarch
- esophageal
- Gluck
- Jackson
- Jackson-Moore
- laminectomy
- laryngofissure
- Lebsche
- Liston
- plaster
- rib (see separate listing)
- Semb
- Shoemaker
- sternum
- Stille
- Weck

sheath
sheath cystoscope
sheath of rectus abdominis muscle
Sheehan chisel
Sheehan osteotome
Sheehan retractor
Sheehy forceps
Sheehy-House prosthesis
Sheehy knife
Sheehy tube
sheepskin dressing
sheet wadding
Sheldon-Pudenz dissector
Sheldon-Pudenz tube
Sheldon retractor
Sheldon-Spatz needle
Sheldon-Swann needle
shelf operation
shelf procedure
shelf reamer

shelf-type eye implant
shell eye implant
shell implant
shelving edge
shelving edge of Poupart's liga-
    ment
shelving incision
shelving operation
shelving portion of ligament
Shepard tube
Shepherd fracture
Sherman plate
Sherman screw
Sherman screwdriver
shield
shield incision
Shier knee prosthesis
Shiley-Bjork tube
Shiley shunt
Shiley tube
shin bone
shin splint
Shiner tube
Shirodkar-Barter cervical cerclage
Shirodkar cerclage
Shirodkar needle
Shirodkar operation
Shirodkar-Page cerclage
Shirodkar procedure
shock
shock position
shock therapy
short-wave diathermy
Shoemaker clamp
Shoemaker rib shears
Shoemaker shears
Shoepinger incision
short-leg brace

short-length tracheal tube
short needle
Shortbent scissors
shortening
shortening of bone
shortening of eyeball
shortening of ocular muscle
shortening of round ligaments
shortening of sacrouterine ligaments
shortening of tendon
shot compressor
shotted sutures
shotty nodes
shoulder arthrodesis
shoulder blade
shoulder joint
shoulder-strap incision
Shrady saw
shred
Shriners Hospital instruments
shriveled
shuffle gait
shunt
    Allen-Brown
    Ames
    arteriovenous
    Cavin
    dialysis
    Dow Corning
    endolymphatic subarachnoid
    Holter
    Javid
    LeVeen dialysis
    LeVeen peritoneal
    peritoneal
    polystan
    Pudenz

shunt *(continued)*
    Ramirez
    Rostan
    Scribner
    Shiley
    s. clamp
    s. operation
    s. tube
    Silastic
    subarachnoid
    Torkildsen
    ventriculoatrial
    ventriculoperitoneal
    winged
Shurly retractor
Shuster forceps
shuttle forceps
sialadenitis
sialitis
sialoadenectomy
sialoadenolithotomy
sialoadenotomy
sialodochoplasty
sialogram
sialography
sialolithotomy
Sichel knife
sickle
sickle-shaped knife
side-biting clamp
side-curved forceps
side-curved rongeur
side-grasping forceps
side mouth gag
side-to-end anastomosis
side-to-side anastomosis
Siebold pubiotomy
Siegle otoscope

Siegle speculum
Sierra-Sheldon tracheotome
sieve
sigmoid
sigmoid anastomosis
sigmoid arteries
sigmoid bladder
sigmoid clamp
sigmoid colon
sigmoid colostomy
sigmoid flexure
sigmoid sinus
sigmoid veins
sigmoideae arteries
sigmoideae veins
sigmoidectomy
sigmoiditis
sigmoidopexy
sigmoidoproctectomy
sigmoidoproctostomy
sigmoidorectostomy
sigmoidorrhaphy
sigmoidoscope
    ACMI proctosigmoidoscope
    Boehm
    Buie
    disposable
    ESI
    fiberoptic
    Frankfeldt
    Kelly
    Kleenspec
    Lieberman
    Montague
    proctosigmoidoscope
    Solow
    Strauss
    Turell

sigmoidoscope *(continued)*
    Tuttle
    Vernon-David
    Welch Allyn
    Yeomans
sigmoidoscopy
sigmoidosigmoidostomy
sigmoidostomy
sigmoidotomy
sigmoidovesical
sign
significant
Sigualt symphysiotomy
Siker laryngoscope
Silastic
Silastic adhesive
Silastic cannula
Silastic catheter
Silastic drain
Silastic eye implant
Silastic grommet
Silastic implant
Silastic implant material
Silastic injection
Silastic mammary prosthesis
Silastic penile prosthesis
Silastic plate
Silastic prosthesis
Silastic shunt
Silastic sponge
Silastic testicular prosthesis
Silastic tube
silicone
silicone cannula
silicone eye implant
silicone implant
silicone plate
silicone prosthesis

silicone rod implant
silicone sponge implant
silicone tube
silk-braided sutures
silk glove sign
silk sutures
silk ties
silkworm gut sutures
Silon pouch chimney
Silva-Costa operation
Silver bunionectomy
silver-fork fracture
Silver osteotome
silver nitrate cautery
silver suture wire
Silverman needle
Simon colpocleisis
Simon dermatome
Simon incision
Simon operation
Simon perineorrhaphy
Simon position
Simon speculum
Simon sutures
simple excision
simple fracture
simple iridectomy
simple mastectomy
simple mastoidectomy
simple microscope
simple operation
simple sinusotomy
simple skull fracture
simple sutures
Simpson curet
Simpson forceps
Simpson-Luikart forceps
Simpson operation

Simpson sound
Simpson splint
Sims anoscope
Sims curet
Sims dilator
Sims-Kelly retractor
Sims plug
Sims position
Sims probe
Sims retractor
Sims scissors
Sims sound
Sims speculum
Sims suction tip
Sims sutures
Sims tenaculum
single-armed sutures
single circular saw
single-guarded osteotome
single injection anesthesia
single-pass pacemaker
single-tooth tenaculum
Singleton incision
Singley clamp
Singley forceps
sino-atrial block
sinus
sinus arrest
sinus arrhythmia
sinus balloon
sinus bradycardia
sinus bur
sinus cannula
sinus chisel
sinus curet
sinus operation
sinus probe
sinus rasp

sinus rhythm
sinus tract
sinusectomy
sinusotomy
siphon
Sippy dilator
sirenomelia
Sistrunk operation
Sistrunk retractor
Sistrunk scissors
sitting position
situs
situs inversus viscerum
situs perversus
situs solitus
sitz bath
Sivash hip replacement
Sivash prosthesis
six-hole stainless steel plate
six-prong rake retractor
Skeele curet
skeletal pin
skeletal series
skeletal traction
skeletonize
Skene catheter
Skene forceps
Skene's glands
Skene spoon
Skene tenaculum
ski needle
skiametry
skid
    bone
    Davis
    hip
    MacAusland
    Meyerding

skid *(continued)*
    Murphy-Lane
    Scudder
    s. curet
    s. retractor
Skillern cannula
Skillern curet
Skillern forceps
Skillern fracture
Skillern probe
Skillman forceps
skin clip
skin crease
skin elevator
skin exfoliation
skin flap
skin flap retractor
skin forceps
skin graft
skin graft hook
skin graft knife
skin hook
skin incision
skin pencil
skin planing
skin retraction
skin splint
skin sutures
skin tag
skin towels
skin traction
skinfold caliper
skinfold incision
skinline incision
Sklar-Schiøtz tonometer
Sklar tonometer
skull bur
skull cone punch

skull fracture
skull plate
skull saw
skull tongs
skull tractor
skull trephine
Slaughter saw
sleeper sutures
sleeve
slice graft
sliding capsule forceps
sliding flap
sliding hernia
sliding skin flap
sliding technique
sling

> ptosis
> s. operation
> s. suspension
> s. sutures
> Supramid ptosis
> Velpeau
> Weil
> Zimmer

slip-knot ties
slit
slit lamp
slit-lamp microscope
slit-lamp study
slitting
sliver
Sloan dissector
Sloan incision
Sloan retractor
Slocum operation
Slocum splint
slot incision
slot-type rim incision

slotted bronchoscope
slotted laryngoscope
slotted plate
slotting bur
slough
sloughing
Sluder-Ballenger tonsillectome
Sluder-Demarest tonsillectome
Sluder guillotine
Sluder hook
Sluder-Jansen mouth gag
Sluder knife
Sluder needle
Sluder retractor
Sluder-Sauer guillotine
Sluder-Sauer tonsillectome
Sluder speculum
Sluder tonsillectome
Sluder tonsillectomy
slush
SMA (superior mesenteric artery)
small bowel
small bowel resection
small bowel series
Small-Carrion penile prosthesis
small intestine
small loop electrode
small pick
Smart forceps
Smart scissors
Smead closure
Smead-Jones closure
Smead-Jones sutures
smear
Smedberg drill
smegma
Smellie hook
Smellie perforator

Smellie scissors
Smeloff-Cutter valve
Smeloff-Cutter valve prosthesis
SMI cannula
smile incision
Smiley-Williams needle
smiling incision
Smillie knife
Smillie meniscotome
Smillie nail
Smillie retractor
Smith-Buie retractor
Smith cartilage stripper
Smith cataract extraction
Smith clamp
Smith clip
Smith dissector
Smith drill
Smith electrode
Smith expressor
Smith-Fisher knife
Smith-Fisher spatula
Smith forceps
Smith fracture
Smith-Green knife
Smith-Green spatula
Smith-Hodge pessary
Smith hook
Smith knife
Smith-Kuhnt-Szymanowski
   operation
Smith lens expressor
Smith operation
Smith pessary
Smith-Petersen chisel
Smith-Petersen curet
Smith-Petersen elevator
Smith-Petersen extractor

Smith-Petersen forceps
Smith-Petersen gouge
Smith-Petersen incision
Smith-Petersen mallet
Smith-Petersen nail
Smith-Petersen nailing
Smith-Petersen operation
Smith-Petersen osteotome
Smith-Petersen pin
Smith-Petersen plate
Smith-Petersen prosthesis
Smith-Petersen reamer
Smith-Petersen retractor
Smith-Petersen rongeur
Smith-Petersen spatula
Smith-Petersen tucker
Smith retractor
Smith speculum
Smithwick clamp
Smithwick clip
Smithwick dissector
Smithwick forceps
Smithwick-Hartmann forceps
Smithwick hook
Smithwick operation
SMO plate
SMO prosthesis
smooth broach
smooth tissue forceps
SMR (submucous resection)
SMR speculum
snap-lock brace
snapping
snare
     Banner
     Bosworth
     Brown
     Bruening

snare *(continued)*
- Buerger
- Castroviejo
- caval
- cold
- Crapeau
- cystoscopic
- Douglas
- ear
- enucleation
- Eves
- Farlow
- Farlow-Boettcher
- Förster
- Frankfeldt
- galvanocaustic
- hot
- Jarvis
- Krause
- laryngeal
- Lewis
- Martin
- Myles
- nasal
- Neivert
- Neivert-Eves
- Nesbit
- Norwood
- polyethylene
- rectal
- Reiner-Beck
- Robert
- Sage
- s. loop
- s. removal
- s. with ratchet
- Storz-Beck
- Stutsman

snare *(continued)*
- tonsil
- Tydings
- Wilde-Bruening
- wire
- Wright

Snellen eye implant
Snellen forceps
Snellen operation
Snellen sutures
Snitman retractor
snuffbox
snugness
Snyder forceps
Snyder hemostat
Snyder hemovac
soap
Soave pull-through procedure
Socin operation
socket
soda-lime mechanism
sodium pentothal
soft cataract aspirator
soft catheter
soft palate retractor
soft rubber curet
soft rubber drain
solar cautery
soleus muscle
solid silicone orbital prosthesis
solid-tip catheter
solitary
Solow sigmoidoscope
soluble bougie
solution
Somers clamp
Somers forceps
Somerset bur

SOMI brace
Sondergaard cleft
Sondergaard groove
Sones cardiac catheterization
Sones catheter
sonic applicator
Sonneberg operation
Sonnenschein speculum
sorbose cushion
Soresi cannula
Soria operation
Sorondo-Ferre amputation
Sotteau operation
sound
    Bellocq
    Bénique
    bronchocele
    Campbell
    Davis
    Dittel
    Ellik
    Fowler
    French
    French-following metal
    full-curve
    Gouley
    graduated
    Guyon
    Guyon-Bénique
    Hunt
    infant
    interlocking
    Jewett
    Kocher
    lacrimal
    LeFort
    McCrea
    meatal

sound *(continued)*
    Mercier
    metal
    Otis
    Pratt
    Ritter
    Simpson
    Sims
    urethral
    uterine
    Van Buren
    Walther
    Winternitz
    Woodward
Sourdille keratoplasty
Sourdille operation
Sourdille ptosis operation
Southbent scissors
Southey cannula
Southey-Leech trocar
Southey-Leech tube
Southey trocar
Southey tube
Southwick clamp
Southwick osteotomy
Souttar cautery
Souttar operation
Souttar skin incision
Souttar tube
SP (status post)
space of Forel
Spaeth operation
Spalding-Richardson hysterec-
    tomy
Spalding-Richardson operation
spasm
spasmodic
spasmodic entropion operation

spastic
spastic ileus
spatula
- Berens
- brain
- Castroviejo
- Cave
- Children's Hospital
- Crile
- Cushing
- cyclodialysis
- Davis
- D'Errico
- Dorsey
- double
- double-ended
- Elschnig
- endarterectomy
- flat
- Freer
- Green
- Gross
- iris
- Jacobson
- Kirby
- Knapp
- Lindner
- Lynch
- malleable
- Mayfield
- McPherson
- McReynolds
- Meller
- microsurgical
- Olivecrona
- Paton corneal
- Peyton brain
- Roux

spatula *(continued)*
- Sachs
- scaphoid
- Schuknecht
- Scoville
- Segond
- Smith-Fisher
- Smith-Green
- Smith-Petersen
- s. needle
- s. spoon
- Tauber
- Tooke
- transplant
- Weary
- Wecker
- Wheeler
- Woodson
- Wullstein
speaking tube
Speas operation
specimen forceps
spectrophotometry
speculum
- Adson
- Allingham
- anal
- anoscope
- Arruga
- Aufricht
- aural
- Auvard
- Auvard-Remine
- Barnes
- Barr
- Barraquer
- Barraquer-Colibri
- Beard

speculum *(continued)*
- Beckman
- Beckman-Colver
- Berens
- Berlind-Auvard
- bivalve
- bivalved
- Bodenheimer
- Bosworth
- Boucheron
- Bozeman
- brain
- Breisky-Navratil
- Brewer
- Brinkerhoff
- Bruening
- Bruner
- Buie-Hirschman
- Buie-Smith
- Carter
- Castallo
- Castroviejo
- Chelsea-Eaton
- Chevalier Jackson
- Clark
- Coakley
- Coldlite
- Coldlite-Graves
- Colibri
- Collin
- Converse
- Cook
- Cottle
- Cusco
- David
- DeLee
- DeVilbiss
- DeVilbiss-Stacey

speculum *(continued)*
- disposable
- Douglas
- Doyen
- duckbill
- Dudley-Smith
- Duplay
- Duplay-Lynch
- ear
- Eaton
- endaural
- endospeculum
- Erhardt
- esophageal
- eye
- eyelid
- Fansler
- Farrior
- Fergusson
- Flannery
- Foster-Ballenger
- Fox
- Fränkel
- Garrigue
- Gerzog
- Gilbert-Graves
- Goldbacher
- Goldstein
- Graefe
- Graves
- Gruber
- Guild-Pratt
- Guist
- Guist-Black
- Guttmann
- Guyton-Maumenee
- Guyton-Park
- Halle

speculum *(continued)*
    Halle-Tieck
    Hardy
    Harrison
    Hartmann
    Hartmann-Dewaxer
    heavy weighted
    Heffernan
    Henrotin
    Higbee
    Hinckle-James
    Hood-Graves
    House
    Huffman
    Huffman-Graves
    infant vaginal
    Ingals
    intranasal antrum
    Ives
    Jackson
    Jonas-Graves
    Kahn-Graves
    Kelly
    Killian
    Klaff
    Kleenspec
    Knapp
    Kogan endospeculum
    Kramer
    Kristeller
    Kyle
    Lancaster
    Lancaster-O'Connor
    Lang
    Lange
    laryngeal
    Lempert-Colver
    lid

speculum *(continued)*
    Lillie
    Lister-Burch
    Luer
    Mahoney
    Martin
    Martin and Davy
    Mason-Auvard
    Mathews
    Matzenauer
    Maumenee-Park
    Mayer
    McHugh
    McLaughlin
    McPherson
    Mellinger
    Miller
    Montgomery
    Mosher
    mucosa
    Mueller
    Murdock
    Murdock-Wiener
    Myles
    nasal
    nasopharyngeal
    National
    Nichols
    Nott
    Nott-Guttmann
    Noyes
    O'Sullivan-O'Connor
    oval
    Park
    Park-Guyton
    Park-Maumenee
    Patton
    Pedersen

speculum *(continued)*
- Pennington
- Picot
- Politzer
- Pratt
- Pritchard
- proctoscopic
- Pynchon
- Ray
- rectal
- Roberts
- Rosenthal
- Sauer
- Schuknecht
- Scott
- self-retaining
- Senturia
- septum
- Siegle
- Simon
- Sims
- Sluder
- Smith
- SMR
- Sonnenschein
- s. forceps
- s. holder
- s. transilluminator
- sphenoidal
- stapes
- stop eye
- Storz
- Sweeney
- Tauber
- Taylor
- Terson
- Toynbee
- Trélat

speculum *(continued)*
- Troeltsch
- tubular vaginal
- urethral
- vaginal
- Vernon-David
- Vienna
- Voltolini
- von Graefe
- Watson
- Weeks
- weighted
- weighted vaginal
- Weisman-Graves
- Welch Allyn
- Wiener
- Williams
- wire bivalve
- Yankauer
- Ziegler

Speed-Boyd operation
Speed operation
Speed prosthesis
Spence-Adson forceps
Spence forceps
Spence urethral meatotomy
Spencer cannula
Spencer forceps
Spencer probe
Spencer punch
Spencer scissors
Spencer-Watson operation
Spencer Wells forceps
sperm
spermatic artery
spermatic cord
spermatocele
spermatocelectomy

spermatocystectomy
spermatocystotomy
spermatozoon (*pl.* spermatozoa)
Spero forceps
sphenoethmoidal suture
sphenofrontal suture
sphenoid
sphenoid bone
sphenoid bur
sphenoid cannula
sphenoid probe
sphenoid punch
sphenoid punch forceps
sphenoid sinusotomy
sphenoidectomy
sphenoidostomy
sphenoidotomy
sphenomaxillary suture
sphenopalatina artery
sphenopalatine artery
sphenoparietal suture
sphenosquamous suture
sphenozygomatic suture
sphere
sphere eye implant
sphere implant
sphere introducer
    Carter
    metallic
spherical eye implant
spherical reamer
sphincter
sphincter ampullae hepato-
    pancreaticae muscle
sphincter ani
sphincter ani externus muscle
sphincter ani internus muscle
sphincter dilator

sphincter ductus choledochi
    muscle
sphincter muscle
sphincter of Oddi
sphincter pupillae muscle
sphincter pylori muscle
sphincter tone
sphincter urethrae muscle
sphincter vesicae urinariae muscle
sphincteral
sphincteral achalasia
sphincteralgia
sphincterectomy
sphincterismus
sphincteritis
sphincterolysis
sphincteroplasty
sphincterorrhaphy
sphincteroscope
sphincteroscopy
sphincterotome
sphincterotomy
sphygmograph
sphygmomanometer
sphygmometry
sphygmoscope
sphygmoscopy
spica bandage
spica cast
spicular
spiculated
spicule
spicule forceps
spiculum (*pl.* spicula)
spider nevus
Spieghel line
Spies punch
spigelian hernia

spike
spike retractor
spinal anesthesia
spinal artery
spinal canal
spinal cord
spinal cord retractor
spinal cordotomy
spinal elevator
spinal epidural space
spinal fusion
spinal fusion chisel
spinal fusion curet
spinal fusion elevator
spinal fusion gouge
spinal fusion osteotome
spinal fusion plate
spinal manometer
spinal muscle
spinal needle
spinal nerves
spinal perforating forceps
spinal puncture
spinal retractor
spinal subarachnoid block
spinal trephine
spinal veins
spinales nerves
spinales veins
spinalis anterior artery
spinalis capitis muscle
spinalis cervicis muscle
spinalis posterior artery
spinalis thoracis muscle
spindle cataract
spine
Spinelli operation
Spinhaler

spinous process
spinous process of vertebra
spinous process spreader
spiral
spiral bandage
spiral drill
spiral forceps
spiral fracture
spiral incision
spiral probe
spiral reamer
spiral reverse bandage
spiral stone dislodger
spiral sutures
spiral-tip bougie
spiral-tip catheter
spiral vein of modiolus
spiral vein stripper
spiralis modioli vein
Spirec drill
spirometry
Spivack cystostomy
Spivack gastrostomy
Spivack operation
splanchnic anesthesia
splanchnic block
splanchnic nerve
splanchnic neurectomy
splanchnic retractor
splanchnicectomy
splanchnici lumbales nerves
splanchnici pelvini nerves
splanchnici sacrales nerves
splanchnicotomy
splanchnicus imus nerve
splanchnicus major nerve
splanchnicus minor nerve
spleen

splenectomize
splenectomy
splenectopia
splenic
splenic artery
splenic flexure
splenic puncture
splenic vein
splenitis
splenius capitis muscle
splenius cervicis muscle
splenius muscle
splenocele
splenocleisis
splenocolic
splenocolic ligament
splenogram
splenography
splenolymph glands
splenolysis
splenomegaly
splenoncus
splenopexy
splenoplasty
splenoportogram
splenoportography
splenoptosis
splenorenal
splenorenal anastomosis
splenorenal ligament
splenorrhagia
splenorrhaphy
splenosis
splenotomy
splenulus
spline
    dorsal plaster

spline *(continued)*
    plaster
    stapes
splint
    abduction
    acrylic
    adhesive aluminum
    adjustable
    adjustable cross
    Agnew
    Airfoam
    airplane
    Alumafoam
    aluminum
    aluminum bridge
    aluminum finger cot
    anchor
    Anderson
    Angle
    anterior
    any-angle
    arm
    Asch
    Ashhurst
    Balkan
    banjo
    baseball finger
    Bavarian
    Baylor
    Böhler
    Böhler-Braun
    Bond
    Bowlby
    bracketed
    Brant
    Brown
    Buck
    Bunnell

splint *(continued)*

- Cabot
- Campbell
- canine-to-canine lingual
- cap
- Carter
- Chandler
- Chatfield-Girdlestone
- clavicle
- clavicular cross
- Clayton
- clear acrylic template
- clubfoot
- coaptation
- cock-up hand
- Colles
- compression
- contact
- countertraction
- Craig
- Cramer
- Culley
- Curry
- Davis
- Denis Browne
- dental
- denture
- DePuy
- DePuy-Pott
- drop-foot
- Dupuytren
- dynamic
- Eggers
- elephant-ear clavicle
- Englemann
- Erich
- Essig-type
- extension

splint *(continued)*

- external
- external nasal
- felt collar
- femoral
- fence
- Fillauer
- finger
- finger cot
- forearm
- forearm and metacarpal
- Forrester
- Fosler
- Fox
- fracture
- Frejka
- functional
- Gibson
- Gilmer
- Gordon
- greenstick fracture
- Gunning
- half-ring leg
- Hammond
- hand
- hand cock-up
- Hanna
- Hart
- Haynes-Griffin
- Hirschtick
- Hodgen
- humerus
- Ilfeld-Gustafson
- infant abduction
- inflatable
- interdental
- intranasal
- jaw

splint *(continued)*
- Jelanko
- Johnson
- Jonell
- Jones
- Joseph
- Kanavel
- Kazanjian
- Keller-Blake
- Kerr
- Kingsley
- Kirschner-wire
- knee
- knuckle-bender
- labial
- Lambrinudi
- leg
- leg extension
- Levis
- Lewin
- Lewin-Stern
- limb
- lingual
- Liston
- live
- Love
- Lytle
- Magnuson
- mandible
- Mason
- Mason-Allen
- Mayer
- McIntire
- metacarpal
- metal
- metatarsal
- Middeldorpf
- Mohr

splint *(continued)*
- molded
- Morris
- nasal
- Neubeiser
- night
- O'Donaghue
- open thimble
- opponens
- outrigger
- padded
- Peabody
- pelvic
- Phelps
- pillow
- plaster
- plastic
- Pond
- poroplastic
- Porzett
- posterior
- Pott
- protecto
- Putti
- radial nerve
- reverse Kingsley
- rocking leg
- Roger Anderson
- rolled Colles
- Rumel
- Sayre
- Scott
- septum
- shin
- Simpson
- skin
- Slocum
- Stader

splint *(continued)*
    stirrup
    Stromeyer
    sugar-tong
    supinator
    surgical
    T-finger
    T-splint
    Taylor
    Teflon
    template
    therapeutic
    thigh
    Thomas
    Tobruk
    Toronto
    ulna
    universal
    utility shoulder
    Valentine
    volar
    Volkmann
    walking
    Weil
    well-leg
    Wertheim
    Wilson
    wire
    Zimfoam
    Zimmer
splinter forceps
splintered fracture
splinting
split
split-heel incision
split sheet
split-thickness
split-thickness graft

split-thickness skin graft
splitter
splitting
splitting chisel
spondylolisthesis
spondylosyndesis
sponge
    cherry
    Ivalon
    Lincoff
    saline-moistened
    Silastic
    s. biopsy
    s. carrier
    s. count
    s. eye implant
    s. forceps
    sponge-holding forceps
    s. implant
    s. stick
    Weck-cel
sponging forceps
spontaneous
spontaneous abortion
spontaneous breech delivery
spontaneous fracture
spontaneous version
spoon
    appendectomy
    brain
    Bunge
    cataract
    Cushing
    Daviel
    Elschnig
    enucleation
    evisceration
    excavator

spoon *(continued)*
    exenteration
    eye
    eye evisceration
    Falk
    Fisher
    gall duct
    gallbladder
    Gross
    Hess
    Hoke
    intracapsular lens
    Kalt
    Kirby
    Knapp
    Kocher
    lens
    marrow
    Moore
    obstetrical
    Ray
    sharp
    Skene
    spatula
    s. excavator
    spoon-shaped forceps
    uterine
    Volkmann
    Wells
    Woodson
spot cautery
sprain fracture
Spratt curet
Spratt rasp
spray bandage
spreader (see also *rib spreader*)
    bladder neck
    Blount

spreader *(continued)*
    bone
    Burford
    Burford-Finochietto
    Cloward vertebral
    ductus
    Gross
    Kimpton
    Kirschner-wire
    Leksell sternal
    Lemmon sternal
    Millin-Bacon
    mitral valve
    rib
    root-canal
    spinous process
    sternal
    tonsil
    Turek
    valve
    vein
    vertebral
    Weinberg
    Wilson
    Wiltberger
    wire
spring clip
spring plate
spring retractor
spring wire retractor
sprinter's fracture
Sprong sutures
spud
    Bennett
    Corbett
    Davis
    Dix
    Ellis

spud *(continued)*
- eye
- Fisher
- foreign-body
- Francis
- Gross
- Hosford
- knife
- Laforce
- Walter

spur
spur crusher
- Mayo-Lovelace
- Stetton
- Warthen

spur-crushing clamp
Spurling forceps
Spurling-Kerrison forceps
Spurling-Kerrison punch
Spurling-Kerrison rongeur
Spurling periosteal elevator
Spurling rongeur
Spurling sign
Sputnik-Federov lens
sputum tube
squamosomastoid suture
squamous bone
squamous cell carcinoma
square punch
square specimen forceps
squint hook
Squire catheter
Ssabanajew-Frank gastrostomy
St. Clair forceps
St. Clair-Thompson curet
St. Clair-Thompson forceps
St. Luke retractor
St. Luke rongeur

St. Marks incision
St. Martin forceps
stab drain
stab incision
stab-wound drain
stab-wound incision
stabilization of joint
Stacke operation
Stader splint
staghorn calculus
stain
stainless steel
stainless steel bobbins
stainless steel cup
stainless steel implant
stainless steel mesh
stainless steel piston
stainless steel prosthesis
stainless steel screw
stainless steel strut
stainless steel stud
stainless steel wire
stainless steel wire prosthesis
stainless steel wire sutures
stalk
Stallard operation
Stallard sutures
Stamey bladder neck suspension
Stamey-Pereyra bladder neck
    suspension
Stamm gastrostomy
Stamm-Kader operation
Stamm operation
Stamm tube
standard bronchoscope
standard laryngoscope
standby
Stanicor pacemaker

Stanischeff operation
Stanton clamp
stapedectomy
stapediolysis
stapediotenotomy
stapedius muscle
stapedius nerve
stapedius tendon knife
stapes
stapes chisel
stapes curet
stapes elevator
stapes forceps
stapes hoe
stapes hook
stapes mobilization
stapes pick
stapes prosthesis
stapes speculum
stapes spline
Staph. aureus (Staphylococcus)
Staphylococcus
staphylectomy
staphyloplasty
staphylorrhaphy
staphylorrhaphy elevator
staphylorrhaphy needle
staphylotomy
staple
staple bronchoscope
staple forceps
staple sutures
stapler
     Blount
     EEA
     GIA
     TA-30
     TA-55

stapler *(continued)*
     Zimaloy
stapling
starch bandage
Starck dilator
Starlinger dilator
Starr-Edwards pacemaker
Starr-Edwards valve
Starr-Edwards valve prosthesis
stasis (*pl.* stases)
stasis dermatitis
stasis ulcer
State colorectal anastomosis
Statham flowmeter
stationary cataract
Staude forceps
Staude-Moore forceps
Staude-Moore tenaculum
stay sutures
steam cautery
steatorrhea
Stedman aspirator
Stedman suction pump
Stedman suction tube
steel mesh
steel plate
steel sutures
steel wire prosthesis
Steele dilator
Steele periosteal elevator
Steele-Stewart operation
steep Trendelenburg position
steeple sign
Stein-Abbe lip flap
Stein cheiloplasty
Stein-Kazanjian flap
Stein perforator
Steinach operation

Steindler arthrodesis
Steindler operation
Steindler stripping
Steinmann nail
Steinmann pin
Steinmann tractor
stellatae renis veins
stellate block
stellate cataract
stellate fracture
stellate ganglion block
stellate incision
stellate veins of kidney
stem
stem pessary
stem prosthesis
stem rasp
stencil wire
stenopeic iridectomy
stenosis (*pl.* stenoses)
stenosis clamp
stenotic
Stensen's duct
stent
stent dressing
stent graft
Stenver position
Stenver view
Stenzel rod
Stenzel rod prosthesis
step-down drill
Stepita clamp
stepladder incision
stercoraceous
stercoral appendicitis
stereoscopic microscope
stereotaxic
stereotaxis procedure

Steri-Drape
sterile
sterile absorbent gauze
sterile compression dressing
sterile dressing
sterile field
sterile fluffs
sterile saline
sterile tape
sterilely
sterilely draped
sterilization
sterilizer
Steri-Strips
Steritapes
Stern-McCarthy electrode
Stern-McCarthy electrotome
Stern-McCarthy panendoscope
Stern-McCarthy resectoscope
stern position
sternal approximator
       Leksell
       Lemmon
       Nunez
sternal blade
sternal muscle
sternal needle
sternal notch
sternal punch
sternal puncture by aspiration
sternal puncture by curettage
sternal puncture needle
sternal retractor
sternal-splitting incision
sternal spreader
sternal trephine
sternal wire sutures
sternalis muscle

sternoclavicular
sternoclavicular articulation
sternoclavicular ligament
sternoclavicular notch
sternocleidomastoid
sternocleidomastoid muscle
sternocleidomastoid vein
sternocleidomastoidea vein
sternocleidomastoideus muscle
sternocostal
sternocostal articulation
sternocostal ligament
sternocostal muscle
sternohyoid
sternohyoid muscle
sternohyoideus muscle
sternomastoid
sternothyroid
sternothyroid muscle
sternothyroideus muscle
sternotomy
sternum
sternum knife
sternum retractor
sternum shears
steroid
stethoscope
Stetton spur crusher
Stevens forceps
Stevens hook
Stevens scissors
Stevenson clamp
Stevenson forceps
Stevenson operation
Stevenson punch
Stevenson retractor
Stevenson scissors
Stewart hook

Stewart incision
Stewart knife
stick
stick-tie sutures
Stieda fracture
Stille-Adson forceps
Stille-Bjork forceps
Stille chisel
Stille clamp
Stille drill
Stille forceps
Stille-French needle holder
Stille-Giertz rib shears
Stille Gigli saw
Stille Gigli-saw guide
Stille gouge
Stille-Horsley forceps
Stille-Leksell rongeur
Stille-Liston forceps
Stille-Luer forceps
Stille-Luer rongeur
Stille osteotome
Stille rib shears
Stille rongeur
Stille shears
Stille trephine
stimulation
stimulus
stimulus response
stirrup anastomosis
stirrup bone
stirrup brace
stirrup-loop curet
stirrup splint
stirrups
stitch scissors
Stitt catheter
Stock operation

Stocker needle
stockinette bandage
stockinette dressing
stocking-seam incision
Stockman clamp
Stoffel operation
Stokes-Adams seizures
Stokes amputation
Stokes-Gritti amputation
Stokes sign
Stolte dissector
Stoltz pubiotomy
stoma (*pl.* stomas or stomata)
stomach
stomach brush
stomach clamp
stomach irrigation tube
stomach magnet
stomach tube
stomal
stomal ulcer
stomata (*sing.* stoma)
stomatitis
stomatoplasty
stomatorrhaphy
stone
stone basket
    Barnes-Dormia
    Browne
    Councill
    Dormia
    Ellik
    Ferguson
    Glassman
    Howard
    Johns Hopkins
    Johnson
    Mitchell

stone basket *(continued)*
    Pfister
    Pfister-Schwartz
    Robinson
    s. b. catheter
    ureteral
Stone bunionectomy
Stone clamp
stone dislodger
    Councill
    Creevy
    Davis
    Dormia
    Howard
    Johnson
    Levant
    Morton
    Ortved
    Robinson
    spiral
    ureteral basket
    woven loop
    Wullen
stone extractor
Stone eye implant
Stone forceps
stone-grasping forceps
Stone-Holcombe clamp
Stoneman forceps
stony hard
Stookey retractor
Stookey rongeur
stool
stooping
stop eye speculum
stop needle
stopcock
Storey forceps

Storz-Beck snare
Storz bronchoscope
Storz-Iglesias resectoscope
Storz magnet
Storz punch
Storz speculum
Storz telescope
strabismus correction
strabismus forceps
strabismus hook
strabismus needle
strabismus operation
strabismus scissors
strabismus tucker
straight arterioles of kidney
straight-blade electrode
straight-blade laryngoscope
straight catheter
straight cautery
straight clamp
straight elevator
straight forceps
straight hemostat
straight incision
straight nerve hook
straight rongeur
straight scissors
straight-stem prosthesis
straight suture needle
Straight tenaculum
straight-tip electrode
straightener
    Asch
    Cottle-Walsham
    Walsham
    septum
strain fracture
straining

Straith operation
strangulated
strangulated hemorrhoid
strangulated hernia
strangulation
strangury
strap muscles
Strap operation
Strassman-Jones operation
Strassman operation
strata (*sing.* stratum)
Stratte clamp
Stratte forceps
Stratte needle holder
stratum (*pl.* strata)
Strauss cannula
Strauss clamp
Strauss needle
Strauss proctoscope
Strauss sigmoidoscope
straw-colored fluid
Strayer knife
Strayer operation
streak retinoscope
Street pin
streptomycin
stress fracture
stress incontinence
stretch
stretching of iris
stretching of muscle
stretching of nerve
stria (*pl.* striae)
striata vein
striate vein
striated
stricture
stridor

stripper

- Babcock vein
- Bartlett
- Brand tendon
- Bunnell tendon
- Cannon
- cartilage
- Clark vein
- clot
- Codman vein
- Cole vein
- Crile
- DeBakey
- disposable
- Doyle vein
- Dunlop
- Emerson vein
- endarterectomy
- endotracheal
- external
- extraluminal
- fascia
- Friedman vein
- intraluminal
- jointed vein
- Joplin
- Keeley vein
- Kurten vein
- Lempka vein
- Linton vein
- loop
- Martin
- Masson fascia
- Matson-Mead
- Matson rib
- Mayo-Myers
- Mayo vein
- Myers

stripper *(continued)*

- Nabatoff vein
- Nelson rib
- Nelson-Roberts
- New Orleans
- periosteum
- polyethylene vein
- Price-Thomas rib
- rib
- rib edge
- Roberts-Nelson rib
- Shaw clot
- Smith cartilage
- spiral vein
- tendon
- thrombus
- Trace
- vagotomy
- vein
- Webb vein
- Wilson
- Wurth vein
- Wylie

stripping
stripping and ligation
stripping of kidney capsule
stripping of vocal cord
stroboscopic microscope
stroma *(pl.* stromata)
Strombeck breast reduction
Strombeck mammoplasty incision
Stromeyer-Little operation
Stromeyer splint
structure
Struempel forceps
Struempel rongeur
Strully curet
Strully hook

Strully-Kerrison rongeur
Strully retractor
Strully scissors
struma
strumectomy
strut
strut bar
strut forceps
strut guide
strut hook
Struyken forceps
Struyken punch
Stryker dermabrader
Stryker dermatome
Stryker drill
Stryker fracture frame
Stryker frame
Stryker saw
Stryker saw trephine
Stryker screw
Stryker screwdriver
Stubbs curet
stump
Sturmdorf amputation of cervix
Sturmdorf colporrhaphy
Sturmdorf needle
Sturmdorf operation
Sturmdorf reamer
Sturmdorf sutures
Stutsman snare
sty
stylet
styletted catheter
styloglossus muscle
stylohyoid muscle
stylohyoideus muscle
styloid process
stylomastoid artery

stylomastoid vein
stylomastoidea artery
stylomastoidea vein
stylopharyngeus muscle
styrofoam dressing
Suarez-Villafranca operation
subacute bacterial endocarditis
   (SBE)
subarachnoid
subarachnoid anesthesia
subarachnoid shunt
subarachnoid ureterostomy
subarcuate fossa
subareolar
subastragalar amputation
subcapital fracture
subcapsular cataract
subcapsular nephrectomy
subclavia artery
subclavia vein
subclavian aortic anastomosis
subclavian artery
subclavian nerve
subclavian triangle
subclavian vein
subclavius muscle
subclavius nerve
subcostal
subcostal artery
subcostal flank incision
subcostal incision
subcostal muscle
subcostal nerve
subcostal vein
subcostales muscles
subcostalis artery
subcostalis nerve
subcostalis vein
subcutaneae abdominis veins

subcutaneous
subcutaneous fracture
subcutaneous operation
subcutaneous saw
subcutaneous tenotomies
subcutaneous tissue
subcutaneous veins of abdomen
subcuticular
subcuticular stitch
subcuticular wire
subdermal implant material
subdural space
subgingival curettage
subglottic forceps
subinguinal incision
subjacent
subjective
sublingual
sublingual artery
sublingual ducts
sublingual glands
sublingual nerve
sublingual vein
sublingualis artery
sublingualis nerve
sublingualis vein
subluxated
subluxation
submammary
submammary incision
submandibular
submandibular duct
submandibular gland
submaxillary
submaxillary duct
submaxillary gland
submaxillary triangle
submental artery

submental vein
submentalis artery
submentalis vein
submucosal implant material
submucous curet
submucous dissection
submucous dissector
submucous elevator
submucous knife
submucous resection (SMR)
submucous retractor
suboccipital incision
suboccipital nerve
suboccipital triangle
suboccipital trigeminal rhizotomy
suboccipitalis nerve
subperiosteal amputation
subperiosteal bone
subperiosteal fracture
subperiosteal implant material
subperiosteally
subphrenic
subphrenic abscess
subpubic hernia
subpyramidal fossa
subscapular
subscapular artery
subscapular muscle
subscapular nerve
subscapular splenectomy
subscapularis artery
subscapularis muscle
subscapularis nerve
subsegmental resection
subserosa
subserous
subsigmoid fossa
substernal

substernal goiter
subtalar articulation
subtend
subtended
subtotal excision
subtotal gastrectomy
subtotal hysterectomy
subtotal laminectomy
subtotal resection
subtotal thyroidectomy
subtrochanteric incision
subumbilical incision
succinyl choline
succulent nodes
succussion
sucker
suction
suction abortion
suction apparatus
suction biopsy needle
suction catheter
suction curet
suction curettage
suction dissector
suction drain
suction elevator
suction evacuator
suction forceps
suction knife
suction ophthalmodynamometer
suction plate
suction pressure pump
suction pump
suction pump aspirator
suction tip (see *tip*)
suction tip curet
suction tube (see also *tube*)
    Adson

suction tube *(continued)*
    Anderson
    angled
    Anthony
    Baron
    bedside
    brain
    Bucy-Frazier
    Buie
    Chaffin
    Chaffin-Pratt
    Cone
    continuous
    Cook County
    Cooley
    coronary sinus
    Cottle
    Coupland
    Davol
    DeBakey
    DeVilbiss
    Emerson
    Fitzpatrick
    flexible
    Frazier
    Frazier-Paparella
    Gomco
    Gwathmey
    Hemovac
    House
    Immergut
    Lennarson
    life-saving
    Lore
    Lukens
    Mason
    mastoid
    Millin

suction tube *(continued)*
    Morse
    Morse-Andrews
    Morse-Ferguson
    Mosher
    Mueller
    Mueller-Frazier
    Mueller-Pool
    Mueller-Pynchon
    Mueller-Yankauer
    nasal
    Pleur-evac
    Pool
    Porto-vac
    Pynchon
    Rosen
    Sachs
    Scott
    Stedman
    suction-tube forceps
    Supramid
    Toomey
    tracheal
    tracheobronchial
    Tucker
    underwater-seal
    Wangensteen
    Weck
    Yankauer
sudoriferous glands
sudorific
sudoriparous glands
Sugar clip
sugar-tong cast
sugar-tong splint
Suggs catheter
sulcus *(pl.* sulci)
sulcus intermedius

Sumner clamp
sump drain
sump tube
sun cautery
Sunday elevator
Sundt clip
sunflower cataract
superficial
superficial fascia
superficial sutures
superior
superior carotid triangle
superior iridotomy
superior maxilla
superior mesenteric-caval
    anastomosis
superior pole of thyroid
superior tracheotomy
supernumerary
superstructure
supination
supination splint
supinator muscle
supine position
Supphose
support
support sutures
suppurate
suppuration
suppurative
suppurative appendicitis
supracervical hysterectomy
supracervical incision
supraclavicular
supraclavicular nerves
supraclaviculares intermedii nerves
supraclaviculares laterales nerves
supraclaviculares mediales nerves

supracondylar
supracondylar fracture
supramalleolar
Supramid implant material
Supramid ptosis sling
Supramid suction tube
Supramid sutures
supraorbital artery
supraorbital nerve
supraorbital vein
supraorbitalis artery
supraorbitalis nerve
supraorbitalis vein
suprapubic
suprapubic bag
suprapubic cannula
suprapubic catheter
suprapubic cystostomy
suprapubic cystotomy
suprapubic drain
suprapubic excision of prostate
suprapubic hemostatic bag
suprapubic incision
suprapubic prostatectomy
suprapubic retractor
suprapubic suction drain
suprapubic trocar
suprapubic urethroplasty
suprarenal arteries
suprarenal gland
suprarenal vein
suprarenales superiores arteries
suprarenalis dextra vein
suprarenalis inferior artery
suprarenalis media artery
suprarenalis sinistra vein
suprascapular artery
suprascapular nerve

suprascapular vein
suprascapularis artery
suprascapularis nerve
suprascapularis vein
suprasellar
supraspinatus muscle
supraspinous fossa
supraspinous muscle
suprasternal
suprasternal notch
supratrochlear artery
supratrochlear nerve
supratrochlear veins
supratrochleares veins
supratrochlearis artery
supratrochlearis nerve
supraumbilical incision
supravaginal hysterectomy
sural arteries
sural nerve
surales arteries
suralis nerve
Surfacaine
surface anesthesia
surface biopsy
surface cooling hypothermia
surface eye implant
Surgaloy sutures
surgery
Surgi-Med clamp
surgical
surgical amputation
surgical anesthesia
surgical correction
surgical dressing
surgical film
surgical flap
surgical gut sutures

surgical linen sutures
surgical microscope
surgical procedure
surgical prosthesis
surgical removal of tooth
surgical silk sutures
surgical splint
surgical steel sutures
surgical stockinette
surgical sutures
Surgicel dressing
Surgicel gauze
Surgiclip
Surgidev lens
Surgiflex bandage
Surgilon sutures
Surgilope sutures
Surital
suspension
suspension apparatus (see
    apparatus)
suspension laryngoscope
suspension of kidney
suspension of uterus
suspension traction
suspensorius muscle
suspensory bandage
suspensory ligament of axilla
suspensory ligament of lens
suspensory muscle
suspicious
Sutton needle
sutural cataract
sutural ligament
suture (see *sutures*)
suture forceps
suture-holding forceps
suture hook

suture-ligated
suture-ligation
suture-ligature
suture needle (see also *needle*)
    atraumatic
    curved
    Dees
    diamond point
    eyed
    eyeless
    eyeless atraumatic
    French
    Henton
    Lane
    noncutting
    reverse cutting
    straight
    taper-point
    tonsil
suture of wound
suture pusher
suture scissors
suture sizes
    1-0, 2-0, 3-0, 4-0, etc.
        or
    0, 00, 000, 0000, 5-0,
      6-0, etc.
suture-tying forceps
suture wire
sutureless valve prosthesis
sutures
    absorbable
    absorbable surgical
    Acutrol
    Albert
    Alcon
    Allison
    alternating

sutures *(continued)*

- Ancap silk
- anchoring
- angle
- Appolito
- apposition
- approximation
- Argyll Robertson
- Arlt
- arterial silk
- atraumatic
- Atroloc
- Axenfeld
- Babcock wire
- back-and-forth
- Barraquer silk
- baseball
- basting stitch
- Béclard
- Bell
- Bertrandi
- black braided
- black silk
- black twisted
- blanket
- blue cotton
- blue twisted cotton
- bolster
- bone wax
- Bonney-type
- Bozeman
- braided
- braided nylon
- braided silk
- braided wire
- bridle
- bronze wire
- bunching

sutures *(continued)*

- Bunnell
- buried
- button
- cable wire
- capitonnage
- cardiovascular
- Cargile
- Carrel
- catgut
- celluloid
- chain
- Chinese twisted silk
- chromic
- chromic catgut
- chromic gut
- circular
- circumcision
- Coakley
- coaptation
- cobbler's
- collagen
- compound
- Connell
- continuous
- continuous interlocking
- continuous loop wire
- continuous over-and-over
- continuous running
- corneoscleral
- cotton
- Cushing
- cushioning
- Custodis
- cutaneous
- cuticular
- Czerny
- Czerny-Lembert

sutures *(continued)*
- Dacron
- Degnon
- dekalon
- deknatel
- delayed
- dermal
- Dermalene
- Dermalon
- Dexon
- double-armed
- double-armed retention
- double black silk
- double-button
- doubly armed
- Dupuytren
- Duvergier
- edge-to-edge
- Edinburgh
- elastic
- Emmet
- end-on mattress
- Equisetene
- Ethibond
- Ethicon
- Ethicon silk
- Ethiflex
- Ethilon
- Ethilon nylon
- everting
- everting interrupted
- far
- far-and-near
- figure-of-eight
- fine chromic
- fine silk
- Finsterer
- fixation

sutures *(continued)*
- flat
- Flaxedil
- Flexiton
- Flexon
- free ligature
- free-tie
- French
- Frost
- furrier's
- Gaillard-Arlt
- Gambee
- gastrointestinal surgical gut
- gastrointestinal surgical linen
- gastrointestinal surgical silk
- Gély
- general closure
- Gibson
- glover's
- Gould
- groove
- Gudebrod
- guide
- Gussenbauer
- gut
- gut chromic
- gut plain
- Guyton-Friedenwald
- Halsted
- Harrington
- Harris
- heavy silk retention
- Heaney
- helical
- hemostatic
- horizontal mattress
- horsehair

sutures *(continued)*

horseshoe
Horsley
imbricated
imbricating
implanted
interlocking
intermaxillary
internasal
interpalpebral
interrupted
interrupted vertical mattress
intradermal mattress
intradermic
inverted
inverting
iodized surgical gut
Ivalon
Jobert
Jobert de Lamballe
Kalt
kangaroo tendon
Kelly
Kessler
Kirby
Kirschner
Kleinert
Kypher
lace
Lacidem
La Roque
Le Dentu
Le Dran
LeFort
Lembert
Lespinasse
ligation
limbal

sutures *(continued)*

linear polyethylene
linen
linen thread
lip
Littre
lock-stitch
locking
Löffler
loop
Lukens catgut
Marlex
mattress
Maunsell
Mayo linen
McGraw
McKissock
McLean
Measuroll
medium chromic
Medrafil wire
Meigs
Mersilene
metal band
monofilament
monofilament wire
multifilament
multistrand
near-and-far
nerve
neurological
Nissen
nonabsorbable
nonabsorbable surgical
noose
Nurolon
nylon
nylon monofilament

sutures *(continued)*
    Oertli silk
    on-edge mattress
    over-and-over
    overlapping
    Owens silk
    Oyloidin
    Pagenstecher linen thread
    Palfyn
    Pancoast
    Paré
    Parker-Kerr
    Parker-Kerr "basting stitch"
    Pearsall silk
    pericostal
    perineal support
    Perma-hand silk
    Petit
    pin
    plain catgut
    plain gut
    plain interrupted
    plain tie
    plastic
    plicating
    plication
    Polydek
    postplaced
    polyester
    polyethylene
    polyfilament
    polypropylene
    postplaced
    presection
    primary
    prolene
    pull-out wire
    pulley

sutures *(continued)*
    Purlon
    pursestring
    pyoktanin
    quilled
    quilt
    quilted
    Ramdohr
    Ramsey County pyoktanin
    reinforcing
    relaxation
    retention
    ribbon gut
    Richardson
    Richter
    Rigal
    right-angle mattress
    Ritisch
    rubber
    running chromic
    running continuous
    running lock
    running subcuticular
    Saenger
    Sani-dril
    secondary
    seminal
    seromuscular
    seroserosal silk
    seroserous
    seton
    shotted
    silk
    silk-braided
    silkworm gut
    silver wire
    Simon
    simple

sutures *(continued)*

- Sims
- single-armed
- skin
- sleeper
- sling
- Smead-Jones
- Snellen
- spiral
- Sprong
- stainless steel
- stainless steel wire
- Stallard
- staple
- stay
- steel
- steel mesh
- sternal wire
- stick-tie
- Sturmdorf
- subcuticular
- superficial
- support
- Supramid
- Surgaloy
- surgical
- surgical gut
- surgical linen
- surgical silk
- surgical steel
- Surgilon
- Surgilope
- suture-ligature
- swaged-on
- tacking
- tantalum-wire
- Taylor
- tendon

sutures *(continued)*

- tension
- Tevdek
- Thermo-flex
- Thiersch
- thread
- through-and-through
- tiger gut
- Tom Jones
- tongue
- tongue-and-groove
- traction
- transfixing
- transfixion
- twenty-day gut
- twisted cotton
- twisted silk
- Tycron
- unabsorbable
- uninterrupted
- vascular silk
- Verhoeff
- vertical mattress
- Vicryl
- virgin silk
- Viro-Tec
- visceroparietal
- whipstitch
- white braided
- white nylon
- white silk
- white twisted
- wing
- wire
- Wölfler
- Woodbridge
- Wysler
- Y-sutures

sutures *(continued)*
    Z-sutures
    Zytor
suturing forceps
suturing needle
swaged needle
swaged-on suture
Swan clamp
Swan-Ganz catheter
swan-neck clamp
swan-neck gouge
Swanson implant
Swanson prosthesis
sweat glands
Sweeney retractor
Sweeney speculum
Sweet-Burford rib spreader
Sweet forceps
Sweet magnet
Sweet punch
Sweet retractor
Sweet rib spreader
Sweet scissors
Sweet trocar
swelling
Swenson operation
Swenson pull-through procedure
Swimmer view
Swiss blade
Swiss bulldog clamp
swivel hook
swivel knife
swivel tracheostomy tube
Sylva irrigator
sylvian artery
symblepharon
Syme amputation
Syme urethrotomy

symmetrical
symmetry
Symmonds vaginal prolapse repair
sympathectomy
sympathectomy hook
sympathectomy scissors
sympathetic block
sympathetic nerve
sympathetic trunk
sympathicodiaphtheresis
sympathicotripsy
symphysiotomy
symphysis (*pl.* symphyses)
symphysis pubis
symptomatic
Syms tractor
synaptic blocking agents
synchondrosis
synchondrotomy
synchronous amputation
synchronous pacemaker
syncongestive appendicitis
syncope
syndactylization
syndactyly
syndectomy
syndesmopexy
syndesmoplasty
syndesmorrhaphy
syndesmotomy
syndrome
synechia (*pl.* synechiae)
synechialysis
synechotomy
synoptoscopy
synosteotomy
synostosis
synovectomy

synovia (*sing.* synovium)
synovial
synovial hernia
synovial membrane
synovitis
synovium (*sing.* synovia)
syphilis
syphilitic
syphilitic cataract
syringe
    air
    Alcock
    Anel lacrimal
    Asepto
    bladder
    chip
    colonoscope
    Davidson
    dental
    disposable
    fountain
    hypodermic
    irrigation
    Kaufman
    lacrimal
    laryngeal
    Lehman

syringe *(continued)*
    Luer
    Luer-Lok
    metal
    Neisser
    Nourse
    Pierce
    plastic
    Pritchard
    Robb
    Rochester
    rubber-bulb
    s. cannula
    Thompson
    tonsil
    Toomey
syringectomy
syringing
syringomyelia
syringotome
syringotomy
systole
systolic ejection murmur (SEM)
Sztehlo clamp
Szymanowski-Kuhnt operation
Szymanowski operation

t

T&A (tonsillectomy and
    adenoidectomy)
T&A suction tip
T-bandage
T-binder
T-binder pressure dressing
T-drain
T-finger splint
T-incision
T-shaped forceps
T-shaped incision
T-splint
T-tube
T-tube drain
T-tube technique
TA-30 stapler
TA-55 stapler
Tabb curet
Tabb elevator
Tabb knife
tabes
table
    Abbott
    Albee
    fracture
    hand
    Maquet
    McPheeters
    Mimer
tachyarrhythmia
tachycardia
tack-and-pin forceps

tack hammer
tack operation
tacking
tactile probe
taenia
Taenia coli
tagliacotian operation
tagliacotian rhinoplasty
tail of pancreas
tail of Spence
tailor bunion
Tait perineoplasty
Takahashi forceps
Takahashi punch
take down of anastomosis
takeoff
talc
tali (*sing.* talus)
talipes correction
talipes equinovarus
Tallerman apparatus
Talma operation
talocalcaneonavicular articulation
talonavicular articulation
talus (*pl.* tali)
tamp
tamper
tampon
tampon tube
tamponade
tandem
tangential clamp

tangential forceps
tangentially
Tanner mesher
Tanner method
Tanner operation
Tansini breast amputation
Tansini gastric resection
Tansini removal of liver cyst
Tansini sign
Tansley operation
tantalum bronchogram
tantalum clip
tantalum eye implant
tantalum mesh
tantalum mesh graft
tantalum mesh implant
tantalum prosthesis
tantalum stapes prosthesis
tantalum wire
tantalum-wire sutures
tap
tap drill
taper jaw rongeur
taper-point needle
taper-point needle holder
taper-point suture needle
Tapercut needle
tapered bougie
tapping hammer
target
Tarnier basiotribe
Tarnier forceps
tarry stool
tarsal arteries
tarsal bones
tarsal folds
tarsal muscle
tarsal plate
tarsal wedge osteotomy

tarsalis inferior muscle
tarsalis superior muscle
tarsals
tarsea lateralis artery
tarseae mediales arteries
tarsectomy
tarsoclasis
tarsometatarsal articulations
tarsoplasty
tarsorrhaphy
tarsotibial amputation
tarsotomy
tarsus
tattoo
tattoo of cornea
tattooing
tattooing needle
Tatum clamp
Tauber catheter
Tauber hook
Tauber spatula
Tauber speculum
Taussig-Morton operation
Taussig operation
taut
tautening
Taylor apparatus
Taylor aspirator
Taylor blade
Taylor brace
Taylor curet
Taylor retractor
Taylor scissors
Taylor speculum
Taylor splint
Taylor sutures
TEA (thromboendarterectomy)
Teale amputation

Teale director
Teale forceps
Teale operation
tear duct
tear sac
teardrop fracture
technetium pertechnetate scan
technetium pyrophosphate
technique
TED hose (thromboembolic
    disease)
Teflon
Teflon bolster
Teflon cannula
Teflon catheter
Teflon-covered needle
Teflon felt
Teflon graft
Teflon implant
Teflon mesh
Teflon patch
Teflon plate
Teflon prosthesis
Teflon splint
Teflon tape
Teflon tube
Teflon-wire piston
Telectronic pacemaker
telecurietherapy
Telepaque
telephone probe
teleradiography
telescope
    ACMI
    Best
    biopsy
    bridge
    Broyles

telescope *(continued)*
    Burns
    clamp-on
    direct forward-vision
    direct vision
    examining
    fiberoptic
    Foroblique
    Holinger
    Hopkins
    Kramer
    McCarthy
    miniature
    Negus
    operating
    retrospective
    right-angle
    Storz
    t. bronchoscope
    transilluminating
    Tucker
    Vest
telescoping guide
television microscope
Telfa
Telfa dressing
Telfa plastic film
TeLinde hysterectomy
TeLinde operation
template
template splint
Temple-Fay retractor
Temple procedure
Temple University nail
Temple University plate
temporal
temporal arteries
temporal bone

temporal fossa
temporal incision
temporal line
temporal muscle
temporal nerves
temporal trephine
temporal veins
temporales profundae arteries
temporales profundae veins
temporales profundi nerves
temporales superficiales veins
temporalis media artery
temporalis media vein
temporalis muscle
temporalis superficialis artery
temporary magnet
temporary transvenous pacemaker
temporomandibular articulation
temporomaxillary articulation
temporoparietal muscle
temporoparietalis muscle
temporozygomatic suture
tenaculum
    Adair
    Barrett
    Braun
    breast
    Brophy
    bullet
    cervical
    cleft palate
    Corey
    Cottle
    DeLee
    double-hook skin
    Duplay
    Emmet
    goiter

tenaculum *(continued)*
    Jackson
    Jacobs
    Jarcho
    Kahn
    Lahey
    Marlex
    Newman
    Potts
    Potts-Smith
    Pozzi
    Ritchie
    Schroeder
    sharp-toothed
    Sims
    single-tooth
    Skene
    Staude-Moore
    Straight
    t. forceps
    t. hook
    Thoms
    tracheal
    traction
    uterine
    Watts
    Weisman
Tenckhoff catheter
tendines (*sing.* tendo)
tendinoplasty
tendinotrochanteric ligament
tendinous
tendo (*pl.* tendines)
    t. Achillis
    t. calcaneus
    t. conjunctivus
    t. cordiformis
    t. cricoesophageus

tendo *(continued)*
    t. oculi
    t. palpebrarum
tendolysis
tendon
    Achilles
    calcaneal
    central t. of diaphragm
    central t. of perineum
    common
    conjoined
    cordiform t. of diaphragm
    coronary
    cricoesophageal
    hamstring
    heel
    intermediate t. of diaphragm
    patellar
    t. advancement
    t. clamp
    t. forceps
    t. graft
    t. implant
    t. of Hector
    t. of Zinn
    t. passer (see separate listing)
    tendon-pulling forceps
    t. sheath
    t. stripper
    t. transfer
    t. tucker (see also *tucker*)
    trefoil
tendon passer
    Brand
    Bunnell
    Carroll
    Gallie
    Joplin

tendon passer *(continued)*
    Ober
tendoplasty
tendotomy
tenectomy
tenectomy of ocular muscle
tenesmus
Tenner cannula
tennis-racket incision
Tennison operation
Tennison-Randall cleft lip repair
tenodesis
tenomyoplasty
tenomyotomy
Tenon's capsule
tenonectomy
tenonometer
tenontoplasty
tenontotomy
tenoplasty
tenorrhaphy
tenosuspension
tenosuture
tenosynovectomy
tenotome
tenotomy
tenotomy hook
tenotomy knife
tenotomy of ocular tendon
tenotomy scissors
Tensilon
Tensilon implant
tensing
tension
tension sutures
tensor fasciae latae muscle
tensor muscle
tensor tympani muscle

tensor veli palatini muscle
tensoris tympani nerve
tensoris veli palatini nerve
tented
teratocarcinoma
teratoma
teres major muscle
teres minor muscle
term pregnancy
terminal cancer
terminal electrode
terminal ileitis
terminal ileum
terminal line
terminal sigmoid colostomy
terminoterminal anastomosis
Terramycin
Terrillon operation
Terson forceps
Terson operation
Terson speculum
tertiary amputation
testes (*sing.* testis)
testicle
testicular artery
testicular vein
testicularis artery
testicularis dextra vein
testicularis sinistra vein
testis (*pl.* testes)
tetracaine hydrochloride
tetracycline
Teufel brace
Tevdek sutures
Texas catheter
thalamostriata vein
thalamostriate vein
thalamotomy

thalamus
thallium scan
Tharies surface hip replacement
Thatcher nail
Thatcher screw
theca (*pl.* thecae)
thecal
thecal whitlow
Theden bandage
Theis retractor
Theis rib spreader
theleplasty
thelerethism
thelitis
thelorrhagia
thenar
thenar eminence
Theobald probe
therapeutic
therapeutic abortion
therapeutic electrode
therapeutic splint
thermal agents
thermal burn
thermistor probe
Thermo-flex sutures
thermogram
thermography
thermophore
thermophore bandage
Thermosector electrosurgical unit
thermotherapy
THI needle
thialbarbitone
thiamylal
thiamylal sodium
thickened
Thiersch-Duplay urethroplasty

Thiersch graft
Thiersch knife
Thiersch operation
Thiersch ring
Thiersch sutures
Thiersch wire
thigh
thigh bone
thigh splint
thin osteotome
thiopental sodium
third-degree burn (3rd degree
    burn)
Thom flap laryngeal reconstruc-
    tion
Thomas brace
Thomas cryoextractor
Thomas cryopter
Thomas curet
Thomas keratome
Thomas magnet
Thomas operation
Thomas pessary
Thomas splint
Thomas-Warren incision
Thomayer sign
Thompson catheter
Thompson curet
Thompson drape
Thompson lithotrite
Thompson operation
Thompson prosthesis
Thompson punch
Thompson rasp
Thompson resectoscope
Thompson syringe
Thompson template
Thoms-Allis forceps

Thoms forceps
Thoms-Gaylor biopsy punch
Thoms-Gaylor forceps
Thoms pelvimeter
Thoms tenaculum
Thomson clamp
Thomson fracture frame
Thomson operation
thoracectomy
thoracentesis
thoracic
thoracic aorta
thoracic artery
thoracic clamp
thoracic drainage tube
thoracic duct
thoracic forceps
thoracic nerve block
thoracic nerves
thoracic scissors
thoracic vein
thoracic vertebrae
thoracica interna artery
thoracica lateralis artery
thoracica lateralis vein
thoracica suprema artery
thoracicae internae veins
thoracici nerves
thoracicoabdominal splenectomy
thoracicus longus nerve
thoracoabdominal incision
thoracoacromial artery
thoracoacromial vein
thoracoacromialis artery
thoracoacromialis vein
thoracocentesis
thoracodorsal
thoracodorsal artery

thoracodorsal nerve
thoracodorsalis artery
thoracodorsalis tibialis nerve
thoracoepigastric veins
thoracoepigastricae veins
thoracolaparotomy
thoracolumbar nerve block
thoracolysis
thoracoplasty
thoracoscope
     Coryllos
     Jacobaeus
     Moore
     Sarot
thoracoscopy
thoracostomy
thoracostomy tube
thoracotome
thoracotomy
thoracotomy incision
thoracotomy tube
Thorek aspirator
Thorek-Feldman scissors
Thorek-Mixter forceps
Thorek operation
Thorek scissors
Thornton nail
Thornton plate
Thornton screw
Thornwald drill
Thornwald irrigator
Thornwald perforator
Thornwald trephine
Thorpe caliper
Thorpe-Castroviejo scissors
Thorpe curet
Thorpe forceps
Thorpe scissors

Thorpe-Westcott scissors
thread
thread sutures
threaded pin
threatened abortion
three-bladed clamp
three-clamp technique
three-flanged nail
three-flanged spike
3M drape
3M dressing
3M Vi-Drape
three-prong retractor
three-step tenotomy
three-way catheter
threshold
thrill
throat
throat forceps
throat irrigation tube
throat scissors
thrombectomy
thrombi (*sing.* thrombus)
thromboangiitis
thromboendarterectomy (TEA)
thromboendarteritis
thrombophlebitis
thrombosed hemorrhoid
thrombosis (*pl.* thromboses)
thrombus (*pl.* thrombi)
thrombus stripper
through-and-through sutures
thumb cushion
thumb forceps
thymectomize
thymectomy
thymic veins
thymicae veins

thymopexy
thymus
thymus retractor
thymusectomy
thyroarytenoid muscle
thyroarytenoideus muscle
thyrocervical
thyrocervical trunk
thyrochondrotomy
thyrocricoidectomy
thyrocricotomy
thyroepiglottic muscle
thyroepiglotticus muscle
thyroglossal
thyroglossal cyst
thyroglossal sinus
thyrohyal
thyrohyoid
thyrohyoid muscle
thyrohyoideus muscle
thyroid
thyroid artery
thyroid drain
thyroid forceps
thyroid gland
thyroid isthmectomy
thyroid lobes
thyroid notch
thyroid retractor
thyroid traction forceps
thyroid uptake
thyroid vein
thyroidal
thyroidal hernia
thyroidea
thyroidea accessoria
thyroidea ima artery
thyroidea inferior artery

thyroidea inferior vein
thyroidea superior artery
thyroidea superior vein
thyroideae mediae veins
thyroidectomize
thyroidectomy
thyroiditis
thyroidorrhaphy
thyroidotomy
thyrolaryngeal fascia
thyromegaly
thyroparathyroidectomy
thyrotomy
thyrotoxic goiter
thyrotoxicosis
thyroxin
tibia
tibia retractor
tibial
tibial artery
tibial muscle
tibial nerve
tibial plafond
tibial plateau
tibial plateau prosthesis
tibial prosthesis
tibial tubercle
tibial tuberosity
tibial veins
tibiales anteriores veins
tibiales posteriores veins
tibialis anterior artery
tibialis anterior muscle
tibialis posterior artery
tibialis posterior muscle
tibiofemoral fossa
tibiofemoral prosthesis
tibiofibular articulation

tie-over dressing
Tiemann catheter
Tiemann-coudé catheter
Tiemann nail
ties (see *sutures*)
tiger gut sutures
Timberlake evacuator
Timberlake obturator
Timberlake resectoscope
Timbrall-Fisher incision
tin-bullet probe
tincture
tincture of benzoin
tingling
tip

    Adson brain suction
    aortographic
    aspiration
    Bard cystoscope
    Bishop-Harmon
    Blasucci
    Bovie coagulation
    brain suction
    cannula
    Clerf aspirating
    cystoscope
    exploratory suction
    Frazier suction
    Grieshaber vitrectomy
    Hanafee catheter
    Hildreth
    irrigating
    nasal suction
    plastic suction
    Sims suction
    suction
    T & A suction
    tonsil suction

tip *(continued)*
    ultrasonic
    vitrectomy
    vitrector
tire eye implant
tire-iron maneuver
Tischler forceps
Tischler punch
tissue
tissue desiccation needle
tissue drain
tissue forceps
tissue-grasping forceps
tissue retractor
titanium prosthesis
Titus needle
Tivnen forceps
to-and-fro anesthesia
Tobey-Ayer maneuver
Tobey rongeur
Tobold apparatus
Tobold-Fauvel forceps
Tobold forceps
Tobold knife
Tobruk splint
tocolysis
Todd button
Todd cautery
Todd gouge
Todd needle
toe
toe bones
toe spreader
toedrop brace
toenail
Toennis scissors
toilet
toilette

toluidine blue
Tom Jones closure
Tom Jones sutures
Toma sign
Tomac catheter
Tomac forceps
Tomac goniometer
tomogram
tomography
tongs
    Barton
    Barton-Cone
    biopsy
    Böhler
    Cherry
    Cohen-Eder
    Crutchfield
    Crutchfield-Raney
    Eder
    Gardner-Wells
    Raney-Crutchfield
    Reynolds
    skull
    traction
    Vinke
tongue
tongue-and-groove sutures
tongue blade
tongue depressor
    Andrews
    Blakesley
    Bosworth
    Dorsey
    Dunn
    Farlow
    Hamilton
    Lewis
    Pynchon

tongue depressor *(continued)*
    Pynchon-Lillie
    Weder
tongue forceps
tongue-seizing forceps
tongue sutures
tongue-tie operation
tongue traction
tonic
tonography
tonometer
    air-puff
    applanation
    Bailliart
    electronic
    Gärtner
    Goldmann
    Harrington
    impression
    Mackay-Marg
    McLean
    Mueller
    Musken
    pneumatic
    Recklinghausen
    Schiøtz
    Sklar
    Sklar-Schiøtz
tonometry
tonsil
tonsil artery forceps
tonsil caliper
tonsil clamp
tonsil compressor
tonsil dissector
tonsil electrode
tonsil elevator
tonsil enucleator

tonsil expressor
tonsil forceps
tonsil guillotine
tonsil hemostat
tonsil-holding forceps
tonsil hook
tonsil knife
tonsil-ligating forceps
tonsil needle
tonsil pillar retractor
tonsil position
tonsil punch
tonsil retractor
tonsil scissors
tonsil screw
tonsil-seizing forceps
tonsil separator
tonsil slitter
tonsil snare
tonsil snare wire
tonsil sponges
tonsil spreader
tonsil suction tip
tonsil suture hook
tonsil suture needle
tonsil-suturing forceps
tonsil-suturing instrument
tonsil syringe
tonsil tampons
tonsillectome
    Ballenger-Sluder
    Beck-Mueller
    Beck-Schenck
    Brown
    Daniels
    guillotine
    hemostatic
    Laforce

tonsillectome *(continued)*
    lingual
    Mack
    Moltz-Storz
    Myles
    Sauer
    Sauer-Sluder
    Searcy
    Sluder
    Sluder-Ballenger
    Sluder-Demarest
    Sluder-Sauer
    Tydings
    Van Osdel
    Whiting
tonsillectomy
tonsillectomy and adenoidectomy
tonsilloadenoidectomy
tonsilloscope
tonsillotome
tonsillotomy
Tooke knife
Tooke spatula
Toomey evacuator
Toomey suction tube
Toomey syringe
tooth band
tooth elevator
tooth-extracting forceps
toothache
toothed forceps
toothed retractor
topectomy
tophus (*pl.* tophi)
topical
topical anesthesia
topical cocaine
Torek-Bevan operation

Torek esophagectomy
Torek operation
Torek orchiopexy
Torkildsen shunt
Torkildsen ventriculo-
    cisternostomy
Toronto splint
TORP (total ossicular replacement
    prosthesis)
Torpin operation
torr units of pressure
torsion
torsion forceps
torsion fracture
torticollis
tortuosity
tortuous
torus fracture
total abdominal hysterectomy
total anesthesia
total breech delivery
total capsulectomy
total cardiopulmonary bypass
total gastrectomy
total hip arthroplasty
total hip prosthesis
total hip replacement
total hysterectomy
total keratoplasty
total knee prosthesis
total laryngectomy
total parenteral nutrition (TPN)
total spinal anesthesia
Totco clips
Toti-Mosher operation
Toti operation
tourniquet
    automatic

tourniquet *(continued)*
    automatic rotating
    Bethune
    cardiovascular
    Carr
    caval
    Conn
    Dupuytren
    Esmarch
    flexible
    Kidde
    Kidde-Robbins
    Linton
    lobectomy
    lung
    pneumatic
    Roberts-Nelson
    Rumel
    Rumel-Belmont
    scalp
    t. clamp
    universal
    Velcro
towel clamp
towel clip
towel forceps
Tower forceps
Tower prong
Tower retractor
Towne view
Townley caliper
Townley forceps
Townley prosthesis
Townley screw
toxemia
toxic
toxic goiter
toxicology

Toynbee otoscope
Toynbee speculum
TPN (total parenteral nutrition)
trabecula (*pl.* trabeculae)
trabeculae lienis
trabeculae of spleen
trabecular
trabeculated
trabeculation
trabeculectomy
trabeculodialysis
trabeculotomy
Trace stripper
trachea
tracheal bistoury
tracheal bougie
tracheal cannula
tracheal catheter
tracheal dilator
tracheal fistula
tracheal forceps
tracheal hemostat
tracheal hook
tracheal knife
tracheal muscle
tracheal retractor
tracheal rings
tracheal scissors
tracheal suction tube
tracheal tenaculum
tracheal tube
tracheal tube with obturator
tracheal veins
tracheales veins
trachealis muscle
trachelectomy
trachelopexy
tracheloplasty

trachelorrhaphy
trachelotome
trachelotomy
tracheobronchial suction tube
tracheocricotomy
tracheoesophageal
tracheoesophageal fistula closure
tracheofissure
tracheogram
tracheography
tracheolaryngotomy
tracheoplasty
tracheorrhaphy
tracheoscope
      Haslinger
      Jackson
tracheoscopy
tracheostomy
tracheostomy button
tracheostomy cannula
tracheostomy hook
tracheostomy scissors
tracheostomy trocar
tracheostomy tube
tracheotome
      Salvatore-Maloney
      Sierra-Sheldon
tracheotomize
tracheotomy
tracheotomy cannula
tracheotomy hook
tracheotomy tube
trachoma
trachoma forceps
tracing
tract
tract signs

traction
- axis
- Bryant
- Buck
- elastic
- external
- halo
- halo-pelvic
- halo-to-bale
- intermaxillary
- internal
- maxillomandibular
- Russell
- skeletal
- skin
- tongue
- t. apparatus
- t. bow
- t. clip
- t. forceps
- t. handle (see separate listing)
- t. splint
- t. sutures
- t. tenaculum
- t. tongs

traction handle
- Barton
- Bill
- Castroviejo-Kalt
- Luikart-Bill

tractor
- Buck
- curved
- extension
- Kirschner-wire
- Lowsley
- Perkins
- prostatic

tractor *(continued)*
- Rankin
- Russell
- Russell-Buck
- skull
- Steinmann
- Syms
- Vinke
- Wells
- wire
- Young

tractotomy
tragicus muscle
tragus
Trainor-Nida operation
tranquilizers
transabdominal colonoscopy
transacral block
transcarpal
transcervical fracture
transcondylar fracture
transduodenal
transduodenal choledocho-
    lithotomy
transfibular arthrodesis
transect
transection
transection incision
transection of artery
transection of nerve roots
transection of nerve tracts
transection of tube
transection of vein
transfer
transfer forceps
transfer of tendon
transference
transference of muscle

transfixing sutures
transfixion
transfixion of iris
transfixion screw
transfixion sutures
transformation
transfusion
transilluminating telescope
transillumination
transilluminator
    Briggs
    Finnoff
    hooded
    rotating
    speculum
    Welch Allyn
transitional cell carcinoma
translumbar aortogram
translumbar aortography
transmeatal incision
transmetatarsal
transmetatarsal amputation
transnasal sphenoidotomy
transorbital leukotomy
transorbital lobotomy
transparent drape
transpericardial pacemaker
transperitoneal cesarean section
transperitoneal nephrectomy
transperitoneal technique
transplant
transplant-grafting forceps
transplant spatula
transplantation
transplantation of muscle
transplantation of ocular muscle
transplantation of tendon
transpleural

transposition
transposition of tendon
transposition operation
transrectus incision
transsacral
transsacral anesthesia
transscrotal
transscrotal orchiopexy
transseptal
transseptal catheter
transthoracic catheter
transthoracotomy
transtracheal anesthesia
transudate
transureteroureteral anastomosis
transureteroureterostomy
transurethral biopsy
transurethral prostatectomy
transurethral resection (TUR)
transurethral resection of prostate
    (TURP)
transvenous
transvenous catheter pacemaker
transvenous pacemaker
transvenous pacemaker catheter
transvenous pacing
transventricular dilator
transventricular valvotomy
transversa colli artery
transversa faciei artery
transversa faciei vein
transversae colli veins
transversalis
transversalis fascia
transverse
transverse amputation
transverse arteriotomy
transverse artery of face

transverse artery of neck
transverse artery of scapula
transverse cesarean section
transverse colon
transverse colostomy
transverse facial fracture
transverse fascia
transverse fracture
transverse humeral ligament
transverse incision
transverse maxillary fracture
transverse muscle
transverse osteotomy
transverse process
transverse saw
transversectomy
transversospinal muscle
transversospinalis muscle
transversostomy
transversus abdominis muscle
transversus auriculae muscle
transversus colli nerve
transversus linguae muscle
transversus menti muscle
transversus nuchae muscle
transversus perinei profundus
    muscle
transversus perinei superficialis
    muscle
transversus situs
transversus thoracis
transvesical prostatectomy
Trantas operation
trap-door incision
trap incision
trapezium
trapezius muscle
trapezoid bone

trapezoid ligament
Trattner catheter
traumatic
traumatic amputation
traumatic capsule
traumatize
Travel jejunostomy
Travel operation
Travenol needle
Travenol twin coil for hemo-
    dialysis
trefoil tendon
Treitz hernia
Treitz ligament
Trélat raspatory
Trélat speculum
tremor
tremulous cataract
Trendelenburg cannula
Trendelenburg-Crafoord clamp
Trendelenburg operation
Trendelenburg position
Trendelenburg pulmonary embo-
    lectomy
Trendelenburg synchondro-
    seotomy
Trendelenburg vein ligation
trephination
trephine
    antrum
    Arruga
    automatic corneal
    Barraquer
    Becker
    Blakesley
    Boiler
    bone
    Brown-Pusey

trephine *(continued)*
- Castroviejo
- chalazion
- corneal
- cranial
- dacryocystorhinostomy
- Damshek
- D'Errico
- DeVilbiss
- Dimitry
- electric
- Elliot
- exploratory
- Franceschetti
- Galt
- Gradle
- Green
- Greenwood
- Grieshaber
- Hand
- Harris
- Hippel
- Horsley
- Iliff
- lacrimal
- Lahey
- Lichtenberg
- Lorie
- Michel
- Mueller
- Paton
- Paufique
- Polley-Bickel
- Schuknecht
- scleral
- Scoville
- Searcy
- septum

trephine *(continued)*
- skull
- spinal
- sternal
- Stille
- Stryker
- temporal
- Thornwald
- Turkel
- Walker
- Wilder

trephining

Treves operation

triad

triaditis

trial cup

trial fracture frame

trial prosthesis

trial reduction

triangle
- Calot's
- carotid
- cephalic
- digastric
- facial
- femoral
- Henke's
- Hesselbach's
- inferior carotid
- infraclavicular
- inguinal
- lumbocostoabdominal
- occipital
- Scarpa's
- subclavian
- submaxillary
- suboccipital
- superior carotid

triangle *(continued)*
    t. of elbow
    t. of election
    t. of necessity
triangular bandage
triangular bone
triangular dressing
triangular muscle
triangular punch forceps
tributaries
triceps brachii muscle
triceps muscle
triceps surae muscle
trichiasis operation
trichloroethylene
tricuspid annuloplasty
tricuspid valve
tri-fin chisel
triflange intramedullary nail
triflow incentive spirometer
triflow oxygen
trigeminal nerve (cranial nerve V)
trigeminal nerve compression
trigeminal retractor
trigeminal rhizotomy
trigeminus
trigeminus scissors
trigone
trigonectomy
trigonitis
tri-leaflet aortic prosthesis
Trilene
trimalleolar fracture
Trimar
trimming
trinocular microscope
tripartite
Tripier amputation

Tripier operation
triple amputation
triple arthrodesis
triple-lumen catheter
triquetral bone
trocar
    Allen
    amniotic
    anasarca
    antrum
    aspirating
    Babcock
    Barnes
    Beardsley
    bladder
    Boettcher
    brain-exploring
    Campbell
    catheter
    cecostomy
    Charlton
    Coakley
    conical
    cricothyroid
    Davidson
    Dean
    Denker
    Douglas
    Duchenne
    Duke
    Durham
    Emmet
    empyema
    Faulkner
    Fein
    fiberglass sleeve
    Frazier
    gallbladder

trocar *(continued)*

    Hargin
    Hunt
    Hurwitz
    hydrocele
    Ingram
    intercostal
    internal decompression
    intestinal decompression
    Judd
    Kidd
    Kolb
    Kreutzmann
    laparoscopic
    Lichtwicz
    Lillie
    Livermore
    Myerson
    Nelson
    nested
    Ochsner
    ovarian
    Patterson
    Pierce
    piloting
    Potain
    prostatic
    pyramidal
    rectal
    Ruskin
    Sewall
    Southey
    Southey-Leech
    suprapubic
    Sweet
    tracheostomy
    tracheotomy
    t. chisel

trocar *(continued)*

    trocar-point needle
    Van Alyea
    Verres
    Walther
    Wangensteen
    Wiener-Pierce
    Wilson
    Yankauer

trochanter
trochanter-holding clamp
trochanter pin
trochanter rasp
trochanter reamer
trochanteric plate
trochanteroplasty
trochlear nerve (cranial nerve IV)
trochlearis nerve
Troeltsch speculum
Tronothane hydrochloride
trophic fracture
trough
trough gouge
Trousseau bougie
Trousseau dilator
Trousseau forceps
Trousseau-Jackson dilator
Troutman-Barraquer needle holder
Troutman chisel
Troutman eye implant
Troutman forceps
Troutman gouge
Troutman scissors
Truc operation
TruCut needle
true aneurysm
truncus brachiocephalicus
truncus celiacus

truncus costocervicalis
truncus pulmonalis
truncus thyrocervicalis
trunk
    celiac
    lumbosacral
    pulmonary
    sympathetic
Trusler clamp
TSH (thyroid stimulating hormone)
TTNB (transient tachypnea of the newborn)
tubal implantation into uterus
tubal insufflation
tubal insufflator
tubal ligation
Tubbs dilator
Tubby knife
Tubby-Steindler operation
tube (see also *suction tube*)
    Abbott
    Abbott-Miller
    Abbott-Rawson
    Abramson
    ACMI-Valentine
    Adson
    air
    Air-Lon
    Andrews-Pynchon
    Anthony
    antrum wash
    Argyle
    Argyle chest
    Argyle-Salem sump
    Armour
    aspirating
    Atkins-Cannard

tube *(continued)*
    Ayer
    Baker
    Bardic
    Beardsley
    Bellocq
    Billroth
    bivalve
    bladder
    Blakemore
    Blakemore-Sengstaken
    bone
    Bonina-Jacobson
    Bonnano
    Bouchut
    Broyles
    Buie
    bypass
    Cantor
    Carabelli
    Carlens
    Carmalt
    Carrel
    Castelli
    Castelli-Paparella collar-button
    Castelli-Paparella myringotomy
    Cattell T-tube
    Celestin
    Chaffin
    Chaffin-Pratt
    Chaffin sump
    Chaoul
    Chaussier
    chest
    Chevalier Jackson
    Clerf

tube *(continued)*
- closed drainage
- closed suction drainage
- collar-button
- collecting
- Collins
- colostomy
- Coolidge
- corneal
- cuffed
- cuffless
- cystostomy
- Dakin
- Davol
- Deaver T-tube
- Debove
- Denker
- Depaul
- Devine
- Diamond
- Donaldson
- double-cuffed
- double-lumen
- drain
- drainage
- dressed
- Duke
- duodenal
- Durham tracheostomy
- Einhorn
- empyema
- encircling
- end
- endobronchial
- endoesophageal
- endolymphatic
- endoscopic
- endotracheal

tube *(continued)*
- esophageal
- esophagoscopic
- Ewald
- extra-long tracheal
- feeding
- fil d'Arion
- flexible rubber
- flush
- forked T-tube
- Frazier
- Fuller
- fusion
- Gabriel Tucker
- gallbladder
- gastric
- gastroduodenal
- gastroenterostomy
- gastrointestinal
- gastrostomy
- gavage
- Gilman-Abrams
- granulation
- Greiling
- grommet drain
- Guisez
- Harris
- Heimlich
- hemodialysis
- Hemovac
- Hilger
- Holinger
- Holter
- Honore-Smathers
- horizontal
- House
- Immergut
- infant feeding

tube *(continued)*
- infusion
- intestinal
- intraluminal
- intranasal
- intratracheal
- intubation
- Jackson
- Javid
- Jergesen
- Jesberg
- Joel-Baker
- Johns Hopkins
- Johnson
- Jones
- Jutte
- Kaslow
- Kehr
- Keidel
- Kelly
- Kidd
- Killian
- Kimpton-Brown
- Kistner
- Kuhn
- lacrimal
- Lahey
- Lanz
- LaRocca
- laryngeal
- laryngectomy
- latex
- Lieter
- Lell
- Lennarson
- Lepley-Ernst
- Levin
- Lewis

tube *(continued)*
- Lindeman-Silverstein
- Linton
- Lloyd
- Lord-Blakemore
- Lore-Lawrence
- Lorenz
- Luer
- Lyon
- MacKenty
- Mackler
- Magill
- Martin
- medullary
- Miller-Abbott
- Millin
- Mixter
- monomer suction biopsy
- Montefiore
- Moore
- Morch
- Mosher
- Moss
- Mueller-Frazier
- Mueller-Pool
- Mueller-Pynchon
- Mueller-Yankauer
- Muldoon
- multiholed
- multiple-lumen
- Murphy
- myringotomy
- Nachlas
- nasal
- nasogastric
- nasogastric feeding
- nasolacrimal
- nasopharyngeal

tube *(continued)*
- nasotracheal
- nephrostomy
- Neuber
- New's
- NG
- Nunez
- O'Beirne
- Ochsner
- O'Dwyer
- open-end aspirating
- orotracheal
- Paparella
- Paul-Mixter
- PE (polyethylene)
- PE (pressure equalization)
- Penrose
- pharyngeal
- Pierce
- Pilling
- plastic
- Pleur-evac
- pleural suction
- Polisar-Lyons
- polyethylene
- polyvinyl
- Pool
- Portex speaking
- postnasal
- pressure-equalization
- Pudenz
- pus
- Pynchon
- pyramidal
- Pyrex
- Quinton
- radiopaque intestinal
- rectal

tube *(continued)*
- red-top
- Rehfuss
- Replogle
- Reuter
- Reynolds
- Rochester
- Rosen
- Rubin
- Rubin-Brandborg
- Rusch
- Ryle
- Sachs
- Salem sump
- salvarsan
- Schall
- Sengstaken
- Sengstaken-Blakemore
- seton
- Shaldon
- Shea
- Sheehy
- Sheldon-Pudenz
- Shepard
- Shiley
- Shiley-Bjork
- Shiner
- short-length tracheal
- shunt
- Silastic
- silicone
- Southey
- Southey-Leech
- Souttar
- speaking
- sphincter
- sputum
- Stamm

tube *(continued)*
    stomach
    stomach irrigation
    suction
    sump
    T-tube
    tampon
    Teflon
    thoracic drainage
    thoracostomy
    thoracotomy
    throat irrigation
    tracheal
    tracheal t. with obturator
    tracheostomy
    tracheotomy
    t. drain
    t. forceps
    t. pedicle graft
    Tucker
    Turkel
    U-tube
    uterine
    Valentine
    valve
    Van Alyea
    velvet-eye
    ventilation
    ventricular ventilation
    Vernon
    vertical
    Voltolini
    Von Eichen
    Wangensteen
    warning stop
    wash
    Webster
    Welch Allyn

tube *(continued)*
    Y-tube
    Yankauer
tuber
tubercle
tuberculosis
tubo-ovarian
tubo-ovarian varicoccle
tuboplasty
tubular
tubular blade
tubular forceps
tubular graft
tubular vaginal speculum
tubularization
tuck
tucker
    Bishop-Black tendon
    Bishop-DeWitt tendon
    Bishop-Peter tendon
    Bishop tendon
    Burch-Greenwood tendon
    Fink tendon
    Green strabismus
    Harrison
    Smith-Petersen
    strabismus
    tendon
Tucker bougie
Tucker bronchoscope
Tucker dilator
Tucker esophagoscope
Tucker forceps
Tucker laryngoscope
Tucker-McLane forceps
Tucker suction tube
Tucker telescope
Tucker tube

tucking
Tudor-Edwards costotome
Tudor-Edwards rib shears
Tuffier operation
Tuffier-Raney retractor
Tuffier retractor
Tuffier rib spreader
Tuffnell bandage
tuft
tuft fracture
tulle gras dressing
tumbling technique
tumefaction
tumor
tumor forceps
tumor screw
tunica (*pl.* tunicae)
tunica abdominalis
tunica adventitia
tunica albuginea
tunica vaginalis
tunicary
tunicary hernia
tuning fork
tunnel
tunneled bougie
tunneled eye implant
tunneler
    Craaford-Cooley
    DeBakey
    Favoloro
tunneling
Tuohy catheter
Tuohy needle
TUR (transurethral resection)
turbid
turbinate bone
turbinate electrode

turbinate forceps
turbinate scissors
turbinates
turbinectomy
Turco operation
Turco procedure
Turek spreader
Turell forceps
Turell proctoscope
Turell sigmoidoscope
turgescence
turgescent
turgid
Turkel needle
Turkel punch
Turkel trephine
Turkel tube
turnbuckle
Turner dilator
Turner elevator
Turner gouge
Turner operation
Turner periosteal elevator
Turner pin
Turner prosthesis
Turner-Warwick urethroplasty
turning fracture frame
TURP (transurethral resection of
    prostate)
Tuttle forceps
Tuttle proctoscope
Tuttle sigmoidoscope
Tuttle test
twenty-day gut sutures
twilight anesthesia
twilight sleep
twin knife
twin-pattern chisel

twist drill
twist drill points
twisted cotton sutures
twisted silk sutures
twisted wire loop
two-bladed dilator
two-clamp anastomosis
two-layer anastomosis
two-prong rake retractor
two-prong stem finger prosthesis
two-pronged retractor
two-stage operation
two-step corneal section
two-way catheter
two-way hemostatic bag
two-wing drain
Twombly operation
Twombly-Ulfelder operation
Tycron sutures
Tydings forceps
Tydings knife
Tydings-Lakeside forceps
Tydings snare
Tydings tonsillectome
tylectomy
tympanectomy
tympanic artery

tympanic bone
tympanic membrane
tympanic nerve
tympanic veins
tympanica anterior artery
tympanica inferior artery
tympanica posterior artery
tympanica superior artery
tympanicae veins
tympanicus nerve
tympanites
tympanogram
tympanography
tympanomastoidectomy
tympanoplastic knife
tympanoplasty (type I, type II, or type III)
tympanosympathectomy
tympanotomy
tympanum
tympanum perforator
tympany
typhlectomy
typhloureterostomy
typical
Tyrrell hook
Tyson's glands

u

U stitch
U.S. Army osteotome
U.S. Army retractor
U-shaped forceps
U-shaped incision
U-tube
Uchida incision
Uchida technique
Uchida tubal ligation
UCI-Barnard valve
UCI prosthesis
UCI total knee replacement
Uebe applicator
ulcer
ulcerating
ulceration
ulcerative colitis
ulectomy
Ulloa operation
Ullrich retractor
ulna
ulna splint
ulnar artery
ulnar nerve
ulnar resection
ulnar veins
ulnares veins
ulnaris artery
ulnaris nerve
ulotomy
ultramicroscope
ultrasonic

ultrasonic diathermy
ultrasonic electrode
ultrasonic microscope
ultrasonic tip
ultrasonogram
ultrasonography
ultrasound
ultraviolet microscope
umbilectomy
umbilical
umbilical artery
umbilical artery catheter
umbilical catheter
umbilical clamp
umbilical clip
umbilical cord
umbilical hernia
umbilical hernia repair
umbilical hernia repair with
    omphalectomy
umbilical hernia repair with
    umbilectomy
umbilical herniorrhaphy
umbilical ligament
umbilical scissors
umbilical tape
umbilical vein catheter
umbilical veins
umbilicalis artery
umbilicalis sinistra vein
umbilicalis vein
umbiliclamp

umbiliclip
umbilicus
umbrella
umbrella-type prosthesis
unabsorbable sutures
unassisted respiration
unbridling
unciform bone
uncinate bone
uncinate process
uncovering
undercut
undermine
undersurface
underwater drainage
underwater seal
underwater-seal tube
underwater suction
undifferentiated
undifferentiated carcinoma
unguis
unguis incarnatus
unilateral
unilateral procedure
uninterrupted sutures
unipolar
unipolar electrode
unit
    Bovie electrosurgical
    Burdick electrosurgical
    Cameron electrosurgical
    cataract suction
    Cavitron-Kelman surgical
    Chaffin-Pratt suction
    cryo-ophthalmic
    electrocautery
    electrosurgical
    Keeler cryophake

unit *(continued)*
    Kreiselman
    Malis coagulating
    Mira
    Thermosector electrosurgical
    Viamonte-Hobbs electro-
     surgical
    Viamonte-Jutzy electro-
     surgical
    Zeiss
universal aspirator
universal conformer
universal cystoscope
universal drill
universal drill points
universal forceps
universal joint device
universal nerve hook
universal retractor
universal saw
universal splint
universal T-adapter
universal tourniquet
University of Illinois needle
Unna boot
Unna extractor
Unna paste
Unna wrap
unroof
unroofing
ununited fracture
upbiting biopsy forceps
up-cutting rongeur
Updegraff hook
Updegraff needle
UPP (urethral pressure profile)
upper abdominal midline incision
upper GI series

upper jaw
upper lobe of lung
upper midline incision
upright position
uptake
upward gaze incision
urachal fossa
urachus (*pl.* urachi)
uraniscoplasty
uraniscorrhaphy
uranoplasty
uranorrhaphy
uranostaphyloplasty
uranostaphylorrhaphy
Urban mastectomy
Urbantschitsch bougie
Urecholine
uremia
ureter
ureter isolation forceps
ureteral basket stone dislodger
ureteral bougie
ureteral catheter
ureteral catheter obturator
ureteral catheterization
ureteral dilation
ureteral dilator
ureteral implant
ureteral meatotome
ureteral meatotomy
ureteral meatotomy electrode
ureteral reflux
ureteral stone
ureteral stone basket
ureteral stone extractor
ureterectasis
ureterectomy
ureterocecostomy

ureterocelectomy
ureterocentesis
ureterocolostomy
ureterocystostomy
ureteroenterostomy
ureteroileobladder anastomosis
ureteroileocutaneous anastomosis
ureteroileostomy
ureterolithotomy
ureterolysis
ureteroneocystostomy
ureteronephrectomy
ureteropelvic junction
ureteropelvic junction stricture
ureteropexy
ureteroplasty
ureteroplication
ureteroproctostomy
ureteropyelogram
ureteropyelography
ureteropyeloplasty
ureteropyelostomy
ureterorrhaphy
ureteroscopy
ureterosigmoidostomy
ureterostomy
ureterotomy
ureterotubal anastomosis
ureteroureteral anastomosis
ureteroureterostomy
ureterovaginal fistula
ureterovesical junction
ureterovesicostomy
uretheral pressure profile
urethra
urethral artery
urethral bougie
urethral catheter

urethral catheterization
urethral dilator
urethral forceps
urethral glands
urethral meatotomy
urethral pressure profile (UPP)
urethral sound
urethral speculum
urethral suspension
urethral whip bougie
urethralis artery
urethrectomy
urethrocystogram
urethrocystography
urethrocystopexy
urethrogram
urethrographic cannula
urethrographic clamp
urethrography
urethrolithotomy
urethropexy
urethroplasty
urethrorectal fistula
urethrorrhaphy
urethroscopy
urethrostomy
urethrotome
    Keitzer
    Maisonneuve
    Otis
urethrotomy
urethrovaginal fistula
urgency
urinalysis
urinary catheter
urinary diversion
urinary incontenence
urine culture

uroflowmeter
urogenital
urogram
urography
urologic catheter
urology
Usher Marlex mesh
Usher Marlex mesh implant
Usher Marlex mesh prosthesis
uterina artery
uterinae veins
uterine artery
uterine artery forceps
uterine aspiration
uterine biopsy forceps
uterine biopsy punch
uterine canal
uterine cannula
uterine cuff
uterine curet
uterine curettage
uterine didelphys
uterine dilator
uterine-dressing forceps
uterine-elevating forceps
uterine elevator
uterine evacuation
uterine fibroidectomy
uterine forceps
uterine hernia
uterine incision
uterine knife
uterine needle
uterine-packing forceps
uterine polyp forceps
uterine probe
uterine prolapse
uterine prolapse operation

uterine radium insertion
uterine scissors
uterine sound
uterine spoon
uterine suction curet
uterine suspension
uterine tenaculum
uterine tenaculum forceps
uterine tenaculum hook
uterine tube
uterine veins
uterine vulsellum forceps
uterocentesis
uterofixation
uteropelvic ligaments
uteropexy

uteroplasty
uterosacral
uterosacral ligament
uterus
utility forceps
utility shoulder splint
utricular nerve
utricularis nerve
utriculoampullaris nerve
uveitis
uvula
uvula retractor
uvulae muscle
uvulectomy
uvulitis
uvulotomy

V

V-blade plate
V-medullary nail
V-shaped incision
V-Y operation
vabra aspirator
vabra cannula
vabra catheter
vabra curettage
vabra endometrial biopsy
vaccination
Vacurette
Vacurette catheter
Vacutainer drain
Vacu-tome knife
vacuum abortion
vacuum aspiration apparatus
vacuum aspirator
vacuum curet
vacuum extraction
vacuum hand pump
vacuum intrauterine cannula
vacuum intrauterine probe
vacuum retractor
vacuuming needle
vagal
vagina
vaginal
vaginal artery
vaginal bag
vaginal celiotomy
vaginal cesarean section
vaginal construction

vaginal cuff
vaginal cuff clamp
vaginal douche
vaginal hernia
vaginal hysterectomy
vaginal hysterectomy forceps
vaginal nerves
vaginal pack
vaginal packing
vaginal prolapse
vaginal radium insertion
vaginal reconstruction
vaginal retractor
vaginal speculum
vaginal vault
vaginalectomy
vaginales nerves
vaginalis artery
vaginectomy
vaginofixation
vaginolabial
vaginolabial hernia
vaginoperineotomy
vaginoplasty
vaginorrhaphy
vaginoscope
        Huffman
        infant
vaginoscopy
vaginotomy
vagotomy
vagotomy retractor

vagotomy stripper
vagus
vagus nerve (cranial nerve X)
Valentine irrigator
Valentine position
Valentine splint
Valentine tube
valgus
Valium
vallecula (*pl.* valleculae)
vallecular
Valsalva maneuver
Valsalva procedure
valvanocautery
valve (see also *prosthesis*)
    ACMI
    aortic
    ball
    ball-type
    Bjork-Shiley
    Carpentier
    Carpentier-Edwards
    Cutter-Smellof disk
    disk
    double-angle
    Gott
    Gott-Daggett
    Harken
    hinged leaflet aortic
    Holter
    Houston
    Hufnagel
    Ionescu-Shiley
    irrigating
    Kay-Shiley
    Magnuson
    mitral
    nonrebreathing

valve *(continued)*
    Pudenz
    reducing
    Schulte
    Smeloff-Cutter
    Starr-Edwards
    UCI-Barnard
    v. dilator
    v. prosthesis
    v. spreader
    v. tube
valvotomy
valvotomy knife
valvula (*pl.* valvulae)
valvula ileocolica
valvula pylori
valvulectomy
valvuloplasty
valvulotome
    Bailey-Glover-O'Neil
    Brock
    curved
    Derra
    Dogliotti
    expansile
    Gohrbrand
    Harken
    Himmelstein
    Longmire
    Malm-Himmelstein
    Niedner
    Potts
    Potts-Riker
    pulmonary
    Sellor
valvulotomy
Van Alyea cannula
Van Alyea trocar

Van Alyea tube
van Buren dilator
van Buren forceps
van Buren operation
van Buren sound
Van Doren forceps
Van Gorder operation
van Hook ureteroureterostomy
van Hoorn maneuver
Van Lint akinesia
Van Lint and Atkinson akinesia
Van Lint and Atkinson block
Van Lint block
Van Millingen operation
Van Osdel guillotine
Van Osdel tonsillectome
Van Struycken forceps
Van Struycken punch
Vanderbilt clamp
Vanderbilt forceps
Vanghetti prosthesis
Vannas knife
Vannas scissors
Varco forceps
varices (*sing.* varix)
varicocele
varicocelectomy
varicose
varicose veins
varicosity
varicotomy
varix (*pl.* varices)
varus
varus osteotomy
vas (*pl.* vasa)
vas clamp
vas deferens
vas hook

vas isolation forceps
vasa (*sing.* vas)
vasa brevia
Vasconcelos amputation
Vasconcelos-Baretto clamp
Vascoray
vascular
vascular anastomosis
vascular clamp
vascular clip
vascular dilator
vascular dissector
vascular forceps
vascular needle holder
vascular nevus
vascular prosthesis
vascular retractor
vascular scissors
vascular silk sutures
vascular tissue forceps
vascularity
vascularization
vascularize
vasculitis
vasectomy
vasectomy forceps
Vaseline dressing
Vaseline gauze
Vaseline gauze dressing
Vaseline petrolatum packing
Vaseline wick dressing
vasoconstriction
vasodepression
vasodilatation
vasodilation
vasoepididymectomy
vasoepididymostomy
vasogram

vasography
vasoligation
vasomotor
vasopressor agents
vasoresection
vasorrhaphy
vasostomy
vasotomy
vasotripsy
vasovasostomy
vasovesiculectomy
vastus intermedius muscle
vastus lateralis muscle
vastus medialis muscle
vastus muscle
Vater ampulla
Vater papilla
vault
VCUG (voiding cystourethrogram)
Veau-Axhausen operation
Veau elevator
Veau operation
Veau palatoplasty
vectis
vectis forceps
vectorcardiogram
vectorcardiography
Veenema-Gusberg needle
Veenema-Gusberg punch
Veenema retractor
vegetation growth
vegetations
veil
vein (veins)
    accompanying v. of hypo-
      glossal nerve
    adrenal

vein (veins) *(continued)**
    anastomotic
    angular
    antebrachial
    appendicular
    arcuate v's of kidney
    auditory
    auricular
    axillary
    azygos
    basal
    basilic
    basivertebral
    brachial
    brachiocephalic
    bronchial
    canaliculus
    cardiac
    carotid
    cavernous v's of penis
    central v's of liver
    central v. of retina
    central v. of suprarenal gland
    cephalic
    cerebellar
    cerebral
    cervical
    choroid
    ciliary
    circumflex femoral
    circumflex iliac
    colic
    conjunctival
    coronary

*v. = vein
 v's = veins

vein (veins) *(continued)**
  cubital
  cutaneous
  cystic
  deep v's of clitoris
  deep v's of penis
  digital
  diploic
  dorsal v's of clitoris
  dorsal v's of penis
  dorsal v's of tongue
  emissary
  epigastric
  episcleral
  esophageal
  ethmoidal
  facial
  femoral
  fibular
  gastric
  gastroepiploic
  genicular
  gluteal
  hemiazygos
  hemorrhoidal
  hepatic
  hypogastric
  ileal
  ileocolic
  iliac
  iliolumbar
  innominate
  intercapital
  intercostal

vein (veins) *(continued)**
  interlobar v's of kidney
  interlobular v's of kidney
  interlobular v's of liver
  interosseous v's of foot
  intervertebral
  jejunal
  jejunal and ileal v's
  jugular
  labial
  labyrinthine
  lacrimal
  laryngeal
  lingual
  lumbar
  mastoid emissary
  maxillary
  mediastinal
  meningeal
  mesenteric
  metacarpal
  metatarsal
  musculophrenic
  nasal
  nasofrontal
  oblique v. of left atrium
  obturator
  occipital
  occipital emissary
  ophthalmic
  ovarian
  palatine
  palpebral
  pancreatic
  pancreaticoduodenal
  paraumbilical
  parietal emissary
  parotid

*v. = vein
 v's = veins

vein (veins) *(continued)**
  perforating
  pericardiac
  pericardiacophrenic
  peroneal
  pharyngeal
  phrenic
  popliteal
  portal
  posterior v. of left ventricle
  prepyloric
  pudendal
  pulmonary
  pyloric
  radial
  ranine
  rectal
  renal
  retromandibular
  sacral
  saphenous
  scrotal
  sigmoid
  spinal
  spiral v. of modiolus
  splenic
  stellate v's of kidney
  sternocleidomastoid
  striate
  stylomastoid
  subclavian
  subcostal
  subcutaneous v's of abdomen
  sublingual
  submental

vein (veins) *(continued)**
  supraorbital
  suprarenal
  suprascapular
  supratrochlear
  temporal
  testicular
  thalamostriate
  thoracic
  thoracoacromial
  thoracoepigastric
  thymic
  thyroid
  tibial
  tracheal
  tympanic
  ulnar
  umbilical
  uterine
  v. anesthesia
  v. graft
  v. hook
  v. ligation and stripping
  v. of aqueduct of vestibule
  v. of bulb of penis
  v. of bulb of vestibule
  v. of cochlear canal
  v. of pterygoid canal
  v. of septum pellucidum
  v. retractor
  v. spreader
  v. stripper
Velcro tapes
Velcro tourniquet
Veley headrest
velour patch
Velpeau bandage
Velpeau dressing

*v. = vein
 v's = veins

Velpeau hernia
Velpeau sling
Velroc dressing
velvet-eye tube
vena (*pl.* venae)*
    v. anastomotica inferior
    v. anastomotica superior
    v. angularis
    v. appendicularis
    v. aqueductus vestibuli
    vv. arcuatae renis
    vv. auriculares anteriores
    v. auricularis posterior
    v. axillaris
    v. azygos
    v. basalis
    v. basilica
    vv. basivertebrales
    vv. brachiales
    vv. brachiocephalicae
      (dextra et sinistra)
    vv. bronchiales
    v. bulbi penis
    v. bulbi vestibuli
    v. canaliculi
    v. canalis pterygoidei
    v. cava inferior
    v. cava superior
    vv. cavae
    vv. cavernosae penis
    vv. centrales hepatis
    v. centralis glandulae supra-
      renalis
    v. centralis retinae
    v. cephalica

*v. = vena [*L.*]
 vv. = venae [*L., pl.*]

vena (*pl.* venae)* *(continued)*
    v. cephalica accessoria
    vv. cerebelli inferiores
    vv. cerebelli superiores
    v. cerebri anterior
    vv. cerebri inferiores
    vv. cerebri internae
    v. cerebri magna
    v. cerebri media profunda
    v. cerebri media superficialis
    vv. cerebri superiores
    v. cervicalis profunda
    v. choroidea
    vv. ciliares
    v. circumflexa ilium pro-
      funda
    v. circumflexa ilium super-
      ficialis
    vv. circumflexae femoris
      laterales
    vv. circumflexae femoris
      mediales
    v. colica dextra
    v. colica media
    v. colica sinistra
    v. comitans nervi hypoglossi
    vv. conjunctivales
    vv. cordis anteriores
    v. cordis magna
    v. cordis media
    vv. cordis minimae
    v. cordis parva
    v. cutanea
    v. cystica
    vv. digitales dorsales pedis
    vv. digitales palmares
    vv. digitales plantares
    v. diploica frontalis

vena *(pl.* venae)* *(continued)*
  v. diploica occipitalis
  v. diploica temporalis
    anterior
  v. diploica temporalis
    posterior
  vv. dorsales clitoridis super-
    ficiales
  vv. dorsales linguae
  vv. dorsales penis super-
    ficiales
  v. dorsalis clitoridis pro-
    funda
  v. dorsalis penis profunda
  v. emissaria condylaris
  v. emissaria mastoidea
  v. emissaria occipitalis
  v. emissaria parietalis
  v. epigastrica inferior
  v. epigastrica superficialis
  vv. epigastricae superiores
  vv. episclerales
  vv. esophageae
  v. facialis
  v. faciei profunda
  v. femoralis
  vv. fibulares
  v. gastrica dextra
  v. gastrica sinistra
  vv. gastricae breves
  v. gastroepiploica dextra
  v. gastroepiploica sinistra
  vv. genus
  vv. gluteae inferiores
  vv. gluteae superiores

*v. = vena [*L.*]
vv. = venae [*L., pl.*]

vena *(pl.* venae)* *(continued)*
  v. hemiazygos
  v. hemiazygos accessoria
  vv. hepaticae
  v. ileocolica
  v. iliaca communis
  v. iliaca externa
  v. iliaca interna
  v. iliolumbalis
  vv. intercapitales
  vv. intercostales anteriores
  vv. intercostales posteriores
    (IV et XI)
  v. intercostalis superior
    dextra
  v. intercostalis superior
    sinistra
  v. intercostalis suprema
  vv. interlobares renis
  vv. interlobulares hepatis
  vv. interlobulares renis
  v. intervertebralis
  vv. jejunales et ilei
  v. jugularis anterior
  v. jugularis interna
  vv. labiales anteriores
  vv. labiales inferiores
  vv. labiales posteriores
  v. labialis superior
  vv. labyrinthi
  v. lacrimalis
  v. laryngea inferior
  v. laryngea superior
  v. lienalis
  v. lingualis
  vv. lumbales (I-IV)
  v. lumbalis ascendens
  vv. maxillares

vena (*pl.* venae)* *(continued)*
- v. mediana antebrachii
- v. mediana basilica
- v. mediana cephalica
- v. mediana cubiti
- vv. mediastinales
- vv. meningeae
- vv. meningeae mediae
- v. mesenterica inferior
- v. mesenterica superior
- vv. metacarpeae dorsales
- vv. metacarpeae palmares
- vv. metatarseae dorsales
- vv. metatarseae plantares
- vv. musculophrenicae
- vv. nasales externae
- v. nasofrontalis
- v. obliqua atrii sinistri
- vv. obturatoriae
- v. occipitalis
- v. ophthalmica inferior
- v. ophthalmica superior
- v. ovarica dextra
- v. ovarica sinistra
- v. palatina externa
- vv. palpebrales
- vv. palpebrales inferiores
- vv. palpebrales superiores
- vv. pancreaticae
- vv. pancreaticoduodenales
- vv. paraumbilicales
- vv. parotideae
- vv. perforantes
- vv. pericardiaceae
- vv. pericardiacophrenicae

*v. = vena [*L.*]
vv. = venae [*L., pl.*]

vena (*pl.* venae)* *(continued)*
- vv. peroneae
- vv. pharyngeae
- vv. phrenicae inferiores
- v. poplitea
- v. portea
- v. posterior ventriculi sinistri cordis
- v. prepylorica
- v. profunda femoris
- v. profunda linguae
- vv. profundae clitoridis
- vv. profundae penis
- v. pudenda interna
- vv. pudendae externae
- v. pulmonalis inferior dextra
- v. pulmonalis inferior sinistra
- v. pulmonalis superior dextra
- v. pulmonalis superior sinistra
- vv. radiales
- vv. rectales inferiores
- vv. rectales mediae
- v. rectalis superior
- vv. renales
- v. retromandibularis
- vv. sacrales laterales
- v. sacralis mediana
- v. saphena accessoria
- v. saphena magna
- v. saphena parva
- vv. scrotales anteriores
- vv. scrotales posteriores
- vv. septi pellucidi
- vv. sigmoideae
- vv. spinales

vena (*pl.* venae)* *(continued)*
   v. spiralis modioli
   vv. stellatae renis
   v. sternocleidomastoidea
   v. striata
   v. stylomastoidea
   v. subclavia
   v. subcostalis
   vv. subcutaneae abdominis
   v. sublingualis
   v. submentalis
   v. supraorbitalis
   v. suprarenalis dextra
   v. suprarenalis sinistra
   v. suprascapularis
   vv. supratrochleares
   vv. temporales profundae
   vv. temporales superficiales
   v. temporalis media
   v. testicularis dextra
   v. testicularis sinistra
   v. thalamostriata
   v. thoracica lateralis
   vv. thoracicae internae
   v. thoracoacromialis
   vv. thoracoepigastricae
   vv. thymicae
   v. thyroidea inferior
   v. thyroidea superior
   vv. thyroideae mediae
   vv. tibiales anteriores
   vv. tibiales posteriores
   vv. tracheales
   v. transversa faciei
   vv. transversae colli

*v. = vena [*L.*]
 vv. = venae [*L., pl.*]

vena (*pl.* venae)* *(continued)*
   vv. tympanicae
   vv. ulnares
   v. umbilicalis
   v. umbilicalis sinistra
   vv. uterinae
vena cava clamp
vena cava clip
vena cava inferior
vena cava scissors
vena cava superior
vena caval umbrella
Venable plate
Venable screw
Venable-Stuck nail
Venable-Stuck pin
venectomy
venesection
venipuncture
venipuncture needle
Venocath
venoclysis
venoclysis cannula
venogram
venography
venoperitoneostomy
venorrhaphy
venotomy
venotripsy
venous
venous anastomosis
venous catheter
venous cutdown
venous stasis
venovenostomy
ventilation
ventilation bronchoscope
ventilation perfusion scan

ventilation tube
Venti-mask
ventral
ventral celiotomy
ventral hernia
ventral hernia repair
ventral herniorrhaphy
ventricle
Ventricor pacemaker
ventricular cannula
ventricular fibrillation
ventricular hypertrophy
ventricular ligament
ventricular needle
ventricular-suppressed pacemaker
ventricular tachycardia
ventricular-triggered pacemaker
ventricular ventilation tube
ventriculoatrial shunt
ventriculocholecystostomy
ventriculocisternostomy
ventriculocordectomy
ventriculogram
ventriculogram retractor
ventriculography
ventriculomyocardiotomy
ventriculoperitoneal shunt
ventriculoperitoneostomy
ventriculopuncture
ventriculoseptopexy
ventriculoseptoplasty
ventriculostomy
ventriculotomy
ventriculovenostomy
ventrocystorrhaphy
ventrofixation of uterus
ventrohysteropexy
ventrosuspension of uterus

Venturi insufflator
Venturimask
VER (visual evoked response)
Verbrugge clamp
verge
Verhoeff forceps
Verhoeff lens expressor
Verhoeff operation
Verhoeff scissors
Verhoeff sclerotomy
Verhoeff sutures
Vermale amputation
vermicular
vermiculation
vermiculous
vermiform
vermiform appendix
vermiform process
vermilion
vermilion border
vermilionectomy
verminous appendicitis
vermis incision
Verneuil operation
Vernon-David proctoscope
Vernon-David sigmoidoscope
Vernon-David speculum
Vernon tube
Verres cannula
Verres needle
Verres trocar
verruca (*pl.* verrucae)
verruca acuminata
verruca digitata
verruca filiformis
verruca plana
verruca plantaris
verruca vulgaris

verrucae (*sing.* verruca)
version
vertebra (*pl.* vertebrae)
vertebrae cervicales
vertebrae coccygeae
vertebrae lumbales
vertebrae sacrales
vertebrae thoracicae
vertebral arteriogram
vertebral artery
vertebral body
vertebral canal
vertebral nerve
vertebral spines
vertebral spreader
vertebralis artery
vertebralis nerve
vertebrated catheter
vertebrated probe
vertex
vertex presentation
vertical
vertical bur hole incision
vertical elliptical incision
vertical incision
vertical lateral parapatellar incision
vertical mattress sutures
vertical muscle
vertical retractor
vertical tube
verticalis linguae muscle
vertigo
verumontanum
Verwey operation
Vesely-Street nail
vesical
vesical arteries
vesical hernia

vesical retractor
vesicales superiores arteries
vesicalis inferior artery
vesicle
vesicocervical fistula
vesicofixation
vesicointestinal
vesicolithotomy
vesicosigmoidostomy
vesicostomy
vesicotomy
vesicourethroplasty
vesicouterine ligament
vesicovaginal fistula
vesicular
vesiculation
vesiculectomy
vesiculogram
vesiculography
vesiculotomy
vessel
vessel band
vessel clamp
vessel forceps
vessel prosthesis
vessel punch
vest-over-pants hernia repair
vest-over-pants technique
Vest telescope
vestibular clamp
vestibular ligament
vestibular osteotomy
vestibule
vestibulocochlear nerve (cranial nerve VIII)
vestibulocochlearis nerve
vestibuloplasty
vestibulotomy

vestigial
Vezien scissors
Vi-Drape
Vi-Drape surgical film
Vi-Spray
viability
Viamonte-Hobbs electrosurgical
    unit
Viamonte-Jutzy electrosurgical
    unit
vibratory hammer
Vibrodilator
Vibrodilator probe
vice-grip pliers
Vicq D'Azyr operation
Vicryl sutures
Victorian collar dressing
Vidal operation for varicocele
vidian nerve
vidianectomy
Vienna speculum
Viers erysiphake
Villard button
villi (*sing.* villus)
villous adenoma
villus (*pl.* villi)
villusectomy
Vim needle
Vim-Silverman needle
Vinamar
Vineberg operation
Vinethene
Vinke tongs
Vinke tractor
vinyl ether
vinyl ethyl ether
Vioform dressing
violaceous

Virchow chisel
Virchow knife
Virden catheter
virgin silk
Viro-Tec sutures
virtual cautery
Virtus forceps
virulent
VISC (vitreous infusion suction
    cutter)
viscera (*sing.* viscus)
viscera forceps
visceral peritoneum
visceral pleura
visceroparietal
visceroparietal suture
visceroperitoneal
visceropleural
visceroptosis
Vischer incision
Vischer lumboiliac incision
viscid
viscidity
viscus (*pl.* viscera)
vise forceps
Vistaril
visual acuity
visual axis
visual evoked response (VER)
visual inspection
visual line
vital signs
Vitallium drill
Vitallium eye implant
Vitallium implant
Vitallium mesh
Vitallium Moore prosthesis
Vitallium nail

Vitallium plate
Vitallium prosthesis
Vitallium screw
vitrectomy
vitrectomy tip
vitrector tip
vitreous hemorrhage
vitreous infusion suction cutter
 (VISC)
vitreous membrane
Vivosil implant
Vladimiroff-Mikulicz amputation
Vladimiroff-Mikulicz operation
vocal cordectomy
vocal cordotomy
vocal cords
vocal ligament
vocal muscle
vocalis muscle
Vogel curet
Vogel operation
voiding cystourethrogram (VCUG)
volar splint
volar surface
volatile agents
Volkmann's canal
Volkmann's contracture
Volkmann curet
Volkmann operation for hydrocele
Volkmann rake
Volkmann retractor
Volkmann splint
Volkmann spoon
Volkovitsch sign
voltage clamp
Voltolini speculum

Voltolini tube
voluminous hernia
Volutrol apparatus
volvulus
vomer
vomer forceps
von Bergmann hernia
von Bergmann operation
von Blaskovics-Doyen operation
von Burow operation
Von Eichen cannula
Von Eichen tube
von Graefe cautery
von Graefe cystotome
von Graefe forceps
von Graefe hook
von Graefe knife
von Graefe needle
von Graefe operation
von Graefe scissors
von Graefe speculum
von Haberer-Aguirre gastrectomy
von Haberer-Finney gastrectomy
von Haberer-Finney gastroenterostomy
von Haberer gastrectomy
von Hackler operation
von Hippel (see Hippel)
von Kraske operation
von Langenbeck operation
von Mondak forceps
von Petz clamp
von Petz clip
von Saal pin
Voorhees needle
Voronoff operation

vortex
V/Q scan (ventilation perfusion scan)
vulcanite dental plate
Vulpius-Compere operation
Vulpius operation
vulsella forceps
vulsellum forceps
vulva
vulvar biopsy
vulvectomy
vulvovaginal
vulvovaginal glands
VY advancement flap

W

W. Dean McDonald clamp
w hernia
W-shaped incision
W-Y operation
Wachenheim-Reder sign
Wachsberger bur
Wachtenfeldt clip
Wachtenfeldt forceps
Wada valve prosthesis
Wadsworth-Todd cautery
Wagner hammer
Wagner punch
Wagner skull resection
Wagoner operation
Wagstaffe fracture
Wahl sign
Walcher position
Waldeau forceps
Waldenberg apparatus
Waldeyer colon
Waldeyer's glands
Waldhauer operation
Wales bougie
Wales dilator
Walker-Apple scissors
Walker-Atkinson scissors
Walker curet
Walker dissector
Walker elevator
Walker forceps
Walker lid everter
Walker needle

Walker pin
Walker retractor
Walker scissors
Walker trephine
walking brace
walking caliper
Walldius knee prosthesis
Walsh curet
Walsh-Ogura orbital decompression
Walsham forceps
Walsham straightener
Walter-Deaver retractor
Walter forceps
Walter spud
Walthardt operation
Walther catheter
Walther clamp
Walther-Crenshaw clamp
Walther dilator
Walther forceps
Walther sound
Walton curet
Walton extractor
Walton forceps
Walton gouge
Walton knife
Walton punch
Walton rib shears
Walton rongeur
Walton-Schubert forceps
Walton-Schubert punch

Walton scissors
wandering pacemaker
Wangensteen apparatus
Wangensteen awl
Wangensteen carrier
Wangensteen clamp
Wangensteen colostomy
Wangensteen dissector
Wangensteen drainage
Wangensteen dressing
Wangensteen forceps
Wangensteen herniorrhaphy
Wangensteen needle
Wangensteen needle holder
Wangensteen operation
Wangensteen suction
Wangensteen suction tube
Wangensteen trocar
Wangensteen tube
Wappler cautery
Wappler cystoscope
Wappler electrode
Ward-French needle
Ward-Mayo operation
Ward needle
Wardill-Kilner operation
Wardill palatoplasty
Warm Springs brace
warning stop tube
Warren incision
Warren operation
wart
Warthen clamp
Warthen spur crusher
wash tube
washings
washout cannula
Wasko probe

wasp-waist laryngoscope
Water cesarean section
water cystometer
water dressing
Water operation
Waterhouse urethroplasty
Waterman bronchoscope
Waterman rib contractor
Waters position
Waters-Waldron position
waterseal drainage
watertight
watertight seal
Watkins operation
Watkins-Wertheim operation
Watson-Cheyne dissector
Watson forceps
Watson-Jones gouge
Watson-Jones incision
Watson-Jones operation
Watson operation
Watson speculum
Watson-Williams forceps
Watson-Williams needle
Watson-Williams punch
Watson-Williams rasp
Watson-Williams rongeur
Watts clamp
Watts tenaculum
Waugh operation
wax bougie
wax-tipped bougie
weakness
Weary hook
Weary spatula
Weavenit graft
Weavenit prosthesis
Weaver clamp

web
web space
Webb bolt
Webb nail
Webb retractor
Webb vein stripper
webbing
Weber catheter
Weber-Fergusson incision
Weber-Fergusson-Longmire
    incision
Weber's glands
Weber implant
Weber insufflator
Weber knife
Weber retractor
Weber scissors
Webril bandage
Webster knife
Webster operation
Webster retractor
Webster tube
Weck-cel sponge
Weck clamp
Weck clip
Weck shears
Weck suction tube
Wecker spatula
Weder retractor
Weder-Solenberger retractor
Weder tongue depressor
wedge biopsy
wedge incision
wedge ostectomy
wedge osteotomy
wedge resection
wedge resection clamp
wedge-shaped

Weekers operation
Weeks needle
Weeks speculum
Wehrbein hypospadias operation
Wehrbein-Smith hypospadias
    operation
weightbearing brace
weighted posterior retractor
weighted speculum
weighted vaginal speculum
Weil forceps
Weil rongeur
Weil sling
Weil splint
Weinberg operation
Weinberg retractor
Weinberg rib spreader
Weinberg spreader
Weingartner forceps
Weingartner rongeur
Weir appendectomy
Weir operation
Weis forceps
Weis operation
Weisenbach forceps
Weisman curet
Weisman forceps
Weisman-Graves speculum
Weisman tenaculum
Weitbrecht's ligament
Weitlaner retractor
Welch Allyn anoscope
Welch Allyn forceps
Welch Allyn hook
Welch Allyn laryngoscope
Welch Allyn otoscope
Welch Allyn probe
Welch Allyn proctoscope

Welch Allyn retinoscope
Welch Allyn sigmoidoscope
Welch Allyn speculum
Welch Allyn transilluminator
Welch Allyn tube
well-defined
well-leg splint
Wellaminski perforator
Wells cannula
Wells clamp
Wells forceps
Wells irrigator
Wells pick
Wells scoop
Wells spoon
Wells tractor
Wermer syndrome
Wertheim clamp
Wertheim-Cullen clamp
Wertheim-Cullen forceps
Wertheim forceps
Wertheim hysterectomy
Wertheim-Navratil needle
Wertheim operation
Wertheim-Reverdin clamp
Wertheim-Schauta operation
Wertheim splint
Wertheim-Taussig operation
Wesolowski prosthesis
Wesson mouth gag
Wesson retractor
West chisel
West gouge
West operation
Westcott scissors
Wester clamp
Wester scissors
wet bandage

wet-field cautery
wet-field coagulator
wet tapes
Weve operation
whalebone filiform bougie
whalebone filiform catheter
Wharton's duct
Wharton operation
Wheeler cystotome
Wheeler eye implant
Wheeler implant
Wheeler knife
Wheeler operation
Wheeler spatula
Wheelhouse operation
wheeze
whip
whip bougie
Whipple incision
Whipple operation
Whipple pancreaticoduodenec-
    tomy
whipstitch sutures
whipstitched
whistle
    Edelmann-Galton
    Galton
    hearing
    w. bougie
    whistle-tip catheter
    whistle-tip drain
Whitcomb-Kerrison punch
white braided sutures
White chisel
White forceps
White-Lillie forceps
White mallet
white matter

white nylon sutures
White operation
White-Oslay forceps
White-Proud retractor
White scissors
White screwdriver
white silk sutures
White-Smith forceps
white twisted sutures
Whitehead hemorrhoidectomy
Whitehead operation
Whiting curet
Whiting rongeur
Whiting tonsillectome
whitlow
Whitman arthroplasty
Whitman astragalectomy
Whitman fracture frame
Whitman operation
Whitver clamp
Wicherkiewicz operation
wick
wide excision
Wiener breast reduction
Wiener hook
Wiener keratome
Wiener operation
Wiener-Pierce rasp
Wiener-Pierce trocar
Wiener rasp
Wiener speculum
Wigand version
Wigmore saw
Wilde-Blakesley forceps
Wilde-Bruening snare
Wilde forceps
Wilde incision
Wilde punch

Wilder cystotome
Wilder dilator
Wilder loupe
Wilder scoop
Wilder trephine
Wildgen-Reck magnet
Wildgen-Reck metal locator
Wilke boot
Wilke brace
Wilkerson bur
Willauer raspatory
Willauer scissors
Willett clamp
Willett forceps
William operation
William pelvimeter
Williams brace
Williams clamp
Williams colpopoiesis
Williams craniotome
Williams dilator
Williams forceps
Williams position
Williams probe
Williams-Richardson operation
Williams screwdriver
Williams speculum
Willis antrum
Willis pancreas
willow fracture
Willy Meyer incision
Wilman clamp
Wilmer chisel
Wilmer operation
Wilmer retractor
Wilmer scissors
Wilms operation
Wilson awl

Wilson bolt
Wilson clamp
Wilson-McKeever operation
Wilson operation
Wilson plate
Wilson retractor
Wilson rib spreader
Wilson splint
Wilson spreader
Wilson stripper
Wilson trocar
Wilson wrench
Wiltberger spreader
Wincor scissors
window operation
window rasp
windowing of cortex
Winer catheter
wing clip
wing sutures
winged catheter
winged shunt
Winiwarter cholecystoenteros-
    tomy
Winiwarter operation
Winslow foramen
Winslow pancreas
Winternitz sound
wire
    arch
    Bunnell
    crimped
    double-woven
    electrode
    guide
    House
    ideal arch
    interdental

wire *(continued)*
    intramedullary
    intraoral
    Ivy
    K-wire
    Kirschner
    ligature
    loop
    monofilament
    multifilament
    pacing electrode
    pull-out
    Risdon
    separating
    stainless steel
    stencil
    subcuticular
    suture
    tantalum
    Thiersch
    tonsil snare
    w. bivalve speculum
    w. brush
    wire-closure forceps
    w. crimper (see separate
        listing)
    wire-crimping forceps
    w. cutter
    wire-cutting scissors
    w. electrode
    w. forceps
    w. guide
    w. knot tightener
    w. loop
    w. mesh
    w. mesh eye implant
    w. mesh implant
    w. passer

wire *(continued)*
    w. piston prosthesis
    w. probe
    w. retractor
    w. ring
    w. saw
    w. scissors
    w. snare
    w. splint
    w. spreader
    w. stapes prosthesis
    w. strut
    w. sutures
    w. tamp
    w. tightener
    wire-tightening clamp
    wire-tightening forceps
    w. tractor
    w. twister
wire crimper
    Caparosa
    McGee
    McGee-Caparosa
wiring
wiring of jaw
Wirsung duct
Wis-Foregger laryngoscope
Wis-Hipple laryngoscope
wisdom tooth
Wise operation
Wishard catheter
Wittner biopsy punch
Wittner forceps
Witzel enterostomy
Witzel gastrostomy
Witzel operation
Wladimiroff tarsectomy
Woakes saw

Wolf catheter
Wolf-Schindler gastroscope
Wolfe forceps
Wolfe graft
Wolfe operation
Wolfe ptosis operation
Wolfenden position
Wölfler gastroenterostomy
Wölfler gastrojejunostomy
Wölfler sign
Wölfler sutures
Wolfson clamp
Wolfson retractor
Wolkowitsch sign
Wood needle
Wood operation
wood tongue blade
Woodbridge sutures
Woodruff catheter
Woodson elevator
Woodson spatula
Woodson spoon
Woodward forceps
Woodward operation
Woodward rasp
Woodward sound
wormy veins
Worth chisel
Worth forceps
Worth operation
wound
wound cautery
wound cleaning
wound clip forceps
wound dehiscence
wound excision
woven bougie
woven-loop stone dislodger

woven-silk catheter
woven-tube vascular prosthesis
wrapping of aneurysm
Wreden sign
wrench
    Allen
    hexagonal
    orthopedic
    Wilson
Wright operation
Wright plate
Wright snare
Wright version
wrist bones
wrist excision
Wullen stone dislodger
Wullstein bur
Wullstein curet
Wullstein forceps
Wullstein-House forceps
Wullstein knife

Wullstein retractor
Wullstein scissors
Wullstein spatula
Wullstein tympanoplasty
Wurd catheter
Wurth vein stripper
Wutzer hernia
Wutzer operation
Wutzler scissors
Wydase
Wyeth amputation
Wylie dilator
Wylie drain
Wylie forceps
Wylie operation
Wylie pessary
Wylie stripper
Wyllys-Andrews operation
Wynn cleft lip operation
Wysler sutures

X

x-ray
x-ray microscope
x-ray template
xanthochromic
xanthomatous
xenograft
xenon
xenon arc photocoagulator
Xeroform dressing
Xeroform gauze
xerogram

xerography
xeromammogram
xeromammography
xiphoid
xiphoid process
xiphoidectomy
Xylocaine
Xylocaine jelly
Xylocaine with epinephrine
xyster
xyster raspatory

y

Y-bandage
Y-bone plate
Y-connector
Y-drain
Y-glass rod
Y-incision
Y-plasty procedure
Y-suture
Y-tube
Y-type incision
Yankauer bronchoscope
Yankauer catheter
Yankauer curet
Yankauer esophagoscope
Yankauer forceps
Yankauer laryngoscope
Yankauer-Little forceps
Yankauer nasopharyngoscope
Yankauer needle
Yankauer operation
Yankauer probe
Yankauer punch
Yankauer scissors
Yankauer speculum
Yankauer suction tube
Yankauer trocar
Yankauer tube
Yasargil clamp
Yasargil clip
Yasargil dissector
Yasargil forceps

Yasargil knife
Yasargil microscope
Yasargil raspatory
Yasargil retractor
Yasargil scissors
Yasargil scoop
Yasargil technique
Yazujian bur
Yellen clamp
yellow-tip aspirator
Yeomans forceps
Yeomans proctoscope
Yeomans punch
Yeomans sigmoidoscope
yoke
Yoshida dissector
Young clamp
Young cystoscope
Young dilator
Young dissector
Young forceps
Young-Millin needle holder
Young needle holder
Young operation
Young prostatectomy
Young prostatic enucleator
Young retractor
Young tractor
Young vasectomy
Yount operation

Z

Z-excision
Z-flap incision
Z-incision
Z-plasty
Z-plasty incision
Z-shaped incision
Z-suture
Zachary-Cope DeMartel clamp
Zahradnicek operation
Zancolli operation
Zavod catheter
Zeiss microscope
Zeiss photocoagulator
Zeiss unit
Zephiran
Zephiran pack
Ziegler cautery
Ziegler dilator
Ziegler forceps
Ziegler-Furniss clamp
Ziegler iridectomy
Ziegler knife
Ziegler needle
Ziegler probe
Ziegler puncture
Ziegler speculum
Zieman hernia repair
Zieman operation
Zimaloy prosthesis
Zimaloy staple
Zimany flap
Zimfoam head halter

Zimfoam splint
Zimmer bolt
Zimmer clamp
Zimmer drill
Zimmer pin
Zimmer prosthesis
Zimmer screw
Zimmer screwdriver
Zimmer sling
Zimmer splint
Zimmerman operation
Zipser clamp
Zoellner hook
Zoellner needle
Zoellner raspatory
Zoellner scissors
Zoll pacemaker
Zollinger-Ellison syndrome
zonular cataract
zonule separator
zonulolysis
zonulysis
zoograft
zoografting
Zuelzer awl
Zuelzer plate
Zutt clamp
Zwanck pessary
Zweifel-DeLee cranioclast
zygoma
zygoma elevator
zygomatic

zygomatic bone
zygomatic muscle
zygomatic nerve
zygomatic process
zygomaticomaxillary suture
zygomaticoorbital artery

zygomaticoorbitalis artery
zygomaticus major muscle
zygomaticus minor muscle
zygomaticus nerve
Zytor sutures